A·N·N·U·A·L E·D·I·T·I·O·N·S

Drugs, Society, and Behavior

Fifteenth Edition

00/01

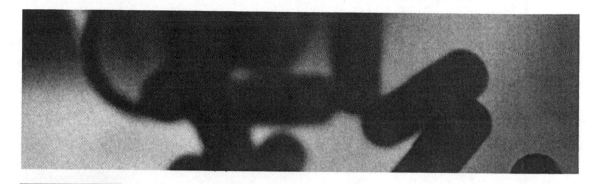

EDITOR

Hugh T. Wilson
California State University, Sacramento

Hugh Wilson received his Bachelor of Arts Degree from California State University, Sacramento, and a Master of Arts degree in Justice Administration and a Doctorate in Public Administration from Golden Gate University in San Francisco. Dr. Wilson is currently a professor of criminal justice at California State University, Sacramento. He has taught drug abuse recognition, enforcement, and policy to police officers and students of criminal justice for more than 20 years.

Dushkin/McGraw-Hill
Sluice Dock, Guilford, Connecticut 06437

Visit us on the Internet
http://www.dushkin.com/annualeditions/

Credits

1. Living with Drugs
Unit photo—© 1996, PhotoDisc, Inc.
2. Understanding How Drugs Work—Use, Dependence, and Addiction
Unit photo—© 1999, PhotoDisc, Inc.
3. The Major Drugs of Use and Abuse
Unit photo—© 1999, CLEO Photograhy.
4. Other Trends and Patterns in Drug Use
Unit photo—United Nations photo by John Robaton.
5. Drugs and Crime
Unit photo—AP/Wide World Photos.
6. Measuring the Social Costs of Drugs
Unit photo—© 1999, CLEO Photograph.
7. Creating and Sustaining Effective Drug Control Policy
Unit photo—© 1999, PhotoDisc, Inc.
8. Prevention and Treatment
Unit photo—© 1999, PhotoDisc, Inc.

Copyright

Cataloging in Publication Data
Main entry under title: Annual Editions: Drugs, Society, and Behavior. 2000/2001.
    1. Drugs—Periodicals. 2. Drug abuse—United States—Periodicals. 3. Alcohol—Periodicals.
4. Drunk driving—Periodicals. I. Wilson, Hugh, *comp.* II. Title: Drugs, society, and behavior.
ISBN 0–07–236538–2   362.2'92'0973'05   87–649280   ISSN 1091–9945

Fifteenth Edition

Cover image © 2000 PhotoDisc, Inc.

Printed in the United States of America   1234567890BAHBAH543210   Printed on Recycled Paper iii

To the Reader

In publishing ANNUAL EDITIONS we recognize the enormous role played by the magazines, newspapers, and journals of the public press in providing current, first-rate educational information in a broad spectrum of interest areas. Many of these articles are appropriate for students, researchers, and professionals seeking accurate, current material to help bridge the gap between principles and theories and the real world. These articles, however, become more useful for study when those of lasting value are carefully collected, organized, indexed, and reproduced in a low-cost format, which provides easy and permanent access when the material is needed. That is the role played by ANNUAL EDITIONS.

New to ANNUAL EDITIONS is the inclusion of related World Wide Web sites. These sites have been selected by our editorial staff to represent some of the best resources found on the World Wide Web today. Through our carefully developed topic guide, we have linked these Web resources to the articles covered in this ANNUAL EDITIONS reader. We think that you will find this volume useful, and we hope that you will take a moment to visit us on the Web at *http://www.dushkin.com* to tell us what you think.

It is difficult to define the framework by which Americans make decisions and develop perspectives on the use of drugs. There is no predictable expression of ideology. A wide range of individual and collective experience defines our national will toward drugs.

One in three Americans has someone close who has been negatively affected by drugs. Presently, there is concern over what many are citing as ambivalent attitudes toward drugs by young persons. Since 1992 drug use by young people has steadily increased following a perceived decline and leveling off. The most recent research suggests that rates of drug use by adults have remained flat since 1992 and that some nefarious threats, such as that which existed with crack cocaine, have waned. There still are, however, an estimated 30 to 40 million chemically dependent people in this country. Social costs from drugs are estimated to exceed $166 billion per year. Subsequently, the prevailing legacies of what we refer to as the drug war or the drug problem will continue to evolve and transform.

Although it is easy to despair and lament the past and present consequences of pervasive, harmful drug use within American society, we must realize the potential for progress as we begin the next millennium. The year 2000 brings with it discoveries, knowledge, understanding, and resolve that may propel us away from the darkness of so many drug-related ills. Scientific discoveries of how the brain transforms as it enters and leaves an addicted state are providing hope never before realized. Hope, literacy, and understanding have always been some of the most powerful tools of progress.

The articles contained in *Annual Editions: Drugs, Society, and Behavior 00/01* are a collection of facts, issues, and perspectives designed to provide the reader with a framework for examining current drug-related issues. The book is designed to offer students something to think about and something with which to think. It is a unique collection of materials of interest to the casual as well as the serious student of drug-related social phenomena. Unit 1 addresses the historical significance that drugs have played in early as well as contemporary American history. It emphasizes the often overlooked reality that drugs, legal and illegal, have remained a pervasive dimension of past as well as present American history. Unit 2 examines the physiological and psychological basis for what we define as use, abuse, dependence, and addiction, and it provides an overview of how drugs produce severe physiological and psychological consequences. Unit 3 examines the major drugs of use and abuse, along with issues relative to understanding the individual impacts of these drugs on society. This unit also illustrates the necessity to perceive the differences and similarities produced by the use of legal and illegal drugs. Unit 4 reviews the dynamic nature of drugs as it relates to changing patterns and trends of use. Unit 5 analyzes the link between drugs and crime. Implications of individual criminal behavior as well as organized, syndicated trafficking are discussed. Unit 6 focuses on the social costs of drug abuse and why the costs overwhelm many American institutions. Unit 7 illustrates the complexity and controversy in creating and implementing drug policy. Unit 8 concludes the book with discussions of current strategies for preventing and treating drug abuse. Can we deter people from harming themselves with drugs, and can we cure people addicted to drugs? What does work and what does not?

We encourage your comments and criticisms on the articles provided and kindly ask for your review on the postage-paid rating form at the end of the book.

Hugh T. Wilson

Hugh T. Wilson
Editor

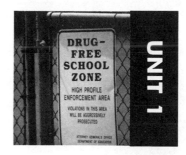

Contents

UNIT 1

Living with Drugs

Seven articles in this
unit examine the past and
present historical evolution of
drugs in the United States.

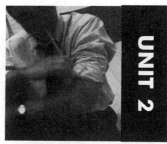

UNIT 2

Understanding How Drugs Work—Use, Dependence, and Addiction

Seven articles in this section examine
the ways drugs affect the mind
and body. The relationship of
pharmacology with dependence
and addiction is described.

The concepts in bold italics are developed in the article. For further expansion please refer to the Topic Guide, the Glossary, and the Index.

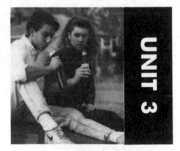

UNIT 3

The Major Drugs of Use and Abuse

This unit addresses some major
drugs of use and abuse.
Cocaine, heroin, marijuana,
alcohol and tobacco, and
methamphetamine are discussed.

The concepts in bold italics are developed in the article. For further expansion please refer to the Topic Guide, the Glossary, and the Index.

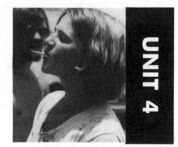

UNIT 4

Other Trends and Patterns in Drug Use

The seven articles in the unit discuss some developing patterns of drug use along with their subsequent implications for society.

The concepts in bold italics are developed in the article. For further expansion please refer to the Topic Guide, the Glossary, and the Index.

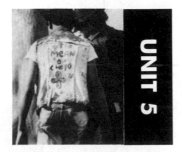

UNIT 5

Drugs and Crime

Five articles review the numbing
social malady caused by criminal
behavior that is created, sustained,
and perpetuated by the use of drugs.

The concepts in bold italics are developed in the article. For further expansion please refer to the Topic Guide, the Glossary, and the Index.

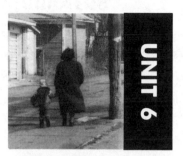

UNIT 6

Measuring the Social Costs of Drugs

Seven articles speak
to the diverse way in which
the impacts of drugs affect and
overwhelm numerous public and
private American institutions.

The concepts in bold italics are developed in the article. For further expansion please refer to the Topic Guide, the Glossary, and the Index.

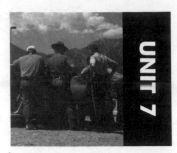

UNIT 7

Creating and Sustaining Effective Drug Control Policy

The eight essays in this unit illustrate the complexity of creating effective drug-related policy.

The concepts in bold italics are developed in the article. For further expansion please refer to the Topic Guide, the Glossary, and the Index.

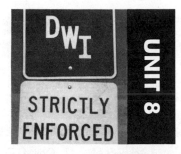

UNIT 8

Prevention and Treatment

Addressing some tough questions concerning previously accepted ideas about drug treatment, the seven unit articles review effectiveness, financial costs, education, and controversial new treatments.

The concepts in bold italics are developed in the article. For further expansion please refer to the Topic Guide, the Glossary, and the Index.

This topic guide suggests how the selections and World Wide Web sites found in the next section of this book relate to topics of traditional concern to students and professionals involved with the study of drugs, society, and behavior. It is useful for locating interrelated articles and Web sites for reading and research. The guide is arranged alphabetically according to topic.

The relevant Web sites, which are numbered and annotated on pages 4 and 5, are easily identified by the Web icon (⊙) under the topic articles. By linking the articles and the Web sites by topic, this ANNUAL EDITIONS reader becomes a powerful learning and research tool.

TOPIC AREA	TREATED IN	TOPIC AREA	TREATED IN
Addiction	1 Opium, Cocaine, and Marijuana in American History 4. One Nation under the Table 5. New Museum Traces History of Drugs in the U.S. 8. Addiction and the Brain—Part 1 11. What Type of Addict Are You? 13. New Pieces Filling In Addiction Puzzle 14. Taping the Horror 15. Resisting Cocaine's Tragic Lure 39. Pregnant, Hooked & Booked 53. Peer Principle: The Key to Addiction Treatment 55. Can Addiction-Related Self-Help/Mutual Aid Groups Lower Demand for Professional Substance Abuse Treatment? ⊙ **1, 2, 3, 4, 5, 6, 7, 8**		7. America's Altered States 17. Heroin and Cocaine—A Global Threat 20. Opium as Cash Drop Is Still Difficult to Beat 22. Big Tobacco Rides East 31. Border Trafficking: Where the U.S. and Mexico Meet, the Drug Smugglers Are Riding High ⊙ **14, 23**
Alcoholism	4. One Nation under the Table 12. Alcoholism: Character or Genetics? 18. Drinking Dilemma 24. Dying for a Drink 25. College Students Drunk on Campus Drinking Lore, Tradition 26. Party Politics 39. Pregnant, Hooked & Booked 40. Alcoholism in Women 41. Facts about Women, Alcohol 52. Outpatient Detoxification 56. Glass Half Empty ⊙ **1, 2, 3, 4, 5, 6, 7, 17, 27**	**Epidemiology**	1. Opium, Cocaine, and Marijuana in American History 5. New Museum Traces History of Drugs in the U.S. 6. Just Don't Say No, Not Us ⊙ **1, 2, 3, 4, 5, 6, 7, 8, 11**
		Etiology	4. One Nation under the Table 12. Alcoholism: Character or Genetics? 13. New Pieces Filling In Addiction Puzzle 41. Facts about Women, Alcohol ⊙ **1, 2, 3, 4, 5, 6, 7, 8, 11**
Amphetamines	7. America's Altered States 23. High in the Heartland 32. Raising the Stakes in U.S.–Mexico Drug Wars 34. Drugs, Crime, Prison and Treatment ⊙ **1, 2, 3, 4, 5, 6, 7, 8, 9, 15, 20, 21, 23, 25, 26, 27**	**Heroin**	1. Opium, Cocaine, and Marijuana in American History 2. Drug Trade Primer for the Late 1990s 3. Hundred-Year Habit 5. New Museum Traces History of Drugs in the U.S. 15. Resisting Cocaine's Tragic Lure 16. Heroin High 17. Heroin and Cocaine—A Global Threat 20. Opium as Cash Drop Is Still Difficult to Beat 33. Charm City Blues 42. Medical Care of Heroin Users ⊙ **1, 2, 3, 4, 5, 6, 7, 8, 19, 20, 21, 23**
Cocaine	1. Opium, Cocaine, and Marijuana in American History 5. New Museum Traces History of Drugs in the U.S. 7. America's Altered States 10. Cocaine Wreaks Subtle Damage on Developing Brains 15. Resisting Cocaine's Tragic Lure 17. Heroin and Cocaine—A Global Threat 33. Charm City Blues 39. Doping Kids 39. Pregnant, Hooked & Booked ⊙ **1, 2, 3, 4, 5, 6, 7, 8**	**Law Enforcement**	1. Opium, Cocaine, and Marijuana in American History 2. Drug Trade Primer for the Late 1990s 5. New Museum Traces History of Drugs in the U.S. 14. Taping the Horror 16. Heroin High 20. Opium as Cash Drop Is Still Difficult to Beat 31. Border Trafficking: Where the U.S. and Mexico Meet, the Drug Smugglers Are Riding High 32. Raising the Stakes in U.S.–Mexico Drug Wars 33. Charm City Blues 34. Drugs, Crime, Prison and Treatment 35. Doping Kids 44. Strange Bedfellows
Drug Economy	2. Drug Trade Primer for the Late 1990s 5. New Museum Traces History of Drugs in the U.S.		

◉ AE: Drugs, Society, and Behavior

The following World Wide Web sites have been carefully researched and selected to support the articles found in this reader. If you are interested in learning more about specific topics found in this book, these Web sites are a good place to start. The sites are cross-referenced by number and appear in the topic guide on the previous two pages. Also, you can link to these Web sites through our DUSHKIN ONLINE support site at *http://www.dushkin.com/online/*.

The following sites were available at the time of publication. Visit our Web site—we update DUSHKIN ONLINE regularly to reflect any changes.

General Information

1. Alcohol and Drug Links
http://www.realsolutions.org/druglink.htm
This is a set of Internet links that provides information on Alcohol and Drug Use and Abuse. These links have been gathered by Real Solutions, a nonprofit organization dedicated to the needs of family and community.

2. Higher Education Center for Alcohol and Other Drug Prevention
http://www.edc.org/hec/
The U.S. Department of Education established the Higher Education Center for Alcohol and Other Drug Prevention to provide nationwide support for campus alcohol and other drug prevention efforts. The Center is working with colleges, universities, and proprietary schools throughout the country to develop strategies for changing campus culture, to foster environments that promote healthy lifestyles, and to prevent illegal alcohol and other drug use among students.

3. National Clearinghouse for Alcohol and Drug Information
http://www.health.org
This site provides information to teens about the problems and ramifications of drug use and abuse. There are numerous links to drug-related informational sites.

Living with Drugs

4. National Council on Alcoholism and Drug Dependence, Inc.
http://www.ncadd.org
According to their Web site, The National Council on Alcoholism and Drug Dependence provides education, information, help, and hope in the fight against the chronic, and sometimes fatal, disease of alcoholism and other drug addictions.

Understanding How Drugs Work— Use, Dependence, and Addiction

5. AMERSA
http://center.butler.brown.edu
AMERSA is an association of multidisciplinary health care professionals in the field of substance abuse. They are dedicated to improving education about alcohol, tobacco, and other drugs.

6. Addiction Research Foundation
http://www.arf.org
According to their Web site, the Addiction Research Foundation (ARF) is one of North America's preeminent facilities for research into alcohol, tobacco, and other drug problems. The foundation's mission is to work with its partners to create and apply knowledge to prevent and reduce the harm associated with alcohol, tobacco, and other drugs in Ontario communities.

7. The National Center on Addiction and Substance Abuse at Columbia University
http://www.casacolumbia.org
According to its Web site, The National Center on Addiction and Substance Abuse at Columbia University is a unique think/action tank that brings together under one roof all of the professional disciplines (health policy, medicine and nursing, communications, economics, sociology and anthropology, law and law enforcement, business, religion, and education) needed to study and combat all forms of substance abuse—illegal drugs, pills, alcohol and tobacco— as they affect all aspects of society.

8. National Institute on Drug Abuse
http://www.nida.nih.gov
NIDA's mission is to lead the nation in bringing the power of science to bear on drug abuse and addiction.

The Major Drugs of Use and Abuse

9. Drug Information
http://area51.upsu.plym.ac.uk/infoserv/drugs/ graphical/main.html
This Web site from the United Kingdom presents the history, effects, dangers, and legal issues surrounding most legal and illegal drugs.

10. QuitNet
http://www.quitnet.org
The QuitNet helps smokers kick their nicotine addiction. This site is a joint project of Join Together, a program of the Boston University School of Public Health, and the Massachusetts Tobacco Control Program.

Other Trends and Patterns in Drug Use

11. Marijuana as a Medicine
http://mojo.calyx.net/~olsen/MEDICAL/medical.html
This site promotes the concept of marijuana as medicine. This is a controversial issue that has been in the news quite a bit over the past two years. At this site, you will find numerous links to other sites that support this idea, as well as information developed specifically for this site.

Drugs and Crime

12. Drug Enforcement Administration
http://www.usdoj.gov/dea/
The mission of the Drug Enforcement Administration is to enforce the controlled substances laws and regulations of the United States.

13. The November Coalition
http://www.november.org
According to its Web site, The November Coalition is a growing body of citizens whose lives have been gravely affected by present drug policy. This group represents convicted prisoners, their loved ones, and others who believe that the U.S. drug policies are unfair and unjust.

14. TRAC DEA Site
http://trac.syr.edu/tracdea/index.html
The Transactional Records Access Clearinghouse (TRAC) is a data gathering, data research, and data distribution organization associated with Syracuse University. According to their Web site, the purpose of TRAC is to provide the American people—and institutions of oversight such as Congress, news organizations, public interest groups, businesses, scholars and lawyers—with comprehensive information about the activities of federal enforcement and regulatory agencies and the communities in which they take place.

Measuring the Social Costs of Drugs

15. DrugText
http://www.drugtext.org
The DrugText library consists of individual drug-related libraries with independent search capabilities.

16. International Powerlifting Federation—Medical Committee
http://www.ipf.com/medical.htm
This site is the IPF Medical Committee Handbook on Drug Control. This information is an example of a steroid-use policy and drug-testing procedure.

17. The National Organization on Fetal Alcohol Syndrome
http://www.nofas.org
NOFAS is a nonprofit organization founded in 1990 dedicated to eliminating birth defects caused by alcohol consumption during pregnancy and improving the quality of life for those individuals and families affected. NOFAS is the only national organization focusing solely on FAS, the leading known cause of mental retardation.

18. National NORML Homepage
http://www.natlnorml.org
This is the homepage for the National Organization for the Reform of Marijuana Laws.

Creating and Sustaining Effective Drug Control Policy

19. The Drug Reform Coordination Network
http://www.drcnet.org
This is the home page of the Drug Reform Coordination Network. According to their home page, the DRC Network is committed to reforming current drug laws in the United States.

20. DrugWatch International
http://www.drugwatch.org
According to their Web site, Drug Watch International is a volunteer nonprofit information network and advocacy organization that promotes the creation of healthy drug-free cultures in the world and opposes the legalization of drugs. The organization upholds a comprehensive approach to drug issues involving prevention, education, intervention/treatment, and law enforcement/interdiction.

21. United Nations International Drug Control Program
http://www.undcp.org
The mission of UNDCP is to work with the nations and the people of the world to tackle the global drug problem and its consequences.

22. Marijuana Policy Project
http://www.mpp.org
According to their Web site, the Marijuana Policy Project's purpose is to develop and promote policies to minimize the harm associated with marijuana.

23. Office of National Drug Control Policy
http://www.whitehousedrugpolicy.gov
The principal purpose of ONDCP is to establish policies, priorities, and objectives for the Nation's drug control program, the goals of which are to reduce illicit drug use, manufacturing, and trafficking; drug-related crime and violence; and drug-related health consequences.

Prevention and Treatment

24. Creative Partnerships for Prevention
http://www.CPPrev.org
The goal of this national initiative is to provide current information, ideas, and resources on how to use the arts and humanities to enhance drug and violence prevention programming, foster resiliency in youth, and implement collaborations within communities to strengthen prevention programs for youth. The materials developed for this initiative have been designed with the guidance of educators, prevention specialists, youth workers, and professionals from cultural institutions (arts and humanities organizations, museums, libraries, etc.).

25. D.A.R.E.
http://www.dare-america.com
According to their Web site, this year 33 million school children around the world—25 million in the U.S.—will benefit from D.A.R.E. (Drug Abuse Resistance Education), the highly acclaimed program that gives kids the skills they need to avoid involvement in drugs, gangs, or violence. D.A.R.E. was founded in 1983 in Los Angeles.

26. Hazelden
http://www.hazelden.org
Hazelden is a nonprofit organization providing high quality, affordable rehabilitation, education, prevention, and professional services and publications in chemical dependency and related disorders.

27. Indiana Prevention Resource Center
http://www.drugs.indiana.edu/home.html
The Indiana Prevention Resource Center at Indiana University is a statewide clearinghouse for prevention, technical assistance, and information about alcohol, tobacco, and other drugs for the state of Indiana.

We highly recommend that you review our Web site for expanded information and our other product lines. We are continually updating and adding links to our Web site in order to offer you the most usable and useful information that will support and expand the value of your Annual Editions. You can reach us at: http://www.dushkin.com/annualeditions/.

www.dushkin.com/online/

Unit 1

Unit Selections

1. **Opium, Cocaine, and Marijuana in American History,** David F. Musto
2. **A Drug Trade Primer for the Late 1990s,** Current History
3. **A Hundred-Year Habit,** Ian Scott
4. **One Nation under the Table,** John Lilly
5. **New Museum Traces History of Drugs in the U.S.,** Christopher S. Wren
6. **Just Don't Say No, Not Us,** Jerry Adler
7. **America's Altered States,** Joshua Wolf Shenk

Key Points to Consider

❖ Why is history important when attempting to understand contemporary drug-related events?

❖ What historical trends are expressed by the use of legal drugs versus illegal drugs?

❖ What are the historical drug-related landmarks of drug prohibition and control?

❖ How is the evolution of drug-related influence on American society like and unlike that occurring in other countries?

❖ What can we learn from these comparisons?

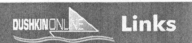 **Links**   **www.dushkin.com/online/**

4. **National Council on Alcoholism and Drug Dependence, Inc.**
   http://www.ncadd.org

These sites are annotated on pages 4 and 5.

When attempting to define the American drug experience, one must examine the past as well as the present. Too often drug use and its associated phenomena are viewed through a contemporary looking glass relative to our personal views, biases, and perspectives. Although today's drug scene is definitely a product of the counterculture of the 1960s and 1970s, the crack trade of the 1980s, and the sophisticated, criminally syndicated, technologically efficient influence of the late 1980s and early 1990s, it is also a product of the past. This past and the lessons it has generated, although largely unknown, forgotten, or ignored, provide one important perspective from which to assess our current status and to guide our future in terms of optimizing our efforts to manage the benefits and control the harm from drugs.

The American drug experience is often defined in terms of a million individual realities, all meaningful and all different. In fact, these realities often originated as pieces of our national, cultural, racial, religious, and personal past that combine to influence significantly present-day drug-related phenomena.

The contemporary American drug experience is the product of centuries of human attempts to alter or sustain consciousness through the use of mind-altering drugs. Early American history is replete with accounts of the exorbitant use of alcohol, opium, morphine, and cocaine.

Heroin and cocaine "epidemics" of the twentieth century are analogous to opiate and cocaine epidemics of the eighteenth and nineteenth centuries. A review of early American history clearly suggests the precedents for our continuing pursuit of stimulant and depressant drugs such as cocaine and heroin. In terms of social costs produced by our historical use of legal and illegal drugs, it is no wonder that some describe us as a nation of addicts. Seldom has history expressed American's collective capacity to use an addictive drug responsibly. On what grounds do we justify 10 percent of the American population as alcoholic and over 1,000 tobacco-related deaths each day? On one hand, we recoil from the consequences of drug use while, on the other, we profess our helplessness to change.

Drug use and its concomitant influences are pervasive. We will all be affected and forced to confront a personally, professionally, or socially troublesome or even tragic event instigated by someone's use of drugs. Drugs are in our homes, our schools, and our workplaces. The most recent survey of illicit drug use in the United States indicates that an estimated 13.6 million Americans have used some form of an illicit drug within 30 days prior to the survey. This number reflects a continued leveling off of illicit drug use by adults. The largest number of adult users was believed to be in 1979 when survey results reported 25 million users. This leveling off is also now reflected, for the first time since 1992, in drug use by those 12 to 17 years of age. Presently, 9.9 percent of this age

group reported using illicit drugs in the last 30 days, a statistically significant decline from last year's 11.4 percent. The usage rate for youths was highest in 1979 at 16.3 percent and lowest in 1992 at 5.3 percent. Since 1992, drug use by youth has climbed steadily. Most survey research suggests the need to continue targeting drug abuse by young persons. Most experts believe parents to be the most important factor in protecting children from drugs. More than two-thirds of teens and two-thirds of their parents report that American culture glamorizes smoking cigarettes and drinking alcohol. It is estimated that 4.1 million or 18.2 percent of youths 12 to 17 years of age are currently cigarette smokers and 10.5 million, aged 12 to 20, are drinkers of alcohol.

Drugs impact our most powerful public institutions on many fronts. Drugs are *the* business of our criminal justice system, and drugs compete with terrorism, war, and other major national security concerns as demanding military issues. Many argue eloquently that drugs pose a "clear and present danger." Just a year ago, five American servicemen and women were killed in a mysterious and little-reported drug reconnaissance flight in Colombia. Drug use is a topic of congressional confirmations and presidential elections. As you read through the pages of this book, the pervasive nature of drug-related influence will become more apparent. Unfortunately, one of the most salient observations one can make is that drug use in our society is a topic about which many Americans have too little knowledge. History suggests that we have continually struggled to respond and react to the influence of drug use in our society. The lessons of our drug legacy are harsh, whether they are the subjects of public health or public policy. Turning an uninformed mind toward a social condition of such importance will only further our inability to address the dynamics of changing drug-related issues and problems.

The articles and graphics contained in unit 1 illustrate the multitude of issues influenced by the historical evolution of drug use in America. The historical development of drug-related phenomena is reflected within the character of all issues and controversies addressed by this book. Drug-related events of yesterday provide important meaning for understanding and addressing drug-related events of today and the future. Creating public policy and controlling crime surface immediately as examples with long-standing historical influences. As you read this and other literature on drug-related events, the dynamics of drug-related historical linkages will become apparent. As you read further, try to identify these historical linkages as they help define the focus at hand. For example, what are the implications for public health resulting from a historical lack of drug-related educational emphasis? What will history reflect 20 years from now? Is there a historical pattern of drug-related educational shortcomings that we should change?

Opium, Cocaine and Marijuana in American History

Over the past 200 years, Americans have twice accepted and then vehemently rejected drugs. Understanding these dramatic historical swings provides perspective on our current reaction to drug use

David F. Musto

DAVID F. MUSTO is professor of psychiatry at the Child Study Center and professor of the history of medicine at Yale University. He earned his medical degree at the University of Washington and received his master's in the history of science and medicine from Yale. Musto began studying the history of drug and alcohol use in the U.S. when he worked at the National Institute of Mental Health in the 1960s. He has served as a consultant for several national organizations, including the Presidential Commission on the HIV epidemic. From 1981 until 1990, Musto was a member of the Smithsonian Institution's National Council.

Dramatic shifts in attitude have characterized America's relation to drugs. During the 19th century, certain mood-altering substances, such as opiates and cocaine, were often regarded as compounds helpful in everyday life. Gradually this perception of drugs changed. By the early 1900s, and until the 1940s, the country viewed these and some other psychoactive drugs as dangerous, addictive compounds that needed to be severely controlled. Today, after a resurgence of a tolerant attitude toward drugs during the 1960s and 1970s, we find ourselves, again, in a period of drug intolerance.

America's recurrent enthusiasm for recreational drugs and subsequent campaigns for abstinence present a problem to policymakers and to the public. Since the peaks of these episodes are about a lifetime apart, citizens rarely have an accurate or even a vivid recollection of the last wave of cocaine or opiate use.

Phases of intolerance have been fueled by such fear and anger that the record of times favorable toward drug taking has been either erased from public memory or so distorted that it becomes useless as a point of reference for policy formation. During each attack on drug taking, total denigration of the preceding, contrary mood has seemed necessary for public welfare. Although such vigorous rejecting may have value in further reducing demand, the long-term effect is to destroy a realistic perception of the past and of the conflicting attitudes toward mood-altering substances that have characterized our national history.

The absence of knowledge concerning our earlier and formative encounters with drugs unnecessarily impedes the already difficult task of establishing a workable and sustainable drug policy. An examination of the period of drug use that peaked around 1900 and the decline that followed it may enable us to approach the current drug problem with more confidence and reduce the likelihood that we will repeat past errors.

Until the 19th century, drugs had been used for millennia in their natural form. Cocaine and morphine, for example, were available only in coca leaves or poppy plants that were chewed, dissolved in alcoholic beverages or taken in some way that diluted the impact of the active agent. The advent of organic chemistry in the 1800s changed the available forms of these drugs. Morphine was isolated in the first decade and cocaine by 1860; in 1874 diacetylmorphine was synthesized from morphine (although it became better known as heroin when the Bayer Company introduced it in 1898).

By mid-century the hypodermic syringe was perfected, and by 1870 it had become a familiar instrument to American physicians and patients [see "The Origins of Hypodermic Medication," by Norman Howard-Jones; SCIENTIFIC AMERICAN, January 1971]. At the same time, the astounding growth of the pharmaceutical industry intensified the ramifications of these accomplishments. As the century wore on, manufacturers grew increasingly adept at exploiting a marketable innovation and moving it into mass production, as well as advertising and distributing it throughout the world.

During this time, because of a peculiarity of the U.S. Constitution, the powerful new forms of opium and cocaine were more readily available in America than in most nations. Under the Constitution, individual states assumed responsibility for health issues, such as regulation of medical practice and the availability of pharmacological products. In fact, America had as many laws regarding health professions as it had states. For much of the 19th century, many states chose to have no controls at all; their legislatures reacted to the claims of contradictory health care philosophies by allowing free enterprise for all practitioners. The federal government limited its concern to communicable diseases and the provision of health care to the merchant marine and to government dependents.

Nations with a less restricted central government, such as Britain and Prussia, had a single, preeminent pharmacy law that controlled availability of dangerous drugs. In those countries, physicians had their right to practice similarly granted by a central authority. Therefore, when we consider consumption of opium, opiates, coca and cocaine in 19th-century America, we are looking at an era of wide availability and unrestrained advertising. The initial enthusiasm for the purified substances was only slightly affected by any substantial doubts or fear about safety, long-term health injuries or psychological dependence.

History encouraged such attitudes. Crude opium, alone or dissolved in some liquid such as alcohol, was brought by European explorers and settlers to North America. Colonists regarded opium as a familiar resource for pain relief. Benjamin Franklin regularly took laudanum—opium in alcohol extract—to alleviate the pain of kidney stones during the last few years of his life. The poet Samuel Taylor Coleridge, while a student at Cambridge in 1791, began using laudanum for pain and developed a lifelong addiction to the drug. Opium use in those early decades constituted an "experiment in nature" that has been largely forgotten, even repressed, as a result of the extremely negative reaction that followed.

Americans had recognized, however, the potential danger of continually using opium long before the availability of morphine and the hypodermic's popularity. The American Dispensatory of 1818 noted that the habitual use of opium could lead to "tremors, paralysis, stupidity and general emaciation." Balancing this danger, the text proclaimed the extraordinary value of opium in a multitude of ailments ranging from cholera to asthma. (Considering the treatments then in vogue—blistering, vomiting and bleeding—we can understand why opium was as cherished by patients as by their physicians.)

Opium's rise and fall can be tracked through U.S. import-consumption statistics compiled while importation of the drug and its derivative, morphine, was unrestricted and carried moderate tariffs. The per capita consumption of crude opium rose gradually during the 1800s, reaching a peak in the last decade of the century. It then declined, but after 1915 the data no longer reflect trends in drug use, because that year new federal laws severely restricted legal imports. In contrast, per capita consumption of smoking opium rose until a 1909 act outlawed its importation.

Americans had quickly associated smoking opium with Chinese immigrants who arrived after the Civil War to work on railroad construction. This association was one of the earliest examples of a powerful theme in the American perception of

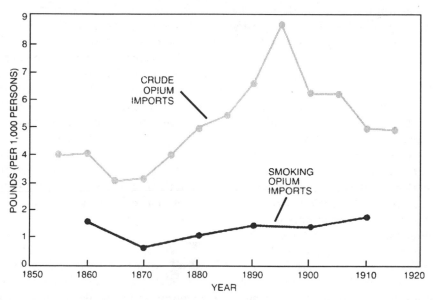

OPIATE CONSUMPTION was documented by the Treasury and the Commerce Departments, starting in the mid-19th century. The importation of smoking opium became illegal in 1909, and crude opium and its derivatives were severely restricted in 1915. After 1915, the data reflected medicinal use.

drugs: linkage between a drug and a feared or rejected group within society. Cocaine would be similarly linked with blacks and marijuana with Mexicans in the first third of the 20th century. The association of a drug with a racial group or a political cause, however, is not unique to America. In the 19th century, for instance, the Chinese came to regard opium as a tool and symbol of Western domination. That perception helped to fuel a vigorous antiopium campaign in China early in the 20th century.

During the 1800s, increasing numbers of people fell under the influence of opiates—substances that demanded regular consumption or the penalty of withdrawal, a painful but rarely life-threatening experience. Whatever the cause—overprescribing by physicians, over-the-counter medicines, self-indulgence or "weak will"—opium addiction brought shame. As consumption increased, so did the frequency of addiction.

At first, neither physicians nor their patients thought that the introduction of the hypodermic syringe or pure morphine contributed to the danger of addiction. On the contrary, because pain could be controlled with less morphine when injected, the presumption was made that the procedure was less likely to foster addiction.

Late in the century some states and localities enacted laws limiting morphine to a physician's prescription, and some laws even forbade refilling these prescriptions. But the absence of any federal control over interstate commerce in habit-forming drugs, of uniformity among the state laws and of effective enforcement meant that the rising tide of legislation directed at opiates—and later cocaine—was more a reflection of changing public attitude toward these drugs than an effective reduction of supplies to users. Indeed, the decline noted after the mid-1890s was probably related

mostly to the public's growing fear of addiction and of the casual social use of habit-forming substances rather than to any successful campaign to reduce supplies.

At the same time, health professionals were developing more specific treatments for painful diseases, finding less dangerous analgesics (such as aspirin) and beginning to appreciate the addictive power of the hypodermic syringe. By now the public had learned to fear the careless, and possibly addicted, physician. In *A Long Day's Journey into Night*, Eugene O'Neill dramatized the painful and shameful impact of his mother's physician-induced addiction.

In a spirit not unlike that of our times, Americans in the last decade of the 19th century grew increasingly concerned about the environment, adulterated foods, destruction of the forests and the widespread use of mood-altering drugs. The concern embraced alcohol as well. The Anti-Saloon League, founded in 1893, led a temperance movement toward prohibition, which later was achieved in 1919 and became law in January 1920.

After overcoming years of resistance by over-the-counter, or patent, medicine manufacturers, the federal government enacted the Pure Food and Drug Act in 1906. This act did not prevent sales of addictive drugs like opiates and cocaine, but it did require accurate labeling of contents for all patent remedies sold in interstate commerce. Still, no national restriction existed on the availability of opiates or cocaine. The solution to this problem would emerge from growing concern, legal ingenuity and the unexpected involvement of the federal government with the international trade in narcotics.

Responsibility for the Philippines in 1898 added an international dimension to the growing domestic alarm about drug abuse. It also revealed that Congress, if given the opportunity, would prohibit nonmedical uses

of opium among its new dependents. Civil Governor William Howard Taft proposed reinstituting an opium monopoly—through which the previous Spanish colonial government had obtained revenue from sales to opium merchants—and using those profits to help pay for a massive public education campaign. President Theodore Roosevelt vetoed this plan, and in 1905 Congress mandated an absolute prohibition of opium for any purpose other than medicinal use.

To deal efficiently with the antidrug policy established for the Philippines, a committee from the Islands visited various territories in the area to see how others dealt with the opium problem. The benefit of controlling narcotics internationally became apparent.

In early 1906 China had instituted a campaign against opium, especially smoking opium, in an attempt to modernize and to make the Empire better able to cope with continued Western encroachments on its sovereignty. At about the same time, Chinese anger at maltreatment of their nationals in the U.S. seethed into a voluntary boycott of American goods. Partly to appease the Chinese by aiding their antiopium efforts and partly to deal with uncontrollable smuggling within the Philippine Archipelago, the U.S. convened a meeting of regional powers. In this way, the U.S. launched a campaign for worldwide narcotics traffic control that would extend through the years in an unbroken diplomatic sequence from the League of Nations to the present efforts of the United Nations.

The International Opium Commission, a gathering of 13 nations, met in Shanghai in February 1909. The Protestant Episcopal bishop of the Philippines, Charles Henry Brent, who had been instrumental in organizing the meeting, was chosen to preside. Resolutions noting problems with opium and opiates were adopted, but they did not constitute a treaty, and no decisions bound the nations attending the commission.

In diplomatic parlance, what was needed now was a conference not a commission. The U.S. began to pursue this goal with determination.

The antinarcotics campaign in America had several motivations. Appeasement of China was certainly one factor for officials of the State Department. The department's opium commissioner, Hamilton Wright, thought the whole matter could be "used as oil to smooth the troubled water of our aggressive commercial policy there." Another reason was the belief, strongly held by the federal government today, that controlling crops and traffic in producing countries could most efficiently stop U.S. nonmedical consumption of drugs.

To restrict opium and coca production required worldwide agreement and, thus, an international conference. After intense diplomatic activity, one was convened in the Hague in December 1911. Brent again presided, and on January 23, 1912, the 12 nations represented signed a convention. Provision was made for the other countries to comply before the treaty was brought into force. After all, no producing or manufacturing nation wanted to leave the market open to nonratifying nations.

The convention required each country to enact domestic legislation controlling narcotics trade. The goal was a world in which narcotics were restricted to medicinal use. Both the producing and consuming nations would have control over their boundaries.

After his return from Shanghai, Wright labored to craft a comprehensive federal antinarcotics law. In his path loomed the problem of states' rights. The health professions were considered a major cause of patient addiction. Yet how could federal law interfere with the prescribing practices of physicians or require that pharmacists keep records? Wright settled on the federal government's power to tax; the result, after prolonged bargaining with pharmaceutical, import, export and medical interests, was the Harrison Act of December 1914.

Representative Francis Burton Harrison's association with the act was an accidental one, the consequence of his introduction of the administration's bill. If the chief proponent and negotiator were to be given eponymic credit, it should have been called the Wright Act. It could even have been called a second Mann Act, after Representative James Mann, who saw the bill through to passage in the House of Representatives, for by that time Harrison had become governor-general of the Philippines.

The act required a strict accounting of opium and coca and their derivatives from entry into the U.S. to dispensing to a patient. To accomplish this control, a small tax had to be paid at each transfer, and permits had to be obtained by applying to the Treasury Department. Only the patient paid no tax, needed no permit and, in fact, was not allowed to obtain one.

Initially Wright and the Department of Justice argued that the Harrison Act forbade indefinite maintenance of addiction unless there was a specific medical reason such as cancer or tuberculosis. This interpretation was rejected in 1916 by the Supreme Court—even though the Justice Department argued that the Harrison Act was the domestic implementation of the Hague Opium Convention and therefore took precedence over states' rights. Maintenance was to be allowed.

That decision was short-lived. In 1919 the Supreme Court, led by Oliver Wendell Holmes and Louis Brandeis, changed its mind by a 5–4 vote. The court declared that indefinite maintenance for "mere addiction" was outside legitimate medical practice and that, consequently, prohibiting it did not constitute interference with a state's right to regulate physicians. Second, because the person receiving the drugs for maintenance was not a bona fide patient but just a recipient of drugs, the transfer of narcotics defrauded the government of taxes required under the Harrison Act.

During the 1920s and 1930s, the opiate problem, chiefly morphine and heroin, declined in the U.S., until much of the problem was confined to the periphery of society and the outcasts of urban areas. There were exceptions: some health professionals and a few others of middle class or higher status continued to take opiates.

America's international efforts continued. After World War I, the British and U.S. governments proposed adding the Hague Convention to the Versailles Treaty. As a result, ratifying the peace treaty meant ratifying the Hague Convention and enacting a domestic law controlling narcotics. This incorporation led to the British Dangerous Drugs Act of 1920, an act often misattributed to a raging heroin epidemic in Britain. In the 1940s some Americans argued that the British system provided heroin to addicts and, by not relying on law enforcement, had almost eradicated the opiate problem. In fact, Britain had no problem to begin with. This argument serves as an interesting example of how the desperate need to solve the drug problem in the U.S. tends to create misperceptions of a foreign drug situation.

The story of cocaine use in America is somewhat shorter than that of opium, but it follows a similar plot. In 1884 purified cocaine became commercially available in the U.S. At first the wholesale cost was very high—$5 to $10 a gram—but it soon fell to 25 cents a gram and remained there until the price inflation of World War I. Problems with cocaine were evident almost from the beginning, but popular opinion and the voices of leading medical experts depicted cocaine as a remarkable, harmless stimulant.

William A. Hammond, one of America's most prominent neurologists, extolled cocaine in print and lectures. By 1887 Hammond was assuring audiences that cocaine was no more habit-forming than coffee or tea. He also told them of the "cocaine wine" he had perfected with the help of a New York druggist: two grains of cocaine to a pint of wine. Hammond claimed that this tonic was far more effective than the popular French coca wine, probably a reference to Vin Mariani, which he complained had only half a grain of cocaine to the pint.

Coca-Cola was also introduced in 1886 as a drink offering the advantages of coca but lacking the danger of alcohol. It amounted to a temperance coca beverage. The cocaine was removed in 1900, a year before the city of Atlanta, Ga., passed an ordinance (and a state statute the following year) prohibiting provision of any cocaine to a consumer without a prescription.

Cocaine is one of the most powerful of the central nervous system euphoriants. This fact underlays cocaine's quickly growing consumption and the ineffectiveness of the early warnings. How could anything that made users so confident and happy be bad? Within a year of cocaine's introduction, the Parke-Davis Company provided coca and cocaine in 15 forms, including coca cigarettes, cocaine for injection and cocaine for sniffing. Parke-Davis and at least one other company also offered consumers a handy cocaine kit. (The Parke-Davis kit contained a hypodermic syringe.) The firm proudly supplied a drug that, it announced, "can supply the place of food, make the coward brave, the silent eloquent and . . . render the sufferer insensitive to pain."

Cocaine spread rapidly throughout the nation. In September 1886 a physician in Puyallup, Washington Territory, reported an adverse reaction to cocaine during an operation. Eventually reports of overdoses and idiosyncratic reactions shifted to accounts of the social and behavioral effects of long-term cocaine use. The ease with which experimenters became regular users and the increasing instances of cocaine being linked

with violence and paranoia gradually took hold in popular and medical thought.

In 1907 an attempt was made in New York State to shift the responsibility for cocaine's availability from the open market to medical control. Assemblyman Alfred E. Smith, later the governor of New York and in 1928 the Democratic party's presidential candidate, sponsored such a bill. The cost of cocaine on New York City streets, as revealed by newspaper and police accounts after the law's enactment, was typically 25 cents a packet, or "deck."

Although 25 cents may seem cheap, it was actually slightly higher than the average industrial wage at that time, which was about 20 cents an hour. Packets, commonly glycine envelopes, usually contained one or two grains (65 to 130 milligrams), or about a tenth of a gram. The going rate was roughly 10 times that of the wholesale price, a ratio not unlike recent cocaine street prices, although in the past few years the street price has actually been lower in real value than what it was in 1910.

Several similar reports from the years before the Harrison Act of 1914 suggest that both the profit margin and the street price of cocaine were unaffected by the legal availability of cocaine from a physician. Perhaps the formality of medical consultation and the growing antagonism among physicians and the public toward cocaine helped to sustain the illicit market.

In 1910 William Howard Taft, then president of the U.S., sent to Congress a report that cocaine posed the most serious drug problem America had ever faced. Four years later President Woodrow Wilson signed into law the Harrison Act, which, in addition to its opiate provisions, permitted the sale of cocaine only through prescriptions. It also forbade any trace of cocaine in patent remedies, the most severe restriction on any habit-forming drug to that date. (Opiates, including heroin, could still be present in small

amounts in nonprescription remedies, such as cough medicines.)

Although the press continued to reveal Hollywood scandals and underworld cocaine practices during the 1920s, cocaine use gradually declined as a societal problem. The laws probably hastened the trend, and certainly the tremendous public fear reduced demand. By 1930 the New York City Mayor's Committee on Drug Addiction was reporting that "during the last 20 years cocaine as an addiction has ceased to be a problem."

Unlike opiates and cocaine, marijuana was introduced during a period of drug intolerance. Consequently, it was not until the 1960s, 40 years after marijuana cigarettes had arrived in America, that it was widely used. The practice of smoking cannabis leaves came to the U.S. with Mexican immigrants, who had come North during the 1920s to work in agriculture, and it soon extended to white and black jazz musicians.

As the Great Depression of the 1930s settled over America, the immigrants became an unwelcome minority linked with violence and with growing and smoking marijuana. Western states pressured the federal government to control marijuana use. The first official response was to urge adoption of a uniform state antinarcotics law. Then a new approach became feasible in 1937, when the Supreme Court upheld the National Firearms Act. This act prohibited the transfer of machine guns between private citizens without purchase of a transfer tax stamp—and the government would not issue the necessary stamp. Prohibition was implemented through the taxing power of the federal government.

Within a month of the Supreme Court's decision, the Treasury Department testified before Congress for a bill to establish a marijuana transfer tax. The bill became law, and until the Comprehensive Drug Abuse Act of 1970, marijuana was legally controlled through a transfer tax for which no stamps or licenses were available to private citizens. Certainly some people were smoking marijuana in the 1930s, but not until the 1960s was its use widespread.

Around the time of the Marijuana Tax Act of 1937, the federal government released dramatic and exaggerated portrayals of marijuana's effects. Scientific publications during the 1930s also fearfully described marijuana's dangers. Even Walter Bromberg, who thought that marijuana made only a small contribution to major crimes, nevertheless reported the drug was "a primary stimulus to the impulsive life with direct expression in the motor field."

Marijuana's image shifted during the 1960s, when it was said that its use at the gigantic Woodstock gathering kept peace—as opposed to what might have happened if alcohol had been the drug of choice. In the shift to drug toleration in the late 1960s and early 1970s, investigators found it difficult to associate health problems with marijuana use. The 1930s and 1940s had marked the nadir of drug toleration in the U.S., and possibly the mood of both times affected professional perception of this controversial plant.

After the Harrison Act, the severity of federal laws concerning the sale and possession of opiates and cocaine gradually rose. As drug use declined, penalties increased until 1956, when the death penalty was introduced as an option by the federal government for anyone older than 18 providing heroin to anyone younger than 18 (apparently no one was ever executed under this statute). At the same time, mandatory minimum prison sentences were extended to 10 years.

After the youthful counterculture discovered marijuana in the 1960s, demand for the substance grew until about 1978, when the favorable attitude toward it reached a peak. In 1972 the Presidential Commission on Marijuana and Drug Abuse rec-

ommended "decriminalization" of marijuana, that is, legal possession of a small amount for personal use. In 1977 the Carter administration formally advocated legalizing marijuana in amounts up to an ounce.

The Gallup Poll on relaxation of laws against marijuana is instructive. In 1980, 53 percent of Americans favored legalization of small amounts of marijuana; by 1986 only 27 percent supported that view. At the same time, those favoring penalties for marijuana use rose from 43 to 67 percent. This reversal parallels the changes in attitude among high school students revealed by the Institute of Social Research at the University of Michigan.

The decline in favorable attitudes toward marijuana that began in the late 1970s continues. In the past few years we have seen penalties rise again against users and dealers. The recriminalization of marijuana possession by popular vote in Alaska in 1990 is one example of such a striking reversal.

In addition to stricter penalties, two other strategies, silence and exaggeration, were implemented in the 1930s to keep drug use low and prevent a recurrence of the decadeslong, frustrating and fearful antidrug battle of the late 19th and early 20th centuries. Primary and secondary schools instituted educational programs against drugs. Then policies shifted amid fears that talking about cocaine or heroin to young people, who now had less exposure to drugs, would arouse their curiosity. This concern led to a decline in drug-related information given during school instruction as well as to the censorship of motion pictures.

The Motion Picture Association of America, under strong public and religious pressure, decided in 1934 to refuse a seal of approval for any film that showed narcotics. This prohibition was enforced with one exception—To the Ends of the Earth, a 1948 film that lauded the Federal Bureau of Narcotics—until Man with a Golden Arm was successfully exhibited in 1956 without a seal.

Associated with a decline in drug information was a second, apparently paradoxical strategy: exaggerating the effects of drugs. The middle ground was abandoned. In 1924 Richmond P. Hobson, a nationally prominent campaigner against drugs, declared that one ounce of heroin could addict 2,000 persons. In 1936 an article in the American Journal of Nursing warned that a marijuana user "will suddenly turn with murderous violence upon whomever is nearest to him. He will run amuck with knife, axe, gun, or anything else that is close at hand, and will kill or maim without any reason."

A goal of this well-meaning exaggeration was to describe drugs so repulsively that anyone reading or hearing of them would not be tempted to experiment with the substances. One contributing factor to such a publicity campaign, especially regarding marijuana, was that the Depression permitted little money for any other course of action.

Severe penalties, silence and, if silence was not possible, exaggeration became the basic strategies against drugs after the decline of their first wave of use. But the effect of these tactics was to create ignorance and false images that would present no real obstacle to a renewed enthusiasm for drugs in the 1960s. At the time, enforcing draconian and mandatory penalties would have filled to overflowing all jails and prisons with the users of marijuana alone.

Exaggeration fell in the face of the realities of drug use and led to a loss of credibility regarding any government pronouncement on drugs. The lack of information erased any awareness of the first epidemic, including the gradually obtained and hard-won public insight into the hazards of cocaine and opiates. Public memory, which would have provided some context for the antidrug laws, was a casualty of the antidrug strategies.

The earlier and present waves of drug use have much in common, but there is at least one major difference.

During the first wave of drug use, antidrug laws were not enacted until the public demanded them. In contrast, today's most severe antidrug laws were on the books from the outset; this gap between law and public opinion made the controls appear ridiculous and bizarre. Our current frustration over the laws' ineffectiveness has been greater and more lengthy than before because we have lived through many years in which antidrug laws lacked substantial public support. Those laws appeared powerless to curb the rise in drug use during the 1960s and 1970s.

The first wave of drug use involved primarily opiates and cocaine. The nation's full experience with marijuana is now under way (marijuana's tax regulation in 1937 was not the result of any lengthy or broad experience with the plant). The popularity and growth in demand for opiates and cocaine in mainstream society derived from a simple factor: the effect on most people's physiology and emotions was enjoyable. Moreover, Americans have recurrently hoped that the technology of drugs would maximize their personal potential. That opiates could relax and cocaine energize seemed wonderful opportunities for fine-tuning such efforts.

Two other factors allowed a long and substantial rise in consumption during the 1800s. First, casualties accumulate gradually; not everyone taking cocaine or opiates becomes hooked on the drug. In the case of opiates, some users have become addicted for a lifetime and have still been productive.

Yet casualties have mounted as those who could not handle occasional use have succumbed to domination by drugs and by drug-seeking behavior. These addicts become not only miserable themselves but also frightening to their families and friends. Such cases are legion today in our larger cities, but the percentage of those who try a substance and acquire a dependence or get into serious legal trouble is not 100 percent. For cocaine, the estimate varies from 3 to 20 percent, or even higher, and so it is a matter of time before cocaine is recognized as a likely danger.

Early in the cycle, when social tolerance prevails, the explanation for casualties is that those who succumb to addiction are seen as having a physiological idiosyncrasy or "foolish trait." Personal disaster is thus viewed as an exception to the rule. Another factor minimizing the sense of risk is our belief in our own invulnerability—that general warnings do not include us. Such faith reigns in the years of greatest exposure to drug use, ages 15 to 25. Resistance to a drug that makes a user feel confident and exuberant takes many years to permeate a society as large and complex as the U.S.

The interesting question is not why people take drugs, but rather why they stop taking them. We perceive risk differently as we begin to reject drugs. One can perceive a hypothetical 3 percent risk from taking cocaine as an assurance of 97 percent safety, or one can react as if told that 3 percent of New York/Washington shuttle flights crash. Our exposure to drug problems at work, in our neighborhood and within our families shifts our perception, gradually shaking our sense of invulnerability.

Cocaine has caused the most dramatic change in estimating risk. From a grand image as the ideal tonic, cocaine's reputation degenerated into that of the most dangerous of drugs, linked in our minds with stereotypes of mad, violent behavior. Opiates have never fallen so far in esteem, nor were they repressed to the extent cocaine had been between 1930 and 1970.

Today we are experiencing the reverse of recent decades, when the technology of drug use promised an extension of our natural potential. Increasingly we see drug consumption as reducing what we could achieve on our own with healthy food and exercise. Our change of attitude about drugs is connected to our concern over air pollution, food adulteration and fears for the stability of the environment.

Ours is an era not unlike that early in this century, when Americans made similar efforts at self-improvement accompanied by an assault on habit-forming drugs. Americans seem to be the least likely of any people to accept the inevitability of historical cycles. Yet if we do not appreciate our history, we may again become captive to the powerful emotions that led to draconian penalties, exaggeration or silence.

FURTHER READING

AMERICAN DIPLOMACY AND THE NARCOTICS TRAFFIC, 1900–1939. Arnold H. Taylor. Duke University Press, 1969.

DRUGS IN AMERICA: A SOCIAL HISTORY, 1800–1980. H. Wayne Morgan. Syracuse University Press, 1981.

DARK PARADISE: OPIATE ADDICTION IN AMERICA BEFORE 1940. David T. Courtwright. Harvard University Press, 1982.

THE AMERICAN DISEASE: ORIGINS OF NARCOTIC CONTROL. Expanded Edition. David F. Musto. Oxford University Press, 1987.

AMERICA'S FIRST COCAINE EPIDEMIC. David F. Musto in Wilson Quarterly, pages 59–65; Summer 1989.

ILLICIT PRICE OF COCAINE IN TWO ERAS: 1908–14 AND 1982–89. David F. Musto in Connecticut Medicine, Vol. 54, No. 6, pages 321–326; June 1990.

A Drug Trade Primer for the Late 1990s

GEOPOLITICAL DRUG WATCH

"As with the effective marketing of any product at the end of the twentieth century, the drug system involves strategies and tactics that bring radically different civilizations, attitudes, and principles into contact. . . . [Yet] the system of producing and marketing drugs is . . . very different from that of any other product, whether legal or not. Everything connected with drugs is at the same time 'modern' and 'traditional,' 'international' and 'local.' In short, drugs are the barely distorted reflection of the problems involved in managing the world at the dawn of the third millennium."

Since the late 1980s, drugs have become public enemy number one in the West, embodying the "new lack of order" that characterizes the post-cold war world. By advancing the theory of "the scourge of drugs," Western nations have above all sought to reemploy the geopolitical tools that had been rusting under the influence of what was perhaps hastily described as the "new world order."

The drug system operates on a global scale that recognizes neither nationality nor borders. It is governed by the rules of supply and demand, dumping, and even bartering. As with the effective marketing of any product at the end of the twentieth century, the drug system involves strategies and tactics that bring radically different civilizations, attitudes, and principles into contact, affecting them in various ways depending on the drugs involved. Although an integral part of local and regional history, the system of producing and marketing drugs is nonetheless very different from that of any other product, whether legal or not. Everything connected with drugs is at the same time "modern" and "traditional," "international" and "local." In short, drugs are the barely distorted reflection of the problems involved in managing the world at the dawn of the third millennium.

THE HYDRA EFFECT

The past two years have been a turning point in several respects, first and foremost because of the changes observed in crime related to drug trafficking. During the 1980s the manufacture, export, and, to a lesser extent, distribution of drugs were mainly carried out by major criminal organizations, some of which had become involved in trafficking on a large scale in the course of the previous decade. These were the Italian criminal organizations, the Colombian cartels, the Turkish mafia, and the Chinese triads. Although the centralized and strictly hierarchical structure of such organizations has often been mythicized, it is true that they monopolized a substantial share of the market and maintained business relations with one another.

In the past two or three years the drug trade has taken on a noticeably different appearance. Admittedly, some large criminal organizations still exist (in Mexico and Burma, for example), as well as midsized outfits (in Colombia, Brazil, and Pakistan), but a massive number of small businesses have sprung up alongside them. In addition to the multi-ton drug shipments occasionally seized by the police—often amid a

From *Current History,* April 1998, pp. 150-153. Adapted from the 1997 report of the Paris-based Geopolitical Drug Watch. The full report may be found at www.ogd.org/rapport/gb/RP03_TENDANCES.html.

blaze of publicity—considerable quantities of drugs are transported in tiny batches. Placed end to end, they would stretch much farther than the large shipments, as the monthly reports issued by the World Customs Organization demonstrate.

There are several reasons for this change. The first and most obvious is that international anti-drug organizations and national police forces have focused on the most visible forms of crime, which have thus become vulnerable. This is especially true in Colombia and Italy, where major criminal organizations have overestimated their own strength and openly attacked the state itself. This has resulted either in the dismantling of the criminal organizations, as happened with the Medellín cartel after the death of drug lord Pablo Escobar in December 1993, or in a withdrawal or tactical change, as in the case of the Cosa Nostra and the Camorra (early 1990s), the Cali cartel (1995–1996), and the organization in Burma led by warlord Khun Sa (1995–1996).

The immediate effect of repression was to disorganize the networks. But by making a virtue of necessity, these large organizations quickly realized that decentralized structures are much less vulnerable and began the process of transforming themselves accordingly. In some cases they even anticipated events. Thus Khun Sa, Burma's "Opium King," gave himself up to the army without a fight in January 1996 in exchange for sharing the market with the military and the possibility of investing in other, licit economic sectors.

Similarly, it is likely that some of the so-called arrests of Cali cartel leaders by the Colombian government were in fact merely disguised surrenders fulfilling agreements with the cartels. Their leaders adopted a strategy of moving into legal business activities after negotiating with Mexican organizations to hand over parts of their export networks to the United States. The Colombian criminal organizations have not disappeared, but they are much more discreet today. They have given rise—if one adds other regional groups, such as the Bogotá and Pereira cartels, to the heirs of the two major cartels—to 40 midsized organizations.

Meanwhile, the withdrawal of the major cartels has enabled small businesses to find their place in the sun without taking too many risks. There might be from 2,000 to 3,000 of these small groups in Colombia, often families or groups of friends who have a relative or other contact in the United States or Europe. The Peruvian and Bolivian organizations, which used to be heavily dependent on their Colombian counterparts, have also taken advantage of the reshuffle to acquire greater independence and, in the case of the Bolivians, to work more closely with Brazilian criminal organizations.

Little is known about the restructuring process involving Cosa Nostra—although researcher Pino Arlachi speculates that the *cupola,* its governing body, has not met for several years—but more information is available about the restructuring of the Camorra. Naples police say that the success of the struggle against the mafia, which can be attributed to the use of "turncoats" that has led to the arrest of the main "godfathers," has caused a breakup of the organization and an increase in the number of smaller groups. In 1983, about a dozen Camorra groups were counted in Naples; there are now believed to be about 100, with a total of some 6,000 members. They are also better equipped, thanks to weapons obtained from the former Yugoslavia. Other chance factors have contributed to this trend. One example is the emergence of African networks—notably Nigerian—which are usually based on family or clan structures.

Clearly, these new types of organizations make the work of the police much more difficult, and in any case the dismantling of a network only affects a tiny part of the quantity of drugs in circulation. But it is not just police efforts that have triggered the traffickers' reshuffle; other factors have caused or allowed organizations connected with the drug trade to undergo major changes.

BOOMING PRODUCTION

In the past 10 years the supply of drugs has seen uninterrupted growth. Most of the older production zones for coca, opium poppies, and cannabis have remained stable or have been extended, while new production zones (poppies in Colombia, coca in Georgia) have been opened and areas previously cultivated for traditional use have been converted to supply the international market (Central Asia, the Caucasus, the Balkans, and Ukraine for poppies and sub-Saharan Africa for cannabis). One of the reasons for this is the internationalization of trade, the effect of which is often augmented by the introduction of structural adjustment programs that have downplayed the role of agriculture in many economies, especially in Latin America and Africa.

To the increase in drug plant cultivation must be added the booming market in synthetic drugs. This growth allows organizations of any size, and even individuals, to obtain drug supplies of all kinds. However, since demand for drugs has at the same time grown and diversified, this profusion on the supply side has not yet resulted in fighting over control of markets.

It was estimated at the end of the 1980s that cocaine hydrochloride production in Latin America ranged between 500 and 700 tons annually; by 1996 this figure was thought to have risen to between 800 and 1,200 tons. In 1988, Burma and Afghanistan were each producing between 800 and 1,000 tons of opium; in 1996 the figure reached about 4,500 tons between the two. Drug production continues to expand in all the countries of Central Asia, the Caucasus, and the Balkans, as well as in China and Vietnam.

Marijuana production is also booming. The amount of land under cannabis cultivation in Morocco rose from 30,000 hectares in 1988 to more than 70,000 in 1996, allowing over 2,000 tons of hashish to be produced. Cultivation in Afghanistan and Pakistan combined yields a similar total weight. Colombia is once more becoming the major marijuana producer it was in the 1970s. Since the United States market is saturated with local crops and imports from Mexico and Jamaica, the Colombians are increasingly turning toward Europe. Seizures of marijuana from Asia, especially Cambodia, are becoming more frequent worldwide. South Africa produces tens of thousands of tons for its own market and is starting to export to Europe. Production is increasing rapidly throughout sub-Saharan Africa, especially in Kenya, Malawi, Nigeria, Ghana, the two Congos, the Ivory Coast, and Senegal. There are many signs that attempts to grow coca and opium poppies are also being made in several of these countries.

Growing global drug production comes in response to booming demand. The large traditional markets, Western Europe and the United States, are relatively stable. But new markets are emerging and expanding rapidly. In the case of cocaine these are Japan and Asia generally, South Africa, and especially Russia and other Eastern European countries. The heroin market is also expanding in the former communist states. In addition, there has been a boom in consumption of all kinds of drugs in the producer countries themselves and, more generally, in the third world. This is especially true with heroin in Asia (especially Pakistan, India, Thailand, and China) and cocaine in Latin America (especially Argentina, Brazil, and Chile). Synthetic drugs are also making major breakthroughs in third world markets in Asia and Africa.

This diversification of both user markets and production zones provides an initial explanation for the growing number of small and midsized businesses—especially given the increasing number of victims of the recession in both the third world and the major urban centers of developed countries, where narcotics production and trafficking and even "utilitarian" drug use can be means of survival.

THE INCREASE IN LOCAL CONFLICTS

The growing number of local conflicts, a side effect of the end of the cold war and the convulsions caused by the collapse of the Soviet Union, have also contributed to the changed nature of the drug system. The major powers, prevented from engaging in direct clashes by nuclear deterrence, previously came into conflict through their allies in the third world. The end of the cold war, far from bringing these local conflicts to a halt, merely highlighted the lack of any true ideological reasons behind them and unleashed forces based on ethnic, religious, and national factors.

The warring factions, no longer able to count on their powerful protectors to finance their causes, have been forced to seek alternative sources of income in trafficking, including drug trafficking. Some of these conflicts, such as those in Colombia, Afghanistan, and Angola, were in progress before the end of the cold war, but the withdrawal of the superpowers means they have acquired a new character, gradually drifting into predatory behavior in the case of the Armed Revolutionary Forces of Colombia (FARC), or ethnic and religious antagonism manipulated by regional forces in the case of the Afghan civil war. In most instances the end of the superpower struggle revealed dissension that the leaden weight of communist regimes had helped to mask; this is what happened in the Yugoslav, Chechen, and Azerbaijani-Armenian conflicts, and in the civil

Growing global drug production comes in response to booming demand.

wars in Georgia and Albania. The protagonists in these clashes were thorough in their search for financial support, trafficking in a host of commodities that included oil, drugs, and strategic metals. Typically they used their diaspora communities and migrants in Western Europe as bridgeheads, with the players setting up networks to earn cash for the cause or sometimes acting autonomously. Secret agents in many countries (Russia, Pakistan, and South Africa, for example) who in earlier times had used the drug trade to finance unofficial operations have often switched to activities with purely criminal ends.

These developments, coupled with the factors mentioned above, have led to an increase in what Geopolitical Drug Watch describes as "short" or "fragmented" networks. The people involved are not trafficking "professionals" and do not specialize in a single product. They work only sporadically and drop their criminal activities once they have achieved their political or economic goals.

EASTERN EUROPE AND SYNTHETIC DRUGS

In another striking development, the mid-1990s saw the countries of the former Soviet bloc enter the drug trade. The main target for these new producers is Western Europe, but there are many signs that they are also taking an interest in more distant markets such as North America, South Africa, and Australia.

To enter the drug trade, local criminal organizations can usually choose to cultivate drug plants or use a deserted chemical factory to make synthetic drugs. In Eastern Europe the latter choice is favored since the basic chemical ingredients are not subjected to close scrutiny; highly qualified and underpaid chemists are in plentiful supply; and drug users in the region (at least in urban areas) have little experience with natural drugs and therefore have no objection to replacements.

In the past few years it appears that synthetic drug production has begun on a large scale in Eastern Europe. German police estimate that between 20 and 25 percent of the amphetamines seized in the country in 1994 came from Poland, while Warsaw authorities estimate that Polish production supplies roughly 10 percent of the European market. University laboratories are suspected of producing drugs and huge numbers of couriers have been arrested at the German and Swedish borders. The Czech Republic vies with Poland for the title of second-largest European producer of psychotropic drugs (after the Netherlands), especially ephedrine, the main precursor chemical in the manufacture of methamphetamines. In 1994, the UN condemned an incident in which 50 tons of Czech ephedrine was sent to clandestine Mexican laboratories by way of Switzerland. The finished product was apparently intended for the United States market.

Various scandals since 1992 have shown that Latvia and Hungary are favored by, notably, Dutch and Scandinavian investors, who finance the production of Ecstasy for European Union countries, as well as the manufacture of amphetamine derivatives in liquid, injectable form. In 1993 the International Narcotics Control Board expressed concern about the existence in Bulgaria of state enterprises manufacturing phenethylamines under the brand name Captagon for export without permission to Nigeria and the Arabian peninsula, by way of Turkey.

Among the former Soviet republics, Azerbaijan has specialized in manufacturing synthetic opiates (methadone, normorphine, 3-methylfentanyl) and methamphetamines in the cities of Gyandzha and Baku. In other parts of the former Soviet Union synthetic ephedrine is extracted from pharmaceutical ingredients and converted into ephedrone (an amphetamine derivative known in the United States as methcathinone). *Ephedra vulgaris,* which is cultivated in Azerbaijan, grows wild in Kyrgyzstan and Kazakhstan's Almaty region.

China also makes the most of its *Ephedra* resources. Clandestine methamphetamine laboratories, supplied with ephedrine appropriated from the pharmaceutical industry, have sprung up in Guangdong and Fujian provinces, for the moment almost exclusively for the Southeast Asian and former Soviet republic markets. In many cases it is the Taiwanese triads, whose members come from southern China, that are behind this production.

A NEW GLOBAL DIVIDE

At the start of the third millennium, synthetic drugs will probably have the dubious merit of standardizing the various divides in drug use: between the better-off and the disadvantaged in rich countries; and between developed countries and the developing world. As with other drugs, the only difference will lie in the quality of the product. But it is also likely that this large-scale drug abuse affecting tens of millions of individuals will merely coexist alongside the "classic" use of drugs derived from plants.

A Hundred-Year Habit

Ian Scott

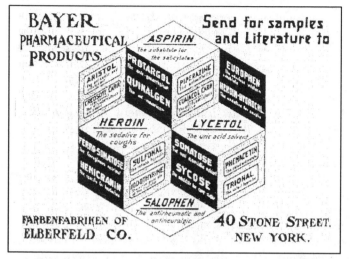

Wonder-drugs: Bayer at the turn of the century advertise their two new over-the-counter products, Heroin and Aspirin.

■ In 1898 a German chemical company launched a new cough medicine called 'Heroin'. A hundred years later, this drug is flooding illegally into Britain in record amounts. The latest Home Office annual figures show a 40 per cent increase in police seizures of heroin. The National Criminal Intelligence Service believes that up to 80 per cent of the heroin currently entering Britain is controlled by Turkish organised criminals based in London and the South East. How, then, did nineteenth-century science come to bequeath this notorious drug of abuse to twentieth-century crime?

In 1863 a dynamic German merchant called Friedrich Bayer (1825–76) set up a factory in Elberfeld to exploit new chemical procedures for making colourful dyes from coal-tar. German coal-tar dye manufacture expanded rapidly, surpassing English or French production six-fold by the mid-1870s. In the mid-1880s, however, price conventions and raw material availability deteriorated in the German dye industry, so the Bayer company invested in scientific research to diversify its product range. In 1888, a new substance synthesised by Bayer chemists became the company's first commercial medicine.

Synthetic chemical medicines were something new. In the early years of the nineteenth century, medicines had been prepared using crude natural materials like opium, the dried milky juice of poppy seed pods. A young German pharmacist called Friedrich Sertürner (1783–1841) had first applied chemical analysis to plant drugs, by purifying in 1805 the main active ingredient of opium. Recalling Morpheus, the Greek god of dreams, Sertürner gave his drug the name 'morphium', which later became morphine. Perhaps appropriately, the discoverer of morphine was in due course nominated for academic honours by the author of 'Faust', Goethe himself.

The possibility of obtaining morphine and other pure drugs from plants brought commercial reward for entrepreneurs such as Georg Merck (1825–73), who turned his family's seventeenth-century pharmacy in Darmstadt into a major supplier of these new products. Morphine was widely used for pain relief in the American Civil War and the Franco-Prussian War, in combination with the hypodermic syringe, which was invented in 1853. In contrast to the old crude preparations, precisely measured doses of the new purified drugs could be administered. Furthermore, drug action in the body could be more scientifically investigated. Pharmacology therefore developed rapidly not least in Germany.

As part of the Prussianisation of Alsace-Lorraine following the Franco-Prussian War, a well-equipped institute was built in Strasbourg in 1872 for the eminent German pharmacologist Oswald Schmiedeberg (1838–1921). One of Schmiedeberg's many talented pupils, Heinrich Dreser (1860–1924), ended up as head of the pharmacological laboratory at the product-hungry Bayer Company in Elberfeld.

Now that plant-derived drugs were available in purified form, chemists could modify them to form new molecules that might prove more effective, or perhaps safer to use. In the late 1890s, Dreser and his colleagues adopted this strategy to produce for Bayer two of the most famous drugs in the world today. Heroin, made by adding two acetyl groups to the morphine molecule, was followed a year later by another acetyl derivative of a painkiller from plants; the second natural drug was salicylic acid and the Bayer derivative was named 'Aspirin'.

Ironically from today's perspective, heroin took its name from the adjective *heroisch* (heroic) sometimes

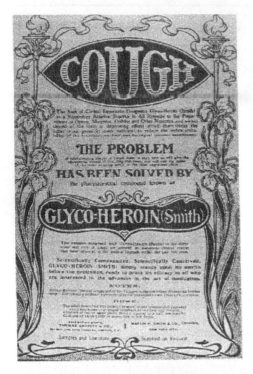
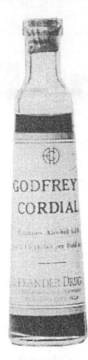

A turn-of-the-century advertisement for New York chemist Smith's Glyco-Heroin compound, 'Superior in All Respects to the Preparations of Opium, Morphine, Codeine and Other Narcotics and withal devoid of the toxic or depressing effects which characterize the latter'. (Right) Godfrey's Cordial—an opium-based tonic for babies.

used by nineteenth-century German doctors for a powerful medicine. Dreser presented his new drug as a cough, chest and lung medicine to the Congress of German Naturalists and Physicians in 1898. Painful respiratory diseases such as pneumonia and tuberculosis ('consumption') were then the leading causes of death, and in the days before antibiotics or the BCG vaccine, doctors could only prescribe narcotics to alleviate the sufferings of patients who otherwise could not sleep. There was, therefore, considerable interest in the highly effective new drug. Today, heroin is known to be a more potent and faster acting painkiller than morphine because it passes more readily from the bloodstream into the brain. Heroin was praised in a number of early clinical trials, and was rapidly adopted in medical establishments in many countries. Bayer advertised the drug in German, English, Italian, Russian and other languages.

Heroin was prescribed in place of morphine or codeine (another constituent of opium, isolated in 1832). In a typical early report of 1898, G. Strube of the Medical University Clinic of Berlin tested oral doses of 5 and 10 mg of heroin on fifty phthisis patients and found it effective in relieving their coughs and producing sleep. He noted no unpleasant reactions; indeed the patients liked it and continued to take the heroin after he ceased to prescribe. The addictive po-

tential of heroin's parent, morphine, was only too well known, and evidence steadily emerged that the new drug was not the hoped-for improvement in this respect. Horatio C. Wood Jr. reported in 1899 that heroin dosages had to be increased with usage to remain effective. Such was the preoccupation with morphine addiction, however, that some doctors, such as A. Morel-Lavallée in 1902, even advocated treatment by heroin in 'demorphinisation'. This practice was criticised by J. Jarrige in 1902, who by then had observed that heroin withdrawal symptoms were even worse than those of morphine.

By 1903 the writing was on the wall: in an article in the *Alabama Medical Journal* entitled 'The Heroin Habit Another Curse', G. E. Pettey declared that of the last 150 people he had treated for drug addiction, eight were dependent on heroin. Nevertheless, other physicians remained reluctant to abandon this highly effective drug. In 1911, J. D. Trawick could still lament in the *Kentucky Medical Journal*: 'I feel that bringing charges against heroin is almost like questioning the fidelity of a good friend. I have used it with good results.'

The United States was the country in which heroin addiction first became a serious problem. By the late nineteenth century, countries such as Britain and Germany had enacted pharmacy laws to control dangerous drugs, but under the US Constitution individual states were responsible for medical regulation. Late in the century some state laws required morphine or cocaine to be prescribed by physician, but drugs could still be obtained from bordering states with laxer legislation. Moreover, this era was the peak of a craze for over-the-counter 'patent' medicines that were still permitted to contain these drugs. At the turn of the century it is believed that over a quarter of a million Americans (from a population of 76 million) were addicted to opium, morphine or cocaine.

After years of resistance, American patent medicine manufacturers were required by the federal Pure Food and Drug Act of 1906 accurately to label the contents of their products. These included 'soothing syrups' for bawling babies, and 'cures' for chronic ills such as consumption or even drug addiction, which previously had not declared (and sometimes denied) their content of opium, cocaine or cannabis. Consumers by this time were becoming fearful of addictive drugs, so the newly labelled patent medicines either declined in popularity or removed their drug ingredients. (The pre-eminent survival from this era is a tonic beverage from Atlanta called 'Coca-Cola'.) Bayer's 1899 launch of Aspirin, moreover, had made available a safe and effective painkiller to replace opium for everyday use.

In 1914 President Woodrow Wilson signed the Harrison Narcotic Act, which exploited the federal government's power to tax as a mechanism for finally enabling federal regulation of medical transactions in opium derivatives or cocaine. The main impetus for national drug laws in the US was diplomatic. As today, China was seen as the greatest emerging market, to which the Americans sought improved access. To help the massive Chinese opium problems, the US had led an international campaign culminating in the Hague Opium Convention of 1912, which required signatories to enact domestic legislation controlling opium trade. After the First World War, the Hague Convention was added to the Treaty of Versailles, requiring the British Dangerous Drugs Act of 1920, despite the absence of a serious drugs problem in this country.

The now familiar association of youthful heroin abusers with underworld suppliers was first noted in New York, where illicit availability was probably greatest due to the proximity of many of the chemical companies that then distributed heroin. In 1910, New York's Bellevue Hospital made its first ever admission for heroin addiction. In 1915, it admitted 425 heroin addicts, who were, according to the *Psychiatric Bulletin of the New York State Hospitals*, 'in many instances members of gangs who congregate on street corners particularly at night, and make insulting remarks to people who pass.' It was noted that 'in practically every case the drug had been tried by one of the members of the gang who then induced the other members to try it.' These early heroin users were mostly between seventeen and twenty-five years old, and took the drug by sniffing.

New York addiction specialist A. Lambert in 1924 described heroin addiction as a 'vice of the underworld' acquired by the young through 'vicious associations'. American drug abusers were completely dependent on black market sources soon after 1919, when legal interpretation of the Harrison Act outlawed medical prescription of narcotics to maintain addicts. At this stage, heroin increased in popularity among drug dealers, who appreciated its black market qualities as a compact and powerful substance that could easily be adulterated. Another development at this time was the discovery by addicts of the enhanced euphoric effects when heroin was injected with the hypodermic syringe.

During the early 1920s a number of New York addicts supported themselves by collecting scrap metal from industrial dumps, so earning the label 'junkies'. Less savoury behavior by heroin addicts was, however, causing concern to the authorities and public. Dr. Lambert claimed that 'heroin destroys the sense of responsibility to the herd'. Heroin addiction was blamed for a number of the 260 murders that occurred in 1922 in New York (which compared with seventeen in London). These concerns led the US Congress to ban all domestic manufacture of heroin in 1924.

Two years later, however, US Narcotic Inspector S. L. Rakusin declared that heroin seemed 'more plentiful than it ever was before'. Organised criminals were still obtaining heroin produced by legitimate pharmaceutical manufacturers in Western Europe, and later Turkey and Bulgaria, until restrictive policies of the League of Nations drove heroin manufacture largely underground by the early 1930s. An exception was militarist Japan and its occupied territories, where pharmaceutical firms produced heroin on a massive scale for the Chinese market until the end of the Second World War. Since then heroin has effectively belonged to the realm of international crime.

Ian Scott is a Lecturer in Biological Sciences in the University of Wales Aberystwyth.

One Nation Under the Table

Reviewed By John Lilly

Drink: A Social History of America

Andrew Barr

Carroll & Graf / 384 pages / $27.95

If *Drink: A Social History of America* can be said to have a central argument, it is as sprawling and disjoint as its subject: that in every sense, the American people have enjoyed a grotesquely abusive relationship with booze, from colonial times to the present day. It's all there in Andrew Barr's book: the first drunken infatuation with spirits, the oft-regretted decision to play the field with wine and beer when things just weren't working out, the trial separations of the temperance movement, the stormy estrangement of Prohibition, the edgy rapprochement of Repeal ... And the bingeing flings throughout, the consequent self-hating hypocrisy, and the violence—bar-smash, car-crash, gangland slaughter. About the only good to have come out of the whole mess, it would seem, has been the creation of some excellent products (bourbon whiskey, California wine), and the birth of the Republic itself.

What roused the eighteenth-century revolutionary rabble was not the liquor, Barr writes, but the opportunity for unmonitored fellowship, as embodied in the institution of the tavern. ("Inside them they had organised the formation of militia; outside they had planted liberty poles," he intones.) We are reminded—more than once, as with so many points in this repetitious book—that Jefferson wrote the first draft of the Declaration of Independence while sipping a pint (!) of Madeira in a Philadelphia tavern. "Pursuit of Happiness," indeed. Of course, at the time, wine (even a wine that packed Madeira's 50-proof fortified wallop) was popularly believed to contain no alcohol.

Whether or not Jefferson was the first alcoholic American writer, the rest of Barr's story is a nearly unmitigated litany of greed, squalor, class warfare, ethnic suspicion, dangerously high-minded campaigning, and intermittent state suppression with all its foreseeably unforeseen consequences. If, for example, the old-line Anglo-Saxons did not like the drinking habits of their newer and poorer Irish and German neighbors—not to mention even more recent immigrants from eastern and southern Europe—the clear solution was to ban the manufacture, transport, and sale of booze altogether. The wretched refuse would lose its right to swill beer, wine, and—particularly—demon whiskey, and the United States would be cleaner, safer, and more sober as a result.

As any schoolchild knows (if not from history class, certainly from reruns of "The Untouchables"), Prohibition did not work out quite as planned. As it will, the market took over in a more ruthless way once supply and demand were driven underground, and Americans ended up downing more hard spirits—the most easily transported form of alcohol—than ever before. Only in New Jersey and Illinois was beer still widely drunk: in "the former through tradition and the latter through the organizational efficiency of Al Capone." Vineyards were reduced to a meager output for the ecclesiastical market, and the production of something called the "wine brick"— a package of pressed grapes "sold to home winemakers, along with a yeast pill and a printed warning not to use it, 'because if you do, this will turn into wine, which would be illegal.' "

Bootleggers proclaimed themselves clerics to take advantage of the legal exception for sacramental wine, then hijacked their own deliveries. The restaurant trade all but died; Manhattan's speakeasies became the only places in town where one could get a decent meal, washed down with bathtub "gin." In any case, "people did not go to speakeasies in order to socialize with the bartender or their fellow customers, but to get drunk." One contemporary observer commented: "No longer is drinking an art with Americans. ... The more quick and fatal the liquor, the better they like it."

If the results of a 1989 survey are anything to go by, the 40 percent of male college students and 34 percent of university women who admitted to drinking habitually in order to get drunk would probably say that not much has changed. Of course, with 1984's passage of the National Minimum Drinking Age Act (a piece of Reagan-era federal legislation that, as Barr points out, betrayed an uncharacteristic hostility toward states' rights), the students in question do inhabit a speakeasy culture: They have become the latter-day subjects of a sort of mini-Prohibition. Having reached their legal majority in every other sense, Americans between 18 and 21 years of age are all unwilling participants in a bit of experimental history. Certainly other factors are at work in the staggering numbers of staggering students, but Barr is right in his conviction that the drinking age has

JOHN LILLY *is co-owner of Liberia Vértice, a bookstore in Seville, Spain.*

almost undeniably taken its toll: Seven years before the imposition of a minimum age of 21, only 25 percent of male students had said they normally drank to get drunk. Five years after the law's passage, that number had risen by 15 points—a 60 percent increase in the number of undergraduate male drunks. As for the population of heavy-drinking coeds, their proportion had zoomed from 10 to 34 percent, for a numerical increase of 240 percent in twelve years. While the proportion of alcohol-related traffic accidents among teenagers has dropped faster than it has among the whole population, in 1996 it still stood at 36.6 percent, down from 63.2 percent in 1982. And as Barr points out, a large chunk of that drop can be attributed to "more strict law enforcement, an increased emphasis on the liability of bartenders, and the introduction of designated driver schemes," as well as the conciousness raising of Mothers Against Drunk Driving, and the elimination of so-called "blood borders" between states with different drinking ages. As for this last factor, Barr reasonably speculates that it "may have nothing to do with the imposition of a minimum drinking age of twenty-one but may simply be explained by the fact that the drinking age has been standardized across the country."

In contrast to the fiasco of American alcohol policy, Barr offers concrete examples of how people handle their drink in other societies, and what drinking could be like in an America freer of meddlesome state supervision. Toward the end of his conclusion, he quotes at length a report on America's "liquor problem" by the Committee of Fifty, a group of nineteenth-century sociologists. They describe in achingly idyllic terms the scene in a Chicago beer garden of the time:

> The waiters, most of them fine-appearing elderly gentlemen, dressed in black, serve beer, wines, and soft drinks to the people out in the open. . . . The garden is brilliantly lighted with Japanese lanterns hanging from the trees. The lights, the trees, the starry heavens above, the moon gliding now and then behind the clouds, soul-stirring music. . . .

And here are entire families, and young lovers, and old men nursing their beer for hours as they philosophize and reminisce. The passage ends:

> A young woman of strong temperance views exclaimed, after spending an hour in this garden for the first time, "Isn't it beautiful? Can it be, is it possible, that after all our ideas are wrong and these people are right?"

A food and wine writer for the London *Times*, Barr admits in his book's introduction to being a polemicist as well, and *Drink: A Social History of America* is, among other things, a polemic. If the book questions one belief more emphatically than any other (and it does question a lot of beliefs), it is the idea of alcohol as a seriously addictive drug. Here Barr is mistaken. Alcohol—as anyone who has ever taken drink will attest, and as he himself admits—is most certainly a drug. And its addictive potential is clear to anyone who has ever truly been in its thrall, or who has ever been close to anyone truly in its thrall, however briefly.

Barr's misapprehension on this point metastasizes throughout the book, as he directs his bile toward even those campaigners whose work has had an undeniably salutary influence and few side-effects. His evident hostility toward Alcoholics Anonymous, for example, would seem to have no other source; it certainly does not proceed from a sincere interest in understanding the tenets of a group which has provided miraculously life-giving results for millions of suffering people.

Barr mistrusts AA's insistence on total abstinence, and indeed, some reformed alcoholics do seem to be able to live a sober life through moderation coupled with counseling. But if "it is true that drinkers who persist in AA remain abstinent," as he admits, then is this not a good thing? He feels these people are duping themselves, but they were unquestionably duping themselves when they were drinking, and with catastrophic consequences for themselves and those around them. If AA works for them, one wonders in what sense they can be said to be wrong: Nowhere in the Twelve Steps and Twelve Traditions does Alcoholics Anonymous claim to understand the etiology of the disease—only that alcoholics have had their lives turned upside-down by an addiction, and that the following things have been found to bring the benefits of sobriety to those who adhere to them. Neither, as Barr implies, do the Twelve Steps absolve their adherents of responsibility for their actions; in fact, they explicitly enjoin members to take full responsibility for the evil they did in their drinking days, and to make amends where possible.

That said, and apart from an overreaching all-inclusiveness that at times crosses the line into digression, Barr's book largely fulfills its ambitious goals, taking a deep and well-researched look at U.S. social history through rosé-tinted glasses. From the first European settlers' attempts to euchre the Indians out of their land by plying them with strong drink, to the Whiskey Rebellion, to latter-day criminal charges of "fetal abuse" leveled against alcoholic mothers, Barr paints an unruly and often unpleasant picture. To anyone from, say, Latin Europe, where people live with alcohol as a normal part of daily life, where beer and wine are taken in moderation with meals and where the vast majority almost never drink to get drunk, it must seem like madness. It probably is.

New Museum Traces

History of Drugs in the U.S.

By CHRISTOPHER S. WREN

WASHINGTON, May 6—Franklin Delano Roosevelt hated fascists. He didn't like drug dealers either, ranking them barely above murderers as the worst sort of criminals.

"In the case of murder, you take away the life of a fellow human being," President Roosevelt said in 1940. "In the case of distributing narcotics, you take away the mind of the individual and make his life intolerable for the good of his own soul."

Roosevelt's sentiment is, not surprisingly, shared by the Drug Enforcement Administration. It has given his remark prominence in its new museum on drugs, which opened this week at the agency's headquarters in Arlington, Va.

The agency, whose personnel spend much of their time pursuing drugs and thugs in secret operations, is not known for operating in the limelight. But Terry Parham, a special agent who is acting chief of public affairs, said the new museum and visitors center is consistent with the agency's mission. "We try to get understanding from the American people on what the problem is all about," he said.

Contrary to early expectations, the museum is short on propaganda celebrating the agency's exploits. Some displays verge on whimsy, like a presentation of the early "tools of the agent's trade"—a Thompson submachine gun and a pair of standard-issue hand grenades. There is

also a clumsy pair of green platform shoes worn by a bell-bottomed agent who infiltrated Detroit's music scene in the 1970's.

An effort to tell the American people 'what the problem is all about.'

The museum's curator, Jill Jonnes, said the museum tries to give context and coherence to the whole national experience with drugs. "This was really lost history," said Ms. Jonnes, the author of "Hepcats, Narcs and Pipe Dreams: A History of America's Romance with Illegal Drugs" (Johns Hopkins University Press, 1999). "Everyone in this country knows of heroin," she said. "Almost nobody knows it was a pharmaceutical product introduced by Bayer" a century ago.

Inside the museum entrance are three storefronts representing changing views of drugs in America. There is a benign drug store in 1940, when people looked at drugs as more of a help than a hindrance. There is a "head shop" displaying rolling papers for marijuana, colored glass bongs, or pipes, and other drug paraphernalia

used in 1970. And there is a crack-house door through which crack cocaine was sold in 1990. Beyond the hole in the reinforced steel door is a bleak photograph of children playing with a pile of crack vials.

The museum entwines three themes: the trends in the popularity of drugs, society's reactions to those trends and the evolution of Federal drug enforcement.

The history of drug use in the United States begins with the opium-smoking of some Chinese immigrants who joined the California gold rush, which started in 1849.

The displays move on to the Civil War, when wounded veterans returned home addicted to morphine, a painkilling opiate, in what was called the "soldier's disease." By the late 19th century, genteel ladies with discreet access to doctors and legal opiates made up the majority of addicts. Laudanum, a form of opium, cost 28 cents for a three-ounce bottle from Sears, Roebuck & Company.

In 1885, cocaine was introduced as an elixir for every ailment from depression to hay fever. A yellow label on display briskly instructed users: "For catarrh and all head diseases, snuff very little up the nose 5 times a day until cured; before bedtime put grease up the nose, wash out with warm water next morning."

Another advertisement urged mothers to give cranky children a dose of Mrs. Winslow's Soothing Syrup, which was laced with morphine. The

From *The New York Times*, May 9, 1999, p. 18. © 1999 by The New York Times Company. Reprinted by permission.

museum displays an ensuing death certificate from Minnesota.

By 1900, one in 200 Americans was addicted to opiates or cocaine, according to the museum. The typical user was a white, middle-class woman who became addicted through well-meaning medical treatment.

"It gives you a sense of how many people were routinely using drugs," Ms. Jonnes said, describing what she called the forgotten epidemic.

Marijuana rose to prominence in the 1930's. The museum offers lyrics for a jazz song extolling marijuana in 1938: "When your throat gets dry, you know you're high, everything is dandy." And there is an enlarged photograph of a marijuana smoke-in by Michigan college students in 1978. By that time, a caption reports, more than one-third of the nation's

adults and one in five teen-agers were frequent drug users.

Drug dealers had more sartorial class in the old days, judging by a display of surveillance photographs of an undercover drug purchase in Baltimore in 1940. The pushers wore jackets, ties and straw boaters.

Exhibits of smuggling devices include a lime-green surfboard hollowed out to conceal packets of drugs, and a cuddly Paddington Bear stuffed with money from drug sales.

The profits of drug smuggling are manifested by the .45-caliber pistol, elaborately engraved and encrusted with diamonds, that Rafael Caro-Quintero, a Mexican drug trafficker, was carrying when he was captured in Costa Rica in 1985. Another such souvenir is a $35,000 chrome Harley-Davidson motorcycle, confiscated

from a Hell's Angel who is in prison for selling drugs.

A gallery shows photographs of rock stars killed by heroin, including Janis Joplin, Jimi Hendrix and, most recently, Kurt Cobain.

"The overall point of the museum is that drugs have exacted a significant toll on us as a society," Ms. Jonnes said, "and we want to tell that story in a very accessible way."

Michael R. Harris, a museum consultant who helped design the displays, said he hoped to put the exhibits on a CD-ROM for schools. "It needs to be brought into the classroom and talked about," he said.

The 2,200-square-foot museum is open from 10 A.M. to 4 P.M., Tuesdays through Fridays, to visitors who make an appointment (202) 307–3463 and clear the metal detector at the entrance to the agency.

Just Don't Say No, Not Us

You can't escape your kids' questions about drugs

BY JERRY ADLER

SUSAN, A LOS ANGELES homemaker and the mother of a 16-year-old son, believes it's never too soon to start lying to your kids about drugs. She began when he was 6 and, all fired up by an elementary-school program, asked if Mommy had done any of those terrible things. "I didn't hesitate to say no," she says, belying a history of marijuana use from the age of 12, LSD at 15 and a two-year addiction to amphetamines. She lied when he asked again five years later, although her husband, with considerably less to hide, confessed. That made her feel even worse. "I lied to him and now he thinks it's so terrific that I never tried drugs," she says. She beats down the impulse to tell the truth. "I think he would feel incredibly betrayed," she reasons.

Susan, and most of the 78 million adult Americans who have used drugs, will never run for president. But they have found that doesn't exempt them from difficult questions about their behavior when, like a certain candidate, they were young and irresponsible. "If you throw a stick into a crowd of people in their 40s, you'll hit at least five who've had to swallow hard and deal with this question," says Bruce Bomier, 52, author of "Marijuana and the Responsible Parent." "We need to confront George W.'s dilemma in our own homes."

It is a dilemma because for most parents, the answers represent a choice of competing hypocrisies. Telling the truth involves admitting you've done things yourself that you won't permit your child to do. But many parents feel uncomfortable lying to their children—especially in the context of asking a child to tell the truth about *his* habits. And there's the practical danger that a college friend will come to dinner and start reminiscing about the time you went to hear Iron Butterfly. "The worst thing is to lie to your kid and have them find out later," says Dr. Pedro Jose Greer, 43, of Miami. (Although he would make an exception about the other question middle-aged parents often face: "I'm a Cuban father. If my daughter asked if I had sex before I was married, I'd tell her I don't even have sex now.")

The best course, experts say, takes into account the child's age and maturity. You don't really have to answer a 6-year-old, says Dr. Steven Berkowitz, a child psychiatrist at Yale. "What they really want to hear is, 'We are going to take care of you, you don't have to worry about it'." With adolescents, "it's useful to say, 'Yeah, I did it.' Then you can say, 'Let's talk about why I was lucky and what happens when you're not'." But the focus of any discussion should be on the child's need for guidance. As a

parent, this is not the occasion to work out your own feelings, and since you're not running for office, your "candor" is not the issue. "You can say, 'I'm simply not prepared to discuss this. It's my personal business from the past'," advises Ariel White-Kovach, executive director of youth services at the Hazelden Foundation.

Some had no choice—like Glenn Loury, 51, the well-known educator who had hopes of being named undersecretary of Education in 1987 but withdrew out of fear that his drug use would come to light. It did, that same year, when he was arrested for possession of cocaine—a charge later dropped after he completed treatment. His children, now 10 and 7, were told about it, because, he reasoned, they would find out eventually anyway. And while "Susan's" son may admire her for saying no, Loury hopes his sons have an even stronger example to guide them: a father who almost blew his career, and even his life, over drugs. You couldn't make up a better answer than that.

WITH JOHN McCORMICK *in Chicago,*
TARA WEINGARTEN *In Los Angeles,*
RENA KIRSCH *in Boston,*
PIPER FOGG *in WASHINGTON* and
CATHARINE SKIPP *in Miami*

AMERICA'S ALTERED STATES

When does legal relief of pain become illegal pursuit of pleasure?
By Joshua Wolf Shenk

My soul was a burden, bruised and bleeding. It was tired of the man who carried it, but I found no place to set it down to rest. Neither the charm of the countryside nor the sweet scents of a garden could soothe it. It found no peace in song or laughter, none in the company of friends at table or in the pleasures of love, none even in books or poetry. . . . Where could my heart find refuge from itself? Where could I go, yet leave myself behind?

—St. Augustine

To suffer and long for relief is a central experience of humanity. But the absence of pain or discomfort or what Pablo Neruda called "the infinite ache" is never enough. Relief is bound up with satisfaction, pleasure, happiness—the pursuit of which is declared a right in the manifesto of our republic. I sit here with two agents of that pursuit: on my right, a bottle from Duane Reade pharmacy; on my left, a bag of plant matter, bought last night for about the same sum in an East Village bar from a group of men who would have sold me different kinds of contraband if they hadn't sniffed cop in my curiosity and eagerness. This being Rudy Giuliani's New York, I had feared they were undercover. But my worst-case scenario was a night or two in jail and theirs a fifteen-year minimum. As I

Joshua Wolf Shenk is a former editor of The Washington Monthly *who writes frequently on drug policy, pharmacology, and mental illness. He lives in New York City.*

exited the bar, I saw an empty police van idling, waiting to be filled with people like me but, mostly, people like them, who are there only because I am.

Fear and suspicion, secrecy and shame, the yearning for pleasure, and the wish to avoid men in blue uniforms. This is (in rough, incomplete terms) an emotional report from the front. The drug wars—which, having spanned more than eight decades, require the plural—are palpable in New York City. The mayor blends propaganda, brute force, and guerrilla tactics, dispatching undercover cops to call "smoke, smoke" and "bud, bud"—and to arrest those who answer. In Washington Square Park, he erected ten video cameras that sweep the environs twenty-four hours a day. Surveillance is a larger theme of these wars, as is the notion that cherished freedoms are incidental. But it is telling that such an extreme manifestation of these ideas appears in a public park, one of the very few common spaces in this city not controlled by, and an altar to, corporate commerce.

Several times a month, I walk through that park to the pharmacy, where a doctor's slip is my passport to another world. Here, altering the mind and body with powders and plants is not only legal but even patriotic. Among the souls wandering these aisles, I feel I have kin. But I am equally at home, and equally ill at ease, among the outlaws. I cross back and forth with wide eyes.

What I see is this: From 1970 to 1998, the inflation-adjusted revenue of major pharmaceutical companies more than quadrupled to $81 billion, 24 percent of that from drugs affecting the central nervous system and sense organs. Sales of herbal medicines now exceed $4 billion a year. Meanwhile, the war on Other drugs escalated dramatically. Since 1970 the federal antidrug budget has risen 3,700 percent and now exceeds $17 billion. More than one and a half million people are arrested on drug charges each year, and 400,000 are now in prison. These numbers are just a window onto an obvious truth: We take more drugs and reward those who supply them. We punish more people for taking drugs and especially punish those who supply them. On the surface, there is no conflict. One kind of drugs is medicine, righting wrongs, restoring the ill to a proper, natural state. These drugs have the sheen of corporate logos and men in white coats. They are kept in the room where we wash grime from our skin and do the same with our souls. Our conception of illegal drugs is a warped reflection of this picture. Offered up from the dirty underworld, they are hedonistic, not curative. They induce artificial pleasure, not health. They harm rather than help, enslave rather than liberate.

There is some truth in each of these extreme pictures. But with my dual citizenship, consciousness split and altered many times over, I come to say this: The drug wars and the drug boom are interrelated, of the same body. The hostility and veneration, the punishment and profits, these come from the same beliefs and the same mistakes.

I.

Before marijuana, cocaine, or "Ecstasy," before nitrous oxide or magic mushrooms, before I had tried any of these, I poked through the foil enclosing a single capsule of fluoxetine hydrochloride. My drug story begins at this point, at the end of a devastating first year of college. For years, I had wrapped myself in an illusion that my lifelong troubles—intense despair, loneliness, anxiety, a relentless inner soundtrack of self-criticism—would dissolve if I could only please the gatekeepers of the Ivy League. By the spring of freshman year, I had been skinned of this illusion and plunged into a deep darkness. From a phone booth in a library basement, I resumed contact with a psychiatrist I'd begun seeing in high school.

I told him how awful I felt, and, after a few sessions, he suggested I consider medication. By now our exchange is a familiar one. This was 1990, three years after Prozac introduced the country to a new class of antidepressants, called selective serotonin reuptake inhibitors. SSRIs were an impressive innovation chemically but a stunning innovation for the market, because, while no more effective than previous generations of

---

WE SAY PROZAC IS GOOD AND COCAINE IS EVIL, BUT GOOD AND EVIL ARE NOT ATTRIBUTES OF MOLECULES

---

antidepressants, SSRIs had fewer side effects and thus could be given to a much broader range of people. (At last count, 22 million Americans have used Prozac alone.) When my doctor suggested I take Prozac, it was with a casual tone. Although the idea of "altering my brain chemistry" unsettled me at first, I soon absorbed his attitude. When I returned home that summer, I asked him how such drugs worked. He drew a crude map of a synapse, or the junction between nerve cells. There is a neurotransmitter called serotonin, he told me, that is ordinarily released at one end of the synapse and, at the other end, absorbed by a sort of molecular pump. Prozac inhibits this pumping process and therefore increases serotonin's presence in the brain. "What we don't understand," he said, looking up from his pad, "is why increased levels of serotonin alleviate depression. But that's what seems to happen."

I didn't understand the importance of this moment until years later, after I had noticed many more sentences in which the distance between the name of a drug—Prozac, heroin, Ritalin, crack cocaine—and its effects had collapsed. For example, the phrase "Prozac eases depression," properly unpacked, actually represents this more complicated thought: "Prozac influences the serotonin patterns in the brain, which for some unknown reason is found to alleviate, more often than would a placebo, a collection of symptoms referred to as depression." What gets lost in abbreviation—Prozac cures! Heroin kills!—is that drugs work because the human body works, and they fail or hurt us because the body and spirit are vulnerable. When drugs spark miracles—prolonging the lives of those with HIV, say, or dulling the edges of a potentially deadly manic depression—we should be thankful.[1] But many of these processes are mysteries that might never yield to science. The psychiatric establishment, for example, still does not understand why serotonin affects mood. According to Michael Montagne of the Massachusetts College of Pharmacy, 42 percent of marketed drugs likewise have no proven mechanism of action. In *Listening to Prozac*, Peter Kramer quotes a pharmacologist explaining the problem this way: "If the human brain were simple enough for us to understand, we would be too simple to understand it." Yet pharmaceutical companies exude certainty. "Smooth and powerful depression relief," reads an ad for Effexor in a recent issue of *The American Journal of Psychiatry*. "Antidepressant efficacy that brings your patients back." In case this message is too subtle, the ad shows an ecstatic mother and child playing together, with a note written in crayon: "I got my mommy back."

The irony is that our *faith* in pharmaceuticals is based on a model of consciousness that science is slowly displacing. "Throughout history," chemist and religious scholar Daniel Perrine writes in *The Chemistry of Mind-Altering Drugs*, "the power that many psychoactive drugs have exerted over the behavior of human beings has been variously ascribed to gods or demons." In a sense, that continues. "We ascribe magical powers to substances," says Perrine, "as if the joy is inside the bottle. Our culture has no sacred realm, so we've assigned a sacred power to these drugs. This is what [Alfred North] Whitehead would call the 'fallacy of misplaced concreteness.' We say, 'The good is in that Prozac powder,' or 'The evil is in that cocaine powder.' But evil and good are not attributes of molecules."

This is a hard lesson to learn. In my gut, where it matters, I still haven't learned it. Back in 1990, I took the Prozac and, eventually, more than two dozen other medications: antidepressants, antipsychotics, antianxiety agents, and so on. The sample pills would be elegantly wrapped. Handing them to me, the doctors would explain the

desired effect: this drug might quiet the voices in my head; this one might make me less depressed and less anxious; this combination might help my concentration and ease my repetitive, obsessive thoughts. Each time I swelled with hope. I've spent many years in therapy and have looked for redemption in literature, work, love. But nothing quite matches the expectancy of putting a capsule on my tongue and waiting to be remade.

But I was not remade. None of the promised benefits of the drugs came, and I suffered still. In 1993, I went to see Donald Klein, one of the top psychopharmacologists in the country. Klein's prestige, underscored by his precipitous fees, again set me off into fantasies of health. He peppered me with questions, listened thoughtfully. After an hour, he pushed his reading glasses onto his forehead and said, "Well, this is what I think you have." He opened the standard psychiatric reference text to a chapter on "disassociative disorders" and pointed to a sublisting called depersonalization disorder, "characterized by a persistent or recurrent feeling of being detached from one's mental processes or body."

I'm still not certain that this illness best describes my experience. I can't even describe myself as "clinically ill," because clinicians don't know what the hell to do with me. But Klein gave me an entirely new way of thinking about my problems, and a grim message. "Depersonalization is very difficult to treat," he said. So I was back where I started, with one exception. During our session, Klein had asked if I used marijuana. Once, I told him, but it didn't do much. After he had given me his diagnosis, he told me the reason he had asked: "A lot of people with depersonalization say they get relief from marijuana." At that time, I happened, for the first time in my life, to be surrounded by friends who liked to smoke pot. So in addition to taking drugs alone and waiting for a miracle, I looked for solace in my own small drug culture. And for a time, I got some. The basic function of antidepressants is to help people with battered inner lives participate in the world around them. This is what pot did for me. It helped me spend time with others, something I have yearned for but also feared; it sparked an eagerness to write and conjure ideas—some of which I found the morning after to be dreamy or naive, but some of which were the germ of something valuable. While high, I could enjoy life's simple pleasures in a way that I hadn't ever been able to and still find

---

[1] *Although I am critical of the exaltation of drugs, it must be noted that a crisis runs in the opposite direction. Only a small minority of people with schizophrenia, bipolar disorder, and major depression—for which medications can be very helpful—receive treatment of any kind.*

maddeningly difficult. Some might see this (and people watching me surely did) as silly and immature. But it's also a reason to keep living.

Sad to say, I quickly found pot's limitations. When my spirits are lifted, pot can help punctuate that. If I smoke while on a downward slope or while idling, I usually experience more depression or anxiety. Salvation, for me at least, is not within that smoked plant, or the granules of a pill, or any other substance. Like I said, it's a hard lesson to learn.

To the more sober-minded among us, it is a source of much consternation that drugs, alcohol, and cigarettes are so central to our collective social lives. It is hard, in fact, to think of a single social ritual that does not revolve around some consciousness-altering substance. ("Should we get together for coffee or drinks?") But drugs are much more than a social lubricant; they are also the centerpiece of many individual lives. When it comes to alcohol, or cigarettes, or any illicit substance, this is seen as a problem. With pharmaceuticals, it is usually considered healthy. Yet the dynamic is often the same.

It begins with a drug that satisfies a particular need or desire—maybe known to us, maybe not. So we have drinks, or a smoke, or swallow a few pills. And we get something from this, a whole lot or maybe just a bit. But we often don't realize that the feeling is inside, perhaps something that, with effort, could be experienced without the drugs or perhaps, as in the psychiatric equivalent of diabetes, something we will always need help with. Yet all too often we project upon the drug a power that resides elsewhere. Many believe this to be a failure of character. If so, it is a failure the whole culture is implicated in. A recent example came with the phrase "pure theatrical Viagra," widely used to describe a Broadway production starring Nicole Kidman. Notice what's happening: Sildenafil citrate is a substance that increases blood circulation and has the side effect of producing erections in men. As a medicine, it is intended to be used as an adjunct to sexual stimulation. As received by our culture, though, the drug *becomes the desired effect, the "real thing" to which a naked woman onstage is compared.*

Such exaltation of drugs is reinforced by the torrent of pharmaceutical ads that now stuff magazines and blanket the airwaves. Since 1994, drug-makers have increased their direct-to-consumer advertising budget seven-fold, to $1.2 billion last year. Take the ad for Meridia, a weight-loss drug. Compared with other drug ads ("We're going to change lives," says a doctor pitching acne cream. "We're going to make a lot of people happy"), it is the essence of restraint. "You do your part," it says in an allusion to exercise and diet. "We'll do ours." The specific intent here is to convince people who are overweight (or believe themselves to be) that they should ask their doctor for Meridia.[2] Like the pitch for Baby Gap that announces "INSTANT KARMA" over a child wrapped in a $44 velvet jacket, drug ads suggest—or explicitly say—that we can solve our problems through magic-bullet consumption. As the old saying goes, "Better living through chemistry."

It's the job of advertisers to try every trick to sell their products. But that's the point: drugs are a commodity designed for profit and not necessarily the best route to health and happiness. The "self help" shelves at pharmacies, the "expert only" section behind the counter, these are promised to contain remedies for all ills. But the wizards behind the curtain are fallible human beings, just like us. Professor Montagne says that despite obvious financial incentives, "there really is an overwhelming belief among pharmacists that the last thing you should do for many problems is take a drug. They'll recommend something when you ask, but there's a good chance that when you're walking out the door they'll be saying, 'Aw, that guy doesn't need a laxative every day. He just needs to eat right. They don't need Tagamet. They just need to cut back on the spicy food.' " It is hard to get worked up about these examples, but they point to the broader pattern of drug worship. With illegal drugs, we see the same pattern, again through that warped mirror.

Not long after his second inauguration, President Clinton signed a bill ear-marking $195 million for an antidrug ad campaign—the first installment of a $1 billion

---

[2] *Fifty-five percent of American adults, or 97 million people, are overweight or obese. It is no surprise, then, that at least forty-five companies have weight-loss drugs in development. But many of these drugs are creatures more of marketing than of pharmacology. Meridia is an SSRI, like Prozac. Similarly, Zyban, a Glaxo Wellcome product for smoking cessation, is chemically identical to the antidepressant Wellbutrin. Admakers exclude this information because they want their products to seem like targeted cures—not vaguely understood remedies like the "tonics" of yesteryear.*

pledge. The ads, which began running last summer, all end with the words "Partnership for a Drug Free America" and "Office of National Drug Control Policy." It is fitting that the two entities are officially joined. The Partnership emerged in 1986, the year basketball star Len Bias died with cocaine in his system and President Reagan signed a bill creating, among many other new penalties, mandatory federal prison terms for possession of an illegal substance. This was the birth of the drug wars' latest phase, in which any drug use at all—not abuse or addiction or "drug-related crime"—became the enemy.[3] Soon the words "drug-free America" began to show up regularly, in the name of a White House conference as well as in legislation that declared it the "policy of the United States Government to create a Drug-Free America by 1995."

Although the work of the Partnership is spread over hundreds of ad firms, the driving force behind the organization is a man named James Burke—and he is a peculiar spokesman for a "drug free" philosophy. Burke is the former CEO of Johnson & Johnson, the maker of Tylenol and other pain-relief products; Nicotrol, a nicotine-delivery device; Pepcid AC, an antacid; and various prescription medications. When he came to the Partnership, he brought with him a crucial grant of $3 million from the Robert Wood Johnson Foundation, a philanthropy tied to Johnson & Johnson stock. Having granted $24 million over the last ten years, RWJ is the Partnership's single largest funder, but the philanthropic arms of Merck, Bristol-Myers Squibb, and Hoffman-La Roche have also made sizable donations.

I resist the urge to use the word "hypocrisy," from the Greek *hypókrisis*, "acting of a part on the stage." I don't believe James Burke is acting. Rather, he embodies a contradiction so common that few people even notice it—the idea that altering the body and mind is morally wrong when done with some substances and salutary when done with others.

This contradiction, on close examination, resolves into coherence. Before the Partnership, Burke was in the business of burnishing the myth of the über-drug, doing his best—as all marketers do—to make some external object the center of existence, displacing the complications of family, community, inner

lives. Now, drawing on the same admakers, he does the same in reverse. (These admakers are happy to work pro bono, having been made rich by ads for pharmaceuticals, cigarettes, and alcohol. Until a few years ago, the Partnership also took money from these latter two industries.) The Partnership formula is to present a problem—urban violence, date rape, juvenile delinquency—and lay it at the feet of drugs. "Marijuana," says a remorseful-looking kid, "cost me a lot of things. I used to be a straight-A student, you know. I was liked by all the neighbors. Never really caused any trouble. I was always a good kid growing up. Before I knew it, I was getting thrown out of my house."

This kid looks to be around seventeen. The Partnership couldn't tell me his real name or anything about him except that he was interviewed through a New York drug-treatment facility. I wanted to talk to him, because I wanted to ask: "Was it *marijuana* that cost you these things? Or was it your *behavior* while using marijuana? Was that behavior caused by, or did it merely coincide with, your marijuana use?"

These kinds of subtleties are crucial, but it isn't a mystery why they are usually glossed over. In Texas, federal prosecutors are seeking life sentences for dealers who supplied heroin to teenagers who subsequently died of overdose. Parents praised the authorities. "We just don't want other people to die," said one, who suggested drug tests for fourth-graders on up. Another said, "I kind of wish all this had happened a year ago so whoever was able to supply Jay that night was already in jail." The desire for justice, and to protect future generations, is certainly understandable. But it is striking to note how rarely, in a story of an overdose, the survivors ask the most important question. It is not: How do we rid illegal drugs from the earth?[4] Despite eighty years of criminal sanctions, stiffened to the point just short of summary executions, markets in this contraband flourish because supply meets demand. Had Jay's dealer been in jail that night, Jay surely would have been able to find someone else—and if not that night, then soon thereafter.

[3] Declared Nancy Reagan, "If you're a casual drug user, you're an accomplice to murder." Los Angeles police chief Daryl Gates told the Senate that "casual drug users should be taken out and shot." And so on.

[4] Many people believe that this is still possible, among them House Speaker Dennis Hastert, who last year co-authored a plan to "help create a drug-free America by the year 2002." In 1995, Hastert sponsored a bill allowing herbal remedies to bypass FDA regulations, thus helping to satisfy Americans' incessant desire for improvement and consciousness alteration.

The real question—why do kids like Jay want to take heroin in the first place?—is consistently, aggressively avoided. Senator Orrin Hatch recently declared that "people who are pushing drugs on our kids ... I think we ought to lock them up and throw away the keys." Implicit in this remark is the idea that kids only alter their consciousness because it is *pushed* upon them.

IS IT MORALLY WRONG TO ALTER THE MIND WITH SOME DRUGS AND SALUTARY TO DO SO WITH OTHERS?

Blaming the alien invader—the dealer, the drug—provides some structure to chaos. Let's say you are a teenager and, in the course of establishing your own identity or quelling inner conflicts, you start smoking a lot of pot. You start running around with a "bad crowd." Your grades suffer. Friction with your parents crescendos, and they throw you out of the house. Later, you regret what you've done— and you're offered a magic button, a way to condense and displace all your misdeeds. So, naturally, you blame everything on the drug. Something maddeningly complicated now has a single name. Psychologist Bruce Alexander points out that the same tendency exists among the seriously addicted. "If your life is really fucked up, you can get into heroin, and that's kind of a way of coping," he says. "You'll have friends to share something with. You'll have an identity. You'll have an explanation for all your troubles." What works for individuals works for a society. ("Good People Go Bad in Iowa," read a 1996 *New York Times* headline, "And a Drug Is Being Blamed.") Why is the wealthiest society in history also one of the most fearful and cynical? What root of unhappiness and discontent spurs thousands of college students to join cults, millions of Americans to seek therapists, gurus, and spiritual advisers? Why has the rate of suicide for people fifteen to twenty-four tripled since 1960? Why would an eleven- and a thirteen-year-old take three rifles and seven handguns to their school, trigger the fire alarm, and shower gunfire on their schoolmates and teachers? Stop searching for an answer. Drug Watch International, a drug "think tank" that regularly consults with drug czar Barry McCaffrey and testifies before Congress, answered the question in an April 1998 press release: "MARIJUANA USED BY JONESBORO KILLERS."[5]

II.

In 1912, Merck Pharmaceuticals in Germany synthesized a type of amphetamine, methylenedioxymethamphetamine, or MDMA. It remained largely unused until 1976, when a bio-chemist at the University of California named Alexander Shulgin, curious about reports from his students, produced and swallowed 120 milligrams of the compound. The result, he wrote soon afterward, was "an easily controlled altered state of consciousness with emotional and sensual overtones."

Shulgin's immediate thought was that the drug might be useful in psychotherapy the way LSD had been. In the two decades after its mind-altering properties were discovered in 1943 by a chemist for Sandoz Laboratories, LSD was widely used as an experimental treatment for alcoholism, depression, and various clinical neuroses. More than a thousand clinical papers discussed the use of LSD among an estimated 40,000 people, and research studies of the drug led to some extraordinary advances—including the discovery of the serotonin system. When LSD experiments were restricted in 1962 and again in 1965, Senator Robert Kennedy held a congressional hearing. "If they were worthwhile six months ago, why aren't they worthwhile now?" he asked officials of the Food and Drug Administration and the National Institute of Mental Health. "Perhaps to some extent we have lost sight of the fact that [LSD] can be very, very helpful in our society if used properly."

The answer to Kennedy's question was that LSD had leaked out of the universities and clinics and into the hands of "recreational users." It had crossed the line that separates

---

[5] *The release describes Andrew Golden and Mitchell Johnson as "reputed marijuana smokers." No reference to Golden and pot could be found in the Nexis database. The Washington* Post *reports that Johnson "said he smoked marijuana. None of his classmates believed him."*

good drugs from bad. LSD was outlawed three years later. In 1970, when a new law devised five categories, or "schedules," of controlled substances, LSD was placed in Schedule I, along with heroin and marijuana. This is the designation for drugs with no accepted medical use and a "high potential for abuse." In 1986, MDMA would be added to that list of demon drugs. The question is: How does a substance get assigned to that category? What separates the good drugs from the bad?

In the nineteenth century, now-illegal substances were commonly used in medicine, tonics, and consumer products. (The Illinois asylum that housed Mary Todd Lincoln in the 1870s offered its patients morphine, cannabis, whiskey, beer, and ale. Sigmund Freud treated himself with cocaine—and, for a time at least, praised it effusively—as did William McKinley and Thomas Edison.) A new era began with the federal Pure Food and Drug Act of 1906, which required the listing of ingredients in medical products. Then, the 1914 Harrison Narcotic Act, ostensibly a tax measure, asserted legal control over distributors and users of opium and cocaine.

On the surface, this might seem progressive, the story of a still-young nation establishing commercial and medical standards. And there was genuine uneasiness about drugs that were intoxicating or that produced dependence; with the disclosure required by the 1906 act, sales of patent medicines containing opium dropped by a third. But the movement for prohibition drew much of its power from a far less savory motive. "Cocaine," warned Theodore Roosevelt's drug adviser, "is often a direct incentive to the crime of rape by the Negroes."[6] As David Musto reports in *The American Disease*, the prohibitions of the early part of the century were all, in part, a reaction to inflamed fears of foreigners or minority groups. Opium was associated with the Chinese. In 1937, the Marijuana Tax Act targeted Mexican immigrants. "I wish I could show you what a small mari-

juana cigarette can do to one of our degenerate Spanish-speaking residents," a Colorado newspaper editor wrote to federal officials in 1936. Even the prohibition of alcohol was underlined by fears of immigrants and exaggerations of the effects of drinking. On the eve of its ban in 1919, a radio preacher told his audience, "The reign of tears is over. The slums will soon be a memory. We will turn our prisons into factories, our jails into storehouses and corncribs. Men will walk upright now, women will smile and the children will laugh. Hell will be forever for rent."

I DON'T MERELY FEEL JUSTIFIED IN USING ILLEGAL DRUGS TO FIND RELIEF; I FEEL ENTITLED

But the federal authorities, temperance advocates, and bigots had reached too far. Whereas alcohol (like coffee and tobacco) has been a demon drug in other cultures, in Western societies its use in medicine, recreation, and religious ceremonies stretches back thousands of years. Most Americans had personal experience with drink and could measure the benefits of Prohibition against the violence (by gangsters and by Prohibition agents, who, according to one estimate, killed 1,000 Americans between 1920 and 1930) and the deaths by "overdose."[7] After Franklin Roosevelt lifted Prohibition, subsequent generations knew that the drug, though often abused and often implicated in crimes, violence, and accidents, differs in its effects depending on the person using it. With outlawed drugs, no such reality check is available. People who use illegal drugs without great harm generally stay quiet.

Alcohol also can be legally used in medicines, such as Nyquil, or used medicinally in a casual way—say, to calm shattered nerves. Demon drugs, on the other hand, are prohibited or seriously limited even in cases of exceptional need. Forty percent of pain specialists admit that they undermedicate pa-

---

[6] *Such propaganda was crucial in convincing the South to allow the Harrison Act's unprecedented extension of federal power. It would be comforting to view this as a sad moment in history, but a prohibition with racist origins continues to have a racist effect: Blacks account for 12 percent of the U.S. population and 15 percent of regular drug users. But they make up 35 percent of arrests for drug possession and 60 percent of the people in state prison on drug offenses.*

[7] *Overdoses always increase in a black market, because drugs are of unknown purity and often include contaminants. Although drug use declined between 1978 and 1994, overdose deaths increased by 400 percent.*

tients to avoid the suspicion of the Drug Enforcement Administration. Their fear is justified: every year about 100 doctors who prescribe narcotics lose their licenses, including, in 1996, Dr. William Hurwitz, a Virginia internist whose more than 200 patients were left with no one to treat them. One of these patients committed suicide, saying in a videotaped message, "Dr. Hurwitz isn't the only doctor that can help. He's the only doctor that will help." Chronic pain, mind you, doesn't mean dull throbbing. "I can't shower," one patient explained to *U.S. News & World Report*, "because the water feels like molten lava. Every time someone turns on a ceiling fan, it feels like razor blades are cutting through my legs." To ease such pain can require massive doses of narcotics. This is what Hurwitz prescribed. This is why he lost his license.

But at least narcotics are acknowledged as a legitimate medical tool. Marijuana is not, despite overwhelming evidence that smoking the cannabis plant is a powerful treatment for glaucoma and seizures, mollifies the effects of AIDS or cancer chemotherapy, and eases anxiety. The editors of *The New England Journal of Medicine*, the American Bar Association, the Institute of Medicine of the National Academy of Sciences, and the majority of voters in California and six other states (plus the District of Columbia) are among those who believe that these uses of marijuana are legitimate. So does the eminent geologist Stephen Jay Gould. He developed abdominal cancer in the 1980s and suffered such intense nausea from intravenous chemotherapy that he came to dread it with an "almost perverse intensity." "The treatment," he remembers, "seem[ed] worse than the disease itself." Gould was reluctant to smoke marijuana, which, as thousands of cancer patients have found, is a powerful antiemetic. When he did, he found it "the greatest boost I received in all my years of treatment." "It is beyond my comprehension," Gould concluded, "and I fancy myself able to comprehend a lot, including much nonsense—that any humane person would withhold such a beneficial substance from people in such great need simply because others use it for different purposes."

This distinction between "people in great need" and those with "different purposes" is crucial to the argument for the medical use of marijuana.[8] Like Gould, many who use marijuana for medical reasons dislike the "high." Many others don't even feel it. But it is a mistake to think that the reason these people can't legally use marijuana is simply that other people use it for purposes other than traditional medical need. Because the very idea of "medical need" is constantly shifting beneath our feet.

I do not have cancer or epilepsy, or a disabling mental disorder such as schizophrenia. The "other purposes" Gould refers to are, in many ways, mine. The qualities of my suffering are (to simplify) anxiety, numbness, and anhedonia. If these were relieved by a legal drug—in other words, if a pharmaceutical helped me relax, feel more alive, have fun—I would be firmly in the mainstream of American medicine. This is my strong preference. But when I returned to see Donald Klein this past summer, hoping that new medications might have emerged in the last five years, he told me that "there are lots of things to try but there's only marginal evidence that any of them would do any good." He also made it clear that I shouldn't get my hopes up. "What you have," he said, "is not a common condition, and it's almost impossible [for pharmaceutical companies] to do a systematic study, let alone make money, on a condition that's not common." And so, yes, I turn sometimes to marijuana and other illicit substances for the (limited) relief they offer. I don't merely feel justified in doing so; I feel entitled, particularly since, every year, the pharmaceutical industry rolls out new products for pleasure, vanity, convenience.

When Viagra emerged, it was not frowned upon by the authorities that lead the drug wars. Instead, President Clinton ordered Medicaid to cover the drug, and the Pentagon budgeted $50 million for fiscal 1999 to supply it to soldiers, veterans, and civilian employees. Pfizer hired Bob Dole to instruct the nation that "it may take a little courage" to use

---

[8] A popular argument against medical marijuana is that it is a ruse for the "real" goal of unrestricted use, but this argument is itself a ruse. We put aside disagreements over immigration to allow amnesty for victims of political torture. We—at least most of us—put aside disagreements over abortion in cases of rape. Medical marijuana use for the seriously ill has the same unambiguous claim to legitimacy. Yet sick people face arrest and punishment. In 1997, there were 606,519 arrests for marijuana possession and 88,682 arrests for sale/manufacture; in the latter category fell an Oklahoma man with severe rheumatoid arthritis who received ninety-three years in prison for growing marijuana in his basement. The prosecutor had told the jury that, in sentencing, they should "pick a number and add two or three zeros to it."

Viagra. This is a medicine whose sole purpose is to allow for sexual pleasure; it was embraced by the black market and is easily available from doctors, including some who perform "examinations" via a three-question form on the Internet. But Viagra's legitimacy was never questioned, because it treats a disease—erectile dysfunction. Before Viagra, when the only treatment options were less-effective pills and awkward injection-based therapies, this condition was referred to as impotence. The change in language is interesting. The "dys" sits on the front of dysfunction like a streak of dirt on a pane of glass. At a level more primal than cognitive, we want it removed. This is what we do with dysfunctions: we fix them. Impotence, on the other hand, meaning "weakness" or "helplessness," is something we all experience at one time or another. Applied to men "incapable of sexual intercourse, often because of an inability to achieve or sustain an erection," the word carries a sense of something unfortunate but part of living, and particularly of growing older.

Viagra falls on the side of legitimacy; a drug that directly induced orgasm would not

---

Thus the advent of Viagra does not simply treat a disease. It changes our conception of disease. This paradigm shift is a common occurrence but is below our radar. Hair loss becomes a disease, not a fact of life. Acid indigestion becomes a disease, not a matter of eating poorly. If these examples seem to make light of the broadening of disease, the ascent of psychopharmaceuticals makes the issue urgent. Outside the realm of the tangibly physical, the power of drugs and drugmakers is far greater. What we now know as "anxiety disorder," for example, existed only in theory from Freud's time through World War II. In the early 1950s, a drug company polled doctors and found that most had no interest in a medication that treated anxiety. But by 1970, one woman in five and one man in thirteen were using a tranquilizer or sedative, and anxiety was a mainstay of psychiatry. The change could be directly attributed to two

drugs, Miltown and Valium, which were released in 1955 and 1963, respectively. The successor to these drugs, Xanax, introduced in 1981, virtually created a disease itself. Donald Klein had already proposed the existence of something called "panic disorder," as opposed to generalized anxiety, some twenty years before. But his theory was widely refuted, and in practice panic anxiety was treated only in the context of a larger problem. Xanax changed that. "With a convenient, effective drug available," writes Peter Kramer, "doctors saw panic anxiety everywhere." Xanax has also become the litmus test for generalized anxiety disorder. "If Xanax doesn't work," instructs *The Essential Guide to Psychiatric Drugs*, "usually the original diagnosis was wrong.[9]

This is not to say that all specific disorders are arbitrary, just that there is a delicate line to be drawn. "The term 'disease'—and the border between health and disease—is a social construct," says Steven Hyman, director of the National Institute of Mental Health. "There are some things we would never argue about, like cancer. But do we call it a disease if you have a few foci of abnormal cells in your body, something that you could live with without any problem? There is a gray zone. With behavior and the brain, the gray zone is much larger." To Hyman's observation, it must be added that, whereas vague dissatisfactions make money for psychic hot lines and interior decorators, diseases make money for pharmaceutical companies. What Peter Kramer calls psychiatric diagnostic creep is not an accident of history but a movement engineered for profit.

We have only begun to grapple with the consequences. The example of Prozac has been chewed over, but it's worth chewing still more—because it is so typical of a new generation of drugs, which are being used to treat debilitating conditions and also by people with far less serious problems. With Lauren Slater, author of the fine memoir *Prozac Diary*, we have a case anyone would regard as serious. Suffering from obsessive-compulsive disorder, severe depression, and anorexia, she had been hospitalized five times, attempted suicide twice, and cut herself with razors. Prescribed Prozac in 1988, she found the drug a

---

[9] *Defining diseases around medication pleases drug companies as well as HMOs. From 1988 to 1997, as general health-care benefits declined 7 percent, mental-health benefits fell 54 percent. Substituting pills for psychotherapy helps cut costs.*

reprieve from a lifetime sentence of serious illness—"a blessing, pure and simple," she writes. The patients described in Peter Kramer's *Listening to Prozac* are quite unlike Lauren Slater. They share, he writes, "something very much like 'neurosis,' psychoanalysis's umbrella term for the mildly disturbed, the near-normal, and those with very little wrong at all." The use of Prozac for these patients is not incidental; they make up a large portion, probably a wide majority, of people on the drug. (One good indication is that only 31 percent of antidepressant prescriptions are written by psychiatrists.)

WE'VE HAD A WAR ON DRUGS AS LONG AS WE'VE HATED OURSELVES FOR WANTING TO GET HIGH

Throughout his book, Kramer flirts with "unsettling" comparisons between Prozac and illegal drugs. Since Prozac can "lend social ease, command, even brilliance," for example, he wonders how its use for this purpose can "be distinguished from, say, the street use of amphetamine as a way of overcoming inhibitions and inspiring zest." The better comparison, I suggested in a conversation with Kramer, is between Prozac and MDMA. Both drugs work by increasing the presence of serotonin in the brain. (Whereas Prozac inhibits serotonin's reuptake, MDMA stimulates its release.) Both can be helpful to the seriously ill as well as to people with more common problems. Most of the objections to MDMA—that it distorts "real" personality, that it rids people of anxiety that may be personally or socially useful, that it induces more pleasure than is natural—have also been marshaled against Prozac. Both these drugs challenge our definitions of normalcy and of the legitimate uses of a mind-altering substance. Yet Kramer rejects the comparison. "The distinction we make," he told me, "is between drugs that give pleasure directly and the drugs that give people the ability to function in society, which can indirectly lead to pleasure. If the medication can make you work well or parent well, and then through your work or parenting you get pleasure, that's fine. But if the drug gives you pleasure by taking it directly, that's not a legitimate use." (Viagra, because it allows men to experience sexual pleasure, falls on the side of legitimacy. But, Kramer said, a drug that directly induced an orgasm would not.)

The line between therapeutic and hedonistic pleasure, however, is awfully hard to draw. I think of a friend of mine who uses MDMA a few times a month. His is a textbook case of "recreational" use. He takes MDMA on weekends, in clubs, for fun. He is not ill and is not in psychotherapy. But he will live for the rest of his life in the shadow of a traumatic experience, which is that for more than two decades he hid his homosexuality. Some might say the drug is an unhealthy escape from "the real world," that the relaxation and intimacy he experiences are illusory. But these experiences give him a point of reference he can use in a "sober" state. His pleasure from the drug is *entirely* social—being and sharing and loving with other people. Is this hedonistic? "I found it astonishing," Kramer writes of Prozac, "that a pill could do in a matter of days what psychiatrists hope, and often fail, to accomplish by other means over a course of years: to restore to a person robbed of it in childhood the capacity to play."

Perhaps I would find restrictions on MDMA more reasonable if they at least carved out an exception for therapeutic use. Keep in mind, that's where this drug started. After Shulgin's experiment word spread, and thousands of doses were taken in a clinical setting. As with LSD, MDMA was seen not as a medicine but as a catalyst to be taken just a few times—or perhaps only once—in the presence of a therapist or "guide." The effects were impressive. Many users found their artifice and defenses stripped away and long-buried emotions rising to the surface. The drug also had the unusual effect of increasing empathy, which helped users trust their therapist—a crucial characteristic of effective healing—and also made it useful in couples therapy. In a collection of first-person accounts of therapeutic MDMA use, *Through the Gateway of the Heart,* published in 1985, a rape victim described working through her fears. Another woman described revelations about her son, her weight problems, and "why angry men are attracted to me."

I can hear the skeptics shuffling their feet, wanting data from double-blind controlled trials. But MDMA research never reached that stage. Mindful of what had happened with LSD, the therapists, scientists, and other adults experimenting with MDMA tried to keep it quiet. Inevitably, though, word spread, and a new mode of use sprang up—at raves, in dance clubs, in dorm rooms. An astute distributor of the drug renamed it Ecstasy to emphasize its pleasurable effects. (" 'Empathy' would be more appropriate," he said later. "But how many people know what that means?")[10]

As the DEA moved to restrict MDMA, advocates of its medical use flooded the agency with testimony, pleading for a chance to subject the drug to methodical study. The agency's administrative-law judge, Francis Young, saw merit in this argument. In a ninety-page decision handed down in 1986, he recommended that the drug be placed in Schedule III, which would allow for it to be prescribed by doctors and tested further. Young cited its history of "currently accepted medical use in treatment in the United States" and argued that "the evidence of record does not establish that . . . MDMA has a 'high potential' for abuse."

DEA officials overruled Young and placed MDMA in Schedule I, with the assurance that its decision would be self-fulfilling. A Schedule I substance cannot be used clinically and can be studied only with great difficulty. So medical use is essentially forever impossible. That leaves illicit use, which, by one common definition, is the abuse for which Schedule I drugs have a "high potential." Since then, government-funded researchers have sought to document MDMA's dangers. Here we come to the truth about the line and how it is maintained. With rare exceptions, everything we know about legal drugs comes from research sponsored by the pharmaceutical industry. Naturally, this work emphasizes the

benefits and downplays the accompanying risks. On the other hand, the National Institute on Drug Abuse, which funds more than 85 percent of the world's health research on illegal drugs, emphasizes the dangers and all but ignores potential benefits.

One recent NIDA-funded study on MDMA was widely reported last fall. Dr. George Ricaurte found, in fourteen men and women who had used MDMA 70 to 400 times in the previous six years, "long-lasting nerve cell damage in the brain." Specifically, Ricaurte found decreases in the number of serotonin-reuptake sites. The study begs three major questions. First, do its conclusions really reflect the experience of heavy MDMA users? British physician Karl Jansen reports that he referred MDMA users who had taken more than 1,000 doses and that "they were told by Ricaurte that they had a clean bill of health" but were excluded from his study. Second, should the brain changes Ricaurte found be called "damage," given that a number of psychiatric medications, Prozac and Zoloft among them, decrease the number of serotonin receptors by blockading them? As psychopharmacologist Julie Holland writes, "This could be interpreted as an adaptive response as opposed to a toxic or 'damaged' response." Third, do Ricaurte's findings have any bearing on the use of MDMA in therapy, which calls for a handful of doses over many months?

In this climate, it's hard to know. Charles Grob, a psychiatrist at Harbor-UCLA Medical Center in Los Angeles, has been trying to restart MDMA research for eight years. He received FDA approval to conduct Phase I trials on human volunteers, to see if MDMA is safe enough to be used as a medicine. But even with his impeccable credentials, the backing of a prestigious research hospital, and an extremely conservative protocol—involving terminal patients—Grob has faced a seemingly interminable wait for permission to begin Phase II, in which he would study efficacy. Grob's struggle explains why he has little company in the research community. "When you have a drug that's popular among young people," Grob says, "that's the kiss of death when it comes to exploring its potential utility in a medical context."

There is another "kiss of death": lack of interest from industry. I asked Lester Grinspoon, a professor of psychiatry at Harvard Medical School, who led the legal challenge to the DEA's scheduling decision, whether he

---

[10] With a street name like Ecstasy, it is hard to take MDMA seriously as a medicine, especially compared with words like painKILLERS, or ANTIdepressants, which signify the elimination of a problem as opposed to the creation of pleasure. But the faux-Latin pharmaceutical names are also designed to suggest the drugs' wonders. David Wood, who used to run the firm that came up with the name Prozac, explains it this way: "It's short and aggressive, the 'Pro' is positive, and the Z indicates efficacy." One of Wood's employees elaborated on good drug names: "Sounds such as 'ah,' or 'ay,' which require that the mouth be open, evoke a feeling of expansiveness and openness." As in Meridia, Viagra, Propecia.

had approached drug companies about supporting the effort. "We didn't even consider it," he said. "No drug company is going to be interested in a drug that's therapeutically useful only once or twice a year. That's a no-brainer for them." When you see the feel-good ads from the Pharmaceutical Research and Manufacturer's Association with the tag line "Leading the way in the search for cures," keep in mind that cures—conditions in which medication is no longer required—are not particularly high on the pharmaceutical companies' priority list.

Market potential isn't the only factor explaining the status of drugs, but its power shouldn't be underestimated. The principal psychoactive ingredient of marijuana, THC, is available in pill form and can be legally prescribed as Marinol. A "new" creation, it was patented by Unimed Pharmaceutical and is sold for about $15 per 10-mg pill. Marinol is considered by patients to be a poor substitute for marijuana, because doses cannot be titrated as precisely and because THC is only one of 460 known compounds in cannabis smoke, among other reasons. But Marinol's profit potential—necessary to justify the up-front research and testing, which can cost upward of $500 million per medication—brought it to market. Opponents of medical marijuana claim that they simply want all medicines to be approved by the FDA, but they know that drug companies have little incentive to overcome the regulatory and financial obstacles for a plant that can't be patented. The FDA is the tail, not the dog.

The market must be taken seriously as an explanation of drugs' status. The reason is that the explanations usually given fall so far short. Take the idea "Bad drugs induce violence." First, violence is demonstrably not a pharmacological effect of marijuana, heroin, and the psychedelics. Of cocaine, in some cases. (Of alcohol, in many.) But if it was violence we feared, then wouldn't we punish that act with the greatest severity? Drug sellers, even people marginally involved in a "conspiracy to distribute," consistently receive longer sentences than rapists and murderers.

Nor can the explanation be the danger of illegal drugs. Marijuana, though not harmless, has never been shown to have caused a single death. Heroin, in long-term "maintenance" use, is safer than habitual heavy drinking. Of course, illegal drugs can do the body great harm. All drugs have some risk, including many legal ones. Because of Viagra's novelty, the 130 deaths it has caused (as of last November) have received a fair amount of attention. But each year, anti-inflammatory agents such as Advil, Tylenol, and aspirin cause an estimated 7,000 deaths and 70,000 hospitalizations. Legal medications are the principal cause of between 45,000 and 200,000 American deaths each year, between 1 and 5.5 million hospitalizations. It is telling that we have only estimates. As Thomas J. Moore notes in *Prescription for Disaster*, the government calculates the annual deaths due to railway accidents and falls of less than one story, among hundreds of categories. But no federal agency collects information on deaths related to legal drugs. (The $30 million spent investigating the crash of TWA Flight 800, in which 230 people died, is six times larger than the FDA's budget for monitoring the safety of approved drugs.) Psychoactive drugs can be particularly toxic. In 1992, according to Moore, nearly 100,000 persons were diagnosed with "poisoning" by psychologically active drugs, 90 percent of the cases due to benzodiazepine tranquilizers and antidepressants. It is simply a myth that legal drugs have been proven "safe." According to one government estimate, 15 percent of children are on Ritalin. But the long-term effects of Ritalin—or antidepressants, which are also commonly prescribed—on young kids isn't known. "I feel in between a rock and a hard place," says NIMH director Hyman. "I know that untreated depression is bad and that we better not just let kids be depressed. But by the same token we don't know what the effects of antidepressants are on the developing brain. . . . We should have humility and be a bit frightened."

These risks are striking, given that protecting children is the cornerstone of the drug wars. We forbid the use of medical marijuana, worrying that it will send a bad message. What message is sent by the long row of pills laid out by the school nurse—or by "educational" visits to high schools by drugmakers? But, you might object, these are medicines—and illegal drug use is purely hedonistic. What, then, about illegal drug use that clearly falls under the category of self-medication? One physician I know who treats women heroin users tells me that each of them suffered sexual abuse as children. According to University of Texas pharmacologist Kathryn Cunningham, 40 to 70 percent of cocaine users have pre-existing depressive conditions.

This is not to suggest that depressed people should use cocaine. The risks of dependence and compulsive use, and the roller-coaster experience of cocaine highs and lows, make for a toxic combination with intense suffering. Given these risks, not to mention the risk of arrest, why wouldn't a depressed person opt for legal treatment? The most obvious answers are economic (many cocaine users lack access to health care) and chemical. Cocaine is a formidable mood elevator and acts immediately, as opposed to the two to four weeks of most prescription antidepressants. Perhaps the most important factor, though, is cultural. Using a "pleasure drug" like cocaine does not signal weakness or vulnerability. Self-medication can be a way of avoiding the stigma of admitting to oneself and others that there is a problem to be treated.

Calling illegal drug use a disease is popular these days, and it is done, I believe, with a compassionate purpose: pushing treatment over incarceration. It also seems clear that drug abuse can be a distinct pathology. But isn't the "disease" whatever the drug users are trying to find relief from (or flee)? According to the Pharmaceutical Research and Manufacturer's Association, nineteen medications are in development for "substance use disorders." This includes six products for "smoking cessation" that contain nicotine. Are these treatments for a disease or competitors in the market for long-term nicotine maintenance?

Perhaps the most damning charge against illegal drugs is that they're addictive. Again, the real story is considerably more complicated. Many illegal drugs, like marijuana and cocaine, do not produce physical dependence. Some, like heroin, do. In any case, the most important factor in destructive use is the craving people experience—craving that leads them to continue a behavior despite serious adverse effects. Legal drugs preclude certain behaviors we associate with addiction—like stealing for dope money—but that doesn't mean people don't become addicted to them. By their own admissions, Betty Ford was addicted to Valium and William Rehnquist to the sleeping pill Placidyl, for nine years. Ritalin shares the addictive qualities of all the amphetamines. "For many people," says NIMH director Hyman, explaining why many psychiatrists will not prescribe one class of drugs, "stopping short-acting high-potency ben-

zodiazepines, such as Xanax, is sheer hell. As they try to stop they develop rebound anxiety symptoms (or insomnia) that seem worse than the original symptoms they were treating." Even antidepressants, although they certainly don't produce the intense craving of classic addiction, can be habit forming. Lauren Slater was first made well by one pill per day, then required more to feel the same effect, then found that even three would not return her to the miraculous health that she had at first experienced. This is called tolerance. She has also been unable to stop taking the drug without "breaking up." This is called dependence. " 'There are plenty of addicts who lead perfectly respectable lives,' " Slater's boyfriend tells her. To which she replies, " 'An addict. . . . You think so?' "

III.

In the late 1980s, in black communities, the Partnership for a Drug Free America placed billboards showing an outstretched hand filled with vials of crack cocaine. It read: "YO, SLAVE! The dealer is selling you something you don't want. . . . Addiction is slavery." The ad was obviously designed to resonate in the black neighborhoods most visibly affected by the wave of crack use. But its idea has a broader significance in a country for which independence of mind and spirit is a primary value.

In *Brave New World*, Aldous Huxley created the archetype of drug-as-enemy-of-freedom: soma. "A really efficient totalitarian state," he wrote in the book's foreword, is one in which the "slaves . . . do not have to be coerced, because they love their servitude." Soma—"euphoric, narcotic, pleasantly hallucinant," with "all the advantages of Christianity and alcohol; none of their defects," and a way to "take a holiday from reality whenever you like, and come back without so much as a headache or a mythology"—is one of the key agents of that voluntary slavery.

In the spring of 1953, two decades after he published this book, Huxley offered himself as a guinea pig in the experiments of a British psychiatrist studying mescaline. What followed was a second masterpiece on drugs and man, *The Doors of Perception*. The title is from William Blake: "If the doors of perception were cleansed every thing would appear to man as it is, infinite—/For man has closed himself up, till he sees all things thro' narrow chinks of his cavern." Huxley found his mescaline experience to be "without question the most extraordinary and significant experience this side of the Beatific vision . . . [I]t opens up a host of philosophical problems, throws intense light and raises all manner of questions in the field of aesthetics, religion, theory of knowledge."

Taken together, these two works frame the dual, contradictory nature of mind-altering substances: they can be agents of servitude or of freedom. Though we are deathly afraid of the first possibility, we are drawn like moths to the light of the second. "The urge to transcend self-conscious selfhood is," Huxley writes, "a principal appetite of the soul. When, for whatever reason, men and women fail to transcend themselves by means of worship, good works and spiritual exercises, they are apt to resort to religion's chemical surrogates."

One might think, as mind diseases are broadened and the substances that alter consciousness take their place beside toothpaste and breakfast cereal, that users of other "surrogates" might receive more understanding and sympathy. You might think the executive taking Xanax before a speech, or the college student on BuSpar, or any of the recipients of 65 million annual antidepressant prescriptions, would have second thoughts about punishing the depressed user of cocaine, or even the person who is not seriously depressed, just, as the Prozac ad says, "feeling blue." In trying to imagine why the opposite has happened, I think of the people I know who use psychopharmaceuticals. Because I've always been up-front about my experiences, friends often approach me when they're thinking of doing so. Every year there are more of them. And yet, in their hushed tones, I hear shame mixed with fear. I think we don't know quite what to make of our own brave new world. The more fixes that become available, the more we realize we're vulnerable. We solve some problems, but add new and perplexing ones.

In the *Odyssey*, when three of his crew are lured by the lotus-eaters and "lost all desire to send a message back, much less return," Odysseus responds decisively. "I brought them back . . . dragged them under the rowing benches, lashed them fast." "Already," writes David Lenson in *On Drugs*, "the high is unspeakable, and already the official response is arrest and restraint." The pattern is set: since

people lose their freedom from drugs, we take their freedom to keep them from drugs.[11] Odysseus' frantic response, though, seems more than just a practical measure. Perhaps he fears his own desire to retire amidst the lotus-eaters. Perhaps he fears what underlies that desire. If we even feel the lure of drugs, we acknowledge that we are not satisfied by what is good and productive and healthy. And that is a frightening thought. "The War on Drugs has been with us," writes Lenson, "for as long as we have despised the part of ourselves that wants to get high."

As Lenson points out, "It is a peculiar feature of history, that peoples with strong historical, physical, and cultural affinities tend to detest each other with the most venom." In the American drug wars, too, animosity runs in both directions. Many users of illegal drugs—particularly kids—do so not just because they like the feeling but because it sets them apart from "straight" society, allows them (without any effort or thought) to join a culture of dissent. On the other side, "straight society" sees a hated version of itself in the drug users. This is not just the 11 percent of Americans using psychotropic medications, or the 6 million who admit to "nonmedical" use of legal drugs, but anyone who fears and desires pleasure, who fears and desires loss of control, who fears and desires chemically enhanced living.

Straight society has remarkable power: it can arrest the enemy, seize assets without judicial review, withdraw public housing or assistance. But the real power of prohibition is that it creates the forbidden world of danger and hedonism that the straights want to distinguish themselves from. A black market spawns violence, thievery, and illnesses—all can be blamed on the demon drugs. For a reminder, we need only go to the movies (in which drug dealers are the stock villains). Or watch *Cops*, in which, one by one, the bedraggled junkies, fearsome crack dealers, and hapless dope smokers are led away in chains. For

---

[11] *In the 1992 campaign, Bill Clinton said, "I don't think my brother would be alive today if it wasn't for the criminal justice system." Roger served sixteen months in Arkansas State Prison for conspiracy to distribute cocaine. Had he been convicted three years later, he would have faced a five-year mandatory minimum sentence, without the possibility of parole. If he had had a prior felony or had sold the same amount of cocaine in crack form, he would have automatically received ten years.*

anyone who is secretly ashamed, or confused, about the explosion in legal drug-taking, here is reassurance: the people in handcuffs are the bad ones. Anything the rest of us do is saintly by comparison.

We are like Robert Louis Stevenson's Dr. Jekyll, longing that we might be divided in two, that "the unjust might go his way... and the just could walk steadfastly and securely on his upward path, doing the good things in which he found his pleasure, and no longer exposed to disgrace and penitence by the hands of this extraneous evil." In his laboratory, Jekyll creates the "foul soul" of Edward Hyde, whose presence heightens the reputation of the esteemed doctor. But Jekyll's dream cannot last. Just before his suicide, he confesses to having become "a creature eaten up and emptied by fever, languidly weak both in body and mind, and solely occupied by one thought: the horror of my other self." To react to an unpleasant truth by separating from it is a fundamental human instinct. Usually, though, what is denied only grows in injurious power. We believe that lashing at the illegal drug user will purify us. We try to separate the "evil" from the "good" of drugs, what we love and what we fear about them, to enforce a drug-free America with handcuffs and jail cells while legal drugs grow in popularity and variety. But we cannot separate the inseparable. We know the truth about ourselves. It is time to begin living with that horror, and that blessing.

Unit Selections

Key Points to Consider

❖ Why are some drugs so reinforcing?

❖ Why do some people become dependent upon certain drugs far sooner than other people?

❖ Is it possible to predict one's personal threshold for becoming drug dependent or addicted?

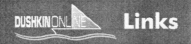 **Links**   **www.dushkin.com/online/**

5. **AMERSA**
   http://center.butler.brown.edu
6. **Addiction Research Foundation**
   http://www.arf.org
7. **The National Center on Addiction and Substance Abuse at Columbia University**
   http://www.casacolumbia.org
8. **National Institute on Drug Abuse**
   http://www.nida.nih.gov

These sites are annotated on pages 4 and 5.

Understanding how drugs act upon the human mind and body is a critical component to the resolution of issues concerning drug use and abuse. An understanding of basic pharmacology is requisite for informed discussion on practically every drug-related issue and controversy. One does not have to look far to find misinformed debate, much of which surrounds the basic lack of knowledge of how drugs work.

Different drugs produce different bodily effects and consequences. All psychoactive drugs influence the central nervous system, which, in turn, sits at the center of how we physiologically and psychologically interpret and react to the world around us. Some drugs, such as methamphetamine and LSD, have great influence on the nervous system, while others, such as tobacco and marijuana, elicit less pronounced reactions. Almost all psychoactive drugs have their effects on the body mitigated by the dosage level of the drug taken, the manner in which it is ingested, and the physiological and emotional state of the user. PCP (phencyclidine) taken in large doses may result in a person's being changed physically and emotionally forever. Cocaine smoked in the form of crack versus snorted as powder produces profoundly different physical and emotional effects on the user. LSD taken by emotionally stable persons in a controlled environment produces a more predictably favorable reaction than use by an emotionally unstable person in an unpredictable physical environment.

Molecular properties of certain drugs allow them to imitate and artificially reproduce certain naturally occurring brain chemicals that provide the basis for the drug's influence. The continued use of certain drugs and their repeated alteration of the body's biochemical structure provide one explanation for the physiological consequences of drug use. For example, heroin use replicates the natural brain chemical endorphin, which supports the body's biochemical defense to pain and stress. The continued use of heroin is believed to deplete natural endorphins, causing the nervous system to produce a painful physical and emotional reaction when heroin is withdrawn.

A word of caution is in order, however, when proceeding through the various explanations for what drugs do and why they do it. Many people, because of an emotional and/or political relationship to the world of drugs, assert a subjective predisposition when interpreting certain drug's effects and consequences. One person's alcoholic is another's social drinker. People often argue, rationalize, and explain the perceived nature of drugs' effects based upon an extremely superficial understanding of diverse pharmacological properties of different drugs. If the 10 percent of the American population suspected of being genetically predisposed to alcoholism were aware of their susceptibility, perhaps rates of alcoholism would be lower. A detached and scientifically sophisticated awareness of drug pharmacology might provide one

sound defense to the negative consequences of drug use.

Drug dependence and addiction is usually a continuum comprised of experimentation, recreational use, regular use, and abuse. The process is influenced by a plethora of physiological, psychological, and environmental factors. It is difficult to predict whether or not a particular individual will become dependent on cocaine after initial experimentation with the drug. The promotion of cocaine as a candidate for a safe recreational drug on the basis that certain people do use it recreationally without undue harm is therefore a misleading statement.

Largely, drugs are described as more addictive or less addictive due to a process described as "reinforcement." Simply explained, reinforcement results from a drug's physiological and psychological influence on behavior that causes repeated introduction of the drug to the body. Cocaine and the amphetamines are known as drugs with high reinforcement potential. Persons addicted to drugs known to be strongly reinforcing typically report that they care more about getting the drug than about anything else.

Reinforcement does not, however, provide the basis for understanding addiction. Addiction is a cloudy term used to describe a multitude of pharmacological and environmental factors that produce a compulsive, nonnegotiable need for a drug. A thorough understanding of addiction requires an awareness of these many factors.

The articles in unit 2 illustrate some of the current research and viewpoints on the ways that drugs act upon the human body. An understanding of these pharmacological processes is critical to understanding the assorted consequences of drug use and abuse. Additionally, recent scientific discoveries have shed new light on the ways drugs alter the brain's natural chemical systems. One of these significant findings concerns the brain's dopamine system and its powerful potential for influencing those areas of the brain that produce and regulate feelings of pleasure. Many experts believe that by understanding the ways drugs artificially stimulate and alter the dopamine system, many age-old questions about addiction will be resolved. Science has taken us closer to understanding that acute drug use changes brain function profoundly, and that these changes may remain with the user long after the drug has left the system. Subsequently, many new issues have emerged for drug and health-related public policy. Increasingly, drug abuse and drug addiction reassert themselves as public enemy number one. Further, the need for a combined biological, behavioral, and social response to this problem becomes more self-evident. In 1997 the National Institute of Health spent more than $5 billion on research on cancer, cardiovascular disease, and AIDS. In the same year, NIH spent $787 million on drug abuse and addiction.

Addiction and the Brain—Part I*

Drug addiction has always created concerns that go beyond the need to understand its causes and develop treatments. As individuals and as a society, we have been unable to decide whether it is a disease, a vice, or a behavior problem—something that people do to themselves or something that happens to them. Now, with the help of scientific innovations that include images of the living brain and detailed molecular analysis of neurons, researchers are beginning to learn about addiction as a biological process. Their discoveries may not only aid in the search for treatments but throw indirect light on these moral, social, and philosophical issues, and even on the nature of desire and habit in general.

The reward system

Unlike most psychiatric disorders, drug addiction can be reliably produced and easily recognized in animals. Healthy laboratory rats will voluntarily take only a few non-nutritious chemicals, the same substances to which human beings become addicted. Even their patterns of intake resemble human addictive patterns, drug by drug. The target of these chemicals is a circuit that runs between the midbrain and the prefrontal region of the cerebral cortex. The central link in the circuit, which joins two regions known as the ventral tegmental area (VTA) and nucleus accumbens (NAC), is known as the medial forebrain bundle. The NAC is part of the basal forebrain, which also contains the seat of planning and judgment in the prefrontal cortex, as well as the amygdala, sometimes described as a factory of the emotions. This circuit serves as a reward system that sets automatic priorities for the organism by guaranteeing the persistence of actions that are useful for survival and reproduction. It tells us what to avoid and what to approach. Stimulation of the NAC gives pleasure and serves as a strong positive reinforcer. Human beings and other animals tend to repeat any action that provides the stimulation, even if it means working hard and long.

Addictive drugs capture this system and subvert its normal functions. Rats will press a lever repeatedly for intravenous injections of cocaine or heroin, just as they do for direct stimulation of the NAC by an implanted electrode. If an experimenter supplies an unlimited amount for a while and then takes the drug away, a rat will press frantically in the hope of receiving more and then give up. After that, for a while, it may not work even for direct stimulation of the brain. It has become temporarily insensitive to normal signals of reward, and no action seems pleasurable.

The role of dopamine

The drugs achieve this effect by suddenly intensifying the activity of the neurotransmitter dopamine (DA) in the medial forebrain bundle. We know that this transmitter is the key to an understanding of addiction because injury or drugs that lower its activity make the reward circuit less sensitive. Addictive drugs take many different routes to their final target. Cocaine blocks the mechanism by which dopamine is reabsorbed into the cells that release it. Amphetamines provoke the release of dopamine. Nicotine acts on a receptor for the neurotransmitter acetylcholine in the reward system and may prevent the enzyme monoamine oxidase from breaking up the dopamine molecule.

Other addictive drugs act more indirectly on neurons that feed impulses into the DA system. Opiates work at receptors for the brain's own morphine-like substances, the endorphins and enkephalins (which may also constitute an alternative reward system). The sedative-hypnotic drugs, including alcohol, barbiturates, and benzodiazepines, act in various parts of the brain on neurons that release the inhibitory transmitter gamma-aminobutyric acid (GABA), which directs neurons to stop firing. In other brain regions, alcohol influences the excitatory transmitter glutamate and certain opioid receptors.

*Editor's note: Please see *the Harvard Mental Health Letter,* July 1998 for Part II.

Reprinted by permission from *Harvard Mental Health Letter,* June 1998, pp. 1-3. © 1998 by President and Fellows of Harvard College.

Dopamine and motivation

The reward system affected by addictive drugs serves the purpose of regulating motivation. Through the prefrontal cortex, we learn about the world and develop expectations based on experience. Through its link to the NAC, these expectations are compared with stimuli the brain is receiving at any given moment. If the reward is greater than expected, dopamine is released in the basal forebrain as a signal for action to continue receiving the stimulus. In this way, we lay down memories of experiences that prove useful for survival, coordinate desires with expectations, and create new motives for action.

By enhancing DA transmission, addictive drugs disturb natural feedback and control in this system and may cause long-lasting changes in its functioning. As the brain adapts to the excess of dopamine, natural production declines and DA receptors become less numerous and sensitive. Tolerance rises, and eventually pleasure is almost absent. But addicts still want the drug and still use it, because most other experiences have become even less rewarding. They need the drug just to feel normal. They have seemingly lost the power to regulate their desire, which they may experience as somehow no longer their own but imposed on them by an external force.

This disturbed state is not the same as the condition that is sometimes called physical dependence and wrongly identified with addiction itself. Addicts withdrawing from heroin may suffer for a week from nausea, tremors, aching muscles, diarrhea, and fever. Alcohol or barbiturate withdrawal can be even more unpleasant, causing seizures, delirium, and in rare cases, death. But stimulant drugs, which are equally addictive, do not cause equally severe physical withdrawal reactions. When mice lacking one type of nerve receptor for dopamine are repeatedly given morphine, they eventually suffer a typical physical withdrawal reaction but have no tendency to go on taking the drug. The vast majority of patients who take high doses of opiates for severe pain respond in the same way. As a well-known study by Lee Robins and her colleagues revealed, so did most soldiers who used heroin in Vietnam. Physical dependence in this sense is not linked to the reward or motivation system, and it is probably evoked in different brain regions by different drugs.

In one experiment, rats were given a choice between plain water and water containing morphine, in a solution either sweetened with sugar or made bitter with quinine. The rats generally drank large amounts of the drug solution in the first few days and then settled at a moderate level that was lower if it contained quinine and higher if it contained sugar. This level tended to rise after a few months. Then the experimenters took the drug out, left it out for several months, and put it back. Now some of the rats took much more than before (in human addicts, this is known as the abstinence violation effect), and their intake was neither reduced by quinine nor increased by sugar. The drug had come to matter more and other objects of desire and aversion less. This transformation occurred only when the rats were originally offered the alternative of pure water. If they were forced to drink the morphine solution, they responded like medical morphine users, with a physical withdrawal reaction but no subsequent urge to take the drug. They were not addicted because they had never chosen to use it and their motivation system was intact.

Relapse

The conscious form taken by the addictive disturbance of motivation is a varying but powerful mixture of feelings and impulses that is sometimes called craving or a protracted withdrawal reaction. The symptoms include irritable restlessness, indeterminate physical discomfort, and mild depression, all creating a tendency to relapse even after long abstinence.

Sometimes a single dose of the drug itself is enough to start a binge and reestablish the addiction, as Alcoholics Anonymous recognizes in its motto, "It's the first drink that gets you drunk." Another cause of relapse is classical conditioning. Members of AA are told to avoid "people, places, and things" associated with alcohol, because any mood or circumstance associated with use of the drug may become a conditioned stimulus. The sight of a crack pipe, bottle, or needle or the onset of anger, sadness, or anxiety can reawaken desire for the drug. A type of classical conditioning often used in animal experiments is place preference. An animal will take the drug more readily when it is returned to the environment where it first developed the addiction—like an alcoholic who passes a familiar bar or a heroin addict who sees the street corner where he used to wait for a connection. At such moments of temptation, brain scans indicate increased activity in the amygdala. It is as though the brain preserves an implicit emotional memory of its predilection that is always available for retrieval by the right cue.

Inside the neuron

Biologists and neurologists are now exploring the interior of neurons to uncover the ultimate sources of addiction. When a neurotransmitter like dopamine locks into receptors on the surface of a cell, it opens channels to the interior and pervasively influences activity within. Molecules known as G-proteins are directed to turn on other molecules, the second messengers, which eventually cause phosphate groups to attach themselves to regulatory proteins. Through this process of phosphorylation, genes in the nucleus are switched on, issuing directions to manufacture substances that neurons need for learning and other normal functions. Neural connections are strengthened and long-term memories are formed. Feedback from the process regulates the sensitivity of receptors and the opening and closing of neuronal access channels. If a drug repeatedly displaces neurotransmitters or modifies their actions, the structure and activity of brain cells themselves can change in pervasive and persistent ways.

Outside influences

The capacity of drugs to disturb the balance of the brain does not depend on their chemical properties alone. Most drug users never become addicts, and many other conditions and circumstances determine whether a particular person uses a particular drug in a compulsive way. Substances are more addictive when taken in pure and concentrated form, and more addictive when smoked or injected directly into the bloodstream than when eaten or drunk.

There are also striking individual differences in susceptibility that arise from heredity, culture, social circumstances, and good or ill fortune. Robins showed that most men who used heroin in Vietnam, even if they took it as much and as often as stateside addicts, had no tendency to relapse into addiction after returning to this country. The men who did relapse usually had drug or alcohol problems and antisocial tendencies before joining the Armed Forces. Even rats have individual personalities that affect their vulnerability to addictions. The leaders of a rat colony, the ones who appear to be admired and imitated, tend to take less than others when they are offered addictive drugs.

FOR FURTHER READING

George Ainslie. Beyond microeconomics: Conflict among interests in a multiple self as a determinant of value. *In: John Elster, ed.* The Multiple Self. *New York: Cambridge University Press, 1985.*

Eliot L. Gardner. Brain reward mechanisms. *In: Joyce H. Lowinson, Pedro Ruiz, Robert B. Millman, and John G. Langrod, eds.* Substance Abuse: A Comprehensive Textbook, *Third Edition. Baltimore: Williams & Wilkins, 1997.*

Steven E. Hyman. Why does the brain prefer opium to broccoli? *Harvard Review of Psychiatry 2: 43–46 (May/June 1994).*

George F. Koob and Eric J. Nestler. Neurobiology of drug addition. *Journal of Neuropsychiatry and Clinical Neuroscience. 9(3): 482–497 (1997).*

Charles P. O'Brien. Recent developments in the pharmacotherapy of substance abuse. *Journal of Consulting and Clinical Psychology 64: 677–686 (August 1996).*

Stanton Peele and Archie Brodsky. The Truth about Addiction and Recovery. *New York: Simon & Schuster, 1991.*

The Mood Controller

A Little Help From Serotonin

Could a single brain chemical hold the key to happiness, high social status and a nice, flat stomach?

BY GEOFFREY COWLEY AND ANNE UNDERWOOD

OR RHESUS MONKEYS, LIFE IN THE WILD IS A little like high school. Some animals—call them losers—slouch around looking aggrieved. They're volatile and bellicose, slow to form alliances and loath to reconcile after a spat. One in five dies during the passage to adulthood. But while the losers scrap over bits of chow, other animals—call them winners—stay busy grooming each other. They maintain wide networks of allies. They deflect challenges without resorting to violence, and 49 out of 50 survive to produce offspring. Why do they fare so well? The answer is no doubt complicated, but the monkeys' spinal fluid provides an intriguing clue. In study after study, researchers at the National Institute on Alcohol Abuse and Alcoholism have found that the winners' nervous systems are loaded with serotonin.

As the 20th century winds down, we humans seem increasingly convinced that serotonin is the key to a good life—and it's easy to see why. This once obscure neurotransmitter is the secret behind Prozac, the drug that revolutionized the pursuit of happiness 10 years ago this winter. Prozac and its mood-altering cousins all work by boosting serotonin's activity in the brain. So do Redux and fenfluramine, the blockbuster diet drugs that were pulled off the market this fall due to safety concerns. Even Imitrex, the hot new migraine treatment, works its magic via serotonin. Somehow serotonin is implicated in just about everything that matters to us—from winning friends and wielding power to managing anxiety and controlling appetites and impulses. So what is serotonin? How does it work? And why is it in such short supply? Those issues are still murky, but science is yielding some clues.

Serotonin is so basic to life that even worms and sea slugs make it. The substance abounds in our bloodstreams, but our brains produce separate supplies via cells known as raphe nuclei. Rooted near the base of the skull, these specialized neurons extend like branching vines through the brain and spinal cord, each one maintaining links with a half-million target cells. When a nerve impulse reaches a branch ending, the neuron releases serotonin into a tiny space, or synapse. Serotonin molecules then lock into receptors on the target cell, transmitting a message that travels through the nervous system. Microseconds later, the neuron that released the chemical takes it back in—a process known as reuptake.

What does serotonin say during its moment in the synapse? It depends on the target. Our nervous systems harbor at least

14 classes of serotonin receptors, each tailored to a distinct piece of the molecule. Since different types of brain cells sport different receptors, their responses to serotonin vary widely. Serotonin excites the motor neurons, which govern muscle activity, but it quiets the sensory neurons that mediate hunger and pain. It also pacifies neurons in the limbic system, the brain's Department of Animal Instincts. "Serotonin puts the brakes on primitive behaviors like sex, aggression and excessive feeding," says Dr. Larry Siever of New York's Mount Sinai School of Medicine.

Small wonder, then, that high serotonin can foster social success. In a classic series of experiments with vervet monkeys, UCLA scientists Michael McGuire and Michael Raleigh found that males who had achieved high rank within a group's social hierarchy had nearly twice as much serotonin in their blood as low-ranking males. But that's not to say they were born leaders; further analysis showed that social standing had as much effect on the animals' serotonin as serotonin had on their status. If an alpha male was displaced by a challenger, his blood count would quickly plummet—and when an upstart came into power, his serotonin level would surge. Raleigh and McGuire found they could deplete a leader's serotonin simply by keeping him behind a one-way mirror, where his peers couldn't acknowledge his dominance displays.

People's social lives are more complicated than monkeys', but not entirely different. When Raleigh and McGuire analyzed blood samples from 48 UCLA fraternity boys, the average serotonin level was nearly 25 percent higher among officers than among members. And when Raleigh compared his own serotonin count with that of his lab director (McGuire), the boss's was 50 percent higher.

Rising to the top may involve some scrapping, but serotonin doesn't foster aggression. "Serotonin provides a restraint mechanism, a kind of behavioral seat belt," says Dr. John Mann of Columbia University. Whether you look at monkeys, dogs, horses or humans, the most aggressive individuals are typically those with the lowest serotonin levels. Drugs that boost serotonin's activity tend to dampen a wide range of impulses (including sexual ones that need no dampening), and they can help violent people get a grip. Yasmin Hamani has seen it happen. When her autistic daughter was 8 years old, her annoying repetitive behaviors turned violent. If Hamani turned her back, the child would sneak up and sink her nails into an exposed piece of flesh with swift pinches that drew blood. She would kick people in church and grab at women's hair in the supermarket. One of her schools confined her to a four-foot pen to protect the other kids. When the child was 11 and increasingly uncontrollable, Dr. Edwin Cook at the University of Chicago tried treating her with Prozac. The drug didn't cure her autism, but violent outbursts stopped. "Everyone loves her now," says Hamani.

In the pink: When serotonin is doing its job, we're apt to feel calm, sociable, alert. Impulses and appetites don't rule us.

Violence is one possible consequence of low serotonin, but there are many others. Without the chemical's leveling effects, we grow more vulnerable to all kinds of impulses—whether to gamble, buy things, steal things or eat things. And low serotonin can have devastating effects on mood. It plays major roles not only in depression and suicide but in premenstrual syndrome (PMS), seasonal affective disorder (SAD) and routine morning grumpiness (RMG).

You might conclude from all this that more serotonin is always better. But just as a serotonin deficiency can unleash destructive impulses, an overly active serotonin system can leave a person paralyzed by obsessions and compulsions. People with compulsive disorders become hyperaware of potential threats—possibly because serotonin is overstimulating the receptors involved in planning and vigilance—and they develop bizarre rituals for managing their anxiety. Incessant cleaning and checking are the classic manifestations, but there are many others. Hypochondria, once dismissed as an annoying bid for sympathy, is now viewed as a type of obsessive-compulsive illness. So is body dysmorphic disorder (BDD), a grim fixation on some flaw in one's appearance. Dr. Eric Hollander of New York's Mount Sinai has seen people undergo two dozen surgeries to correct perceived defects. "This isn't a trivial illness," he says. "There is a high rate of suicide among these patients."

Prozac would seem an unlikely remedy. Its job, after all, is to amplify serotonin's effect, by slowing its removal from the synapse. Yet Prozac and the other "selective serotonin reuptake inhibitors" (SSRIs) are proving as useful against compulsive disorders as they are against impulsive ones. How could the same drugs alleviate such disparate problems? Most experts credit the body's drive to maintain equilibrium. If a neuron is responding poorly to serotonin, blocking reuptake may simply compensate for the shortfall. But if a neuron is already overstimulated, it may compensate for the extra exposure by responding less vigorously. "It's a leap to think 'I hate my nose so I'll take Prozac'," says Dr. Katharine Phillips of Butler Hospital in Providence, R.I., "But it can make a difference."

SSRI therapy won't give you a new nose, but it can change your waistline. Fenfluramine (brand name Pondimin) and dexfenfluramine (Redux), the wildly popular weight-loss drugs that were pulled off the market in September, had chemical actions very similar to Prozac's. By boosting serotonin activity in particular brain regions, they helped dieters feel sated *before* downing that third bowl of Chunky Monkey. But the fenfluramines packed a double whammy: besides slowing serotonin's removal from the synapse, they forced neurons to release more of it. And unlike Prozac, they seemed to cause a dangerous buildup of waxy material on people's heart valves. The cause of that problem is still unknown; it was seen mainly in people who took "fen-phen," a combination of fenfluramine and the stimulant phentermine. But it was serious enough to send Redux and Pondimin into oblivion.

Obesity specialists despaired at the time, but they're now finding safer ways to protect people from their cravings. The FDA recently approved a new diet pill called Meridia, which (like Prozac) enhances serotonin's activity without stimulating its release. Researchers are finding that Prozac itself can safely promote weight loss when combined with phentermine. And enthusiasts are now touting various strategies for boosting serotonin without resorting to drugs at all.

If the brain weren't so well insulated, we could simply pop some serotonin when our spirits or our bellies started to sag. But serotonin can't enter the nervous system from outside. The brain makes its own supply from tryptophan, an amino acid found in protein-rich foods such as meat, fish and milk. The tryptophan in a hamburger *can* enter the brain, but as you've probably noticed, hamburgers don't cure depression. That's because tryptophan-rich foods are packed with a variety of amino acids that compete for passage across the blood-brain barrier. Picture a crowd in front of a department store with a single revolving door, says University of Pittsburgh pharmacologist John Fernstrom. "Tryptophan wants to get in, but it has to stand in line."

Back in the 1970s Fernstrom and Dr. Richard Wurtman of MIT discovered that the best way to shorten that line is simply to eat a carbohydrate. Carbs enter the bloodstream as glucose—and any rise in blood glucose causes the pancreas to secrete insulin. Insulin pushes glucose and various amino acids out of the blood and into fat and muscle cells. But it doesn't mop up tryptophan. So when insulin sweeps through the bloodstream, the crowd at the revolving door disperses and tryptophan glides freely into the brain, where it can be used to make serotonin.

After showing that carb-munching could increase brain serotonin in rats, Wurtman and his wife, Judith, a nutritional scientist at MIT, started thinking about people. Is it possible, they wondered, that people who binge on cookies, chips and candy are unconsciously seeking serotonin? Encouraged by clinical studies showing that obese people draw most of their excess calories from such carb-rich snacks, Judith Wurtman developed a theory of weight management. In books like "The

Out of control: Studies suggest that a killer or arsonist with low serotonin is more likely to strike again after serving time in jail

Carbohydrate Craver's Diet" and "The Serotonin Solution," she claims that a regimen of low-fat, high-carb snacks (toast, pretzels, rice cakes) can quash your cravings without making you fat. It's an interesting idea, but she has yet to document its advantages. In an unpublished study, she compared her diet with a conventional weight-loss plan in 27 obese women. The results didn't differ much—volunteers lost 10 to 12 pounds on her regimen, versus 8 to 9 on the other one—but she says her program left people feeling happier and more vigorous. Fernstrom, the Wurtmans' former collaborator, is skeptical. "There's a lot of hype with this stuff," he says, "and people are making money based on it."

Supplement makers are hoping to get their share. They used to do a brisk business in L-tryptophan, an amino acid that people took orally to keep the brain adequately supplied. That product was banned in the 1980s, after a contaminated batch caused widespread illness and several deaths. But tryptophan is now returning to health-food stores in a new form called 5-HTP (5-hydroxytryptophan). It crosses the blood-brain barrier as readily as L-tryptophan, and once inside the brain it's more readily converted into serotonin. Small studies in Europe have found 5-HTP helpful in treating depression. It performed as well as the SSRI Luvox in one Swiss experiment and caused fewer side effects. If that finding holds, 5-HTP could be a godsend for depressed people who find that drugs spoil their sleep, sex and appetite. St. John's wort, the popular herb, shows similar promise.

But don't assume that supplements or drugs will make you lean, charming and powerful. Our serotonin systems are affected not only by what we ingest but by our genes, experiences and attitudes—and by the countless other chemicals racing through our brains. Scientists may someday learn how all these forces interact, but a good life will still take work. "Your serotonin system doesn't rule you," says Siever. "If you have vulnerabilities associated with low serotonin functioning—guilt, submissiveness, low self-esteem—you can learn to compensate for them." And if you're lucky, you'll be rewarded with a rise in serotonin.

With KAREN SPRINGEN

NEURODEVELOPMENT

Cocaine Wreaks Subtle Damage on Developing Brains

It had started to look like yesterday's scare story. Beginning about a decade ago, countless reports on television and in newspapers and magazines presented the image of the sickly, inattentive, and inconsolable "crack baby." The fear was that the infants, who had been exposed to cocaine when their mothers abused the drug while pregnant, had suffered severe, irreversible damage, including reduced intelligence and social skills. But in recent years the news has swung to the opposite extreme: In several follow-up studies conducted on preschoolers and school-age children, researchers could link no significant reductions in intelligence to cocaine exposures in the womb.

Now that conclusion, too, is looking oversimplified. As researchers find ways to sort out the confounding factors that had weakened earlier studies, they are learning that cocaine leaves its mark on developing brains after all. At a meeting* held last month in Washington, D.C., scientists reported that the latest studies of school-aged children reveal that exposure to cocaine during fetal development may lead to subtle, but significant, deficits later on, especially with behaviors crucial to success in the classroom, such as concentrating for long periods of time and blocking out distractions.

"Cocaine is not a sledgehammer in the developing brain," as some originally feared, says Barry Kosofsky, a developmental neuroscientist at Massachusetts General Hospital and Harvard Medical School in Boston. "Exposed infants are, in general, doing well. But looking at more subtle characteristics, there seem to be some real differences in many exposed children."

Studies of animals exposed to cocaine before they were born buttressed that conclusion. Not only did the researchers find behavioral changes similar to those in the

children, but they also found specific and permanent changes in the animals' brains. In areas of the brain involved in attention, for example, the animals' brain cells have developed abnormally and respond less efficiently to certain neurotransmitters. Together, say researchers, the epidemiology and the laboratory studies strengthen the case for reducing or preventing prenatal cocaine exposure. They will also enable doctors, parents, and teachers to identify cocaine-exposed children and help them, instead of writing them off as hopelessly damaged.

Snowy picture. Pinning down cocaine's effects on the fetus has been difficult not just because they are often subtle, but because they have to be separated out from those that might be caused by a host of other assaults on the child that often accompany maternal drug abuse. Women who use cocaine during pregnancy are also many times more likely to abuse alcohol, tobacco, and other drugs. They are less likely to get proper prenatal care, and are more likely to give birth to underweight and premature babies. Because the fear of prosecution or separation from their baby makes many women reluctant to admit that they have used cocaine, researchers have a hard time sorting cases from controls. And even in known users, documenting how much cocaine they consume and when is impossible.

Now, however, researchers are using complex statistical methods to sort through the confounding factors, and they are analyzing the hair and urine of infants and mothers as well as newborn feces (meconium) to identify cocaine users and their babies more reliably. These more rigorous studies are beginning to show significant—and consistent—results.

One study comes from pediatrician Ira Chasnoff of the University of Illinois College of Medicine in Chicago, who was among the first to report the effects of cocaine on behavior in newborns. At the meeting, he described his prospective study of nearly 200 children in inner-city Chicago. The team recruited pregnant mothers in drug-treatment programs and conducted ran-

dom drug tests throughout pregnancy. During follow-up studies, the researchers collected information on the home environment, including the mother's current drug use. They correlated these data with intelligence quotient (IQ) test results and a detailed assessment of the children's behavior from questionnaires filled out by the child's primary caregiver and teacher.

When he and his colleagues did a careful statistical analysis of the correlations, they found support for the idea that prenatal cocaine exposure may have a limited impact on intelligence. The home environment—in particular whether the mother was currently using drugs—turned out to be the strongest predictor of IQ, overwhelming any prenatal effects of cocaine. As Chasnoff puts it, "The greatest impediment to cognitive development in young children is poverty."

The team also found, however, that children exposed to cocaine prenatally have significantly more behavioral problems. Their mothers and their teachers reported that as a group, cocaine-exposed children were more aggressive, had more trouble paying attention and staying focused, and were more likely to be impulsive. At the same time, they were more anxious and depressed.

Developmental pediatrician Linda Mayes of Yale University reported similar results in direct tests of children. She heads a team that has been following a group of 475 children in inner-city New Haven for 6 years. About half of their mothers either admitted to using cocaine or had a drug-positive urine test while pregnant. The researchers decided to focus on attention and arousal, she says, because cocaine affects the brain's dopamine and serotonin systems, which play key roles in regulating those behaviors.

The team began detecting cocaine-related effects in infants as young as 3 to 6 months. The cocaine-exposed babies were more irritable than those in the comparison group (babies exposed to alcohol, tobacco, and other drugs, but not cocaine) on standard assessments of infant development—a conclu-

---

*The meeting, "Cocaine: Effects on the Developing Brain," was held from 16 to 19 September and sponsored by the New York Academy of Sciences and Allegheny University of the Health Sciences.

sion supported by other researchers. At a year or a year and a half, the cocaine-exposed children began showing signs that they were having trouble focusing their attention. When given a box of toys, for example, they spent less time exploring the new toys than did the control children. Instead they would look aimlessly around the room or hold a toy without exploring it, Mayes says.

The latest data, from 125 children who are now 4-and-a-half years old, shows that their problems with focusing and blocking out distractions have persisted. When the researchers asked the children to hit a button whenever a certain picture, say of a car, flashed on a computer screen, the cocaine-exposed children actually responded faster than their peers. But when the researchers complicated the game by adding pictures of houses or people, which the children were instructed to ignore, the cocaine-exposed children had much more trouble. While they still reacted faster than control groups, they responded to the distracting pictures more often. This suggests, says Mayes, that cocaine-exposed kids are more impulsive and more easily distracted than their peers. At the same time, they are less easily startled by a sudden noise.

The overall picture, Mayes says, is of a child who has a higher threshold for arousal, but once aroused, is harder to control. Chicago's Chasnoff agrees. "The kids are more fragile," he says. Although these deficits do not directly impact intelligence, they are a severe handicap in the classroom. "It's much harder for these children to concentrate on what their teacher is saying when there are competing stimuli," such as a sunbeam through a window or a strange noise, says neuroscientist John Harvey of Allegheny University of the Health Sciences in Philadelphia.

Similar cocaine-induced behavioral problems are also cropping up in lab animals, which opens the way to drawing precise links between the behavioral effects and changes in the brain. Some of this work comes from Harvey's team. In one test, for example, the researchers trained cocaine-exposed and control rabbits to blink in response to a warning tone or light, which preceded a puff of air aimed into the rabbits' eyes. As long as the task was kept simple, the cocaine group had no problem learning the response. In fact, just like the children, they reacted faster than controls did.

But when the researchers made the task more complicated by adding a different neu-

tral tone that was not followed by the puff of air, the cocaine-exposed animals "just fell apart," Harvey says. They had trouble paying attention to the correct tone, especially if the neutral tone was louder or longer—more "salient"—than the real warning. Although rabbit and human brains are quite different, all of this sounded very familiar, says Chasnoff, who heard Harvey's talk at the meeting. "I wanted to jump up and say, 'You're talking about our children!'" he says. "I didn't expect it to be so similar."

Cellular clues. Other researchers at the meeting presented clues to how cocaine might cause such specific behavior changes. Although the drug has many global effects—constricting blood vessels, for example—its specific action is to prevent neurons from taking up certain neurotransmitters, such as serotonin and dopamine, after these chemicals have been dumped into the spaces between the cells. This causes brain levels of the neurotransmitters to surge. Studies in rabbits and mice now suggest that by exposing the brain to such high levels of the transmitters early on, cocaine causes it to undergo permanent changes in an attempt to compensate.

For example, Harvey's Allegheny colleague, Eitan Friedman, reported that the number of cell surface receptors for dopamine in cocaine-exposed rabbit brains is normal, but these receptors do not transmit their signal into the cells as efficiently as do those in normal brains. In studies of one particular type of dopamine receptor, designated D1, the Allegheny team found a clue as to why the receptor efficiency is reduced. The D1 receptor in neurons relays the dopamine signal into a cell by associating with a protein called G_S. In cocaine-exposed brains, however, that association is weakened.

No one has yet made a direct connection between the weakened signaling that results and the changes in the animals' behavior. But the finding is consistent with other changes seen in the brains of rabbits exposed to cocaine. When the dopamine binds to the D1 receptor in normal brains during development, it inhibits the growth of the neuronal extensions called dendrites. In cocaine-exposed brains, however, this growth limiter may not be working properly, as Pat Levitt of the University of Pittsburgh School of Medicine found.

Levitt studied the same rabbit model as the Allegheny team used, looking carefully at the development of brain cells in the anterior cingulate cortex, a part of the brain known to be involved in attention and learn-

ing. In cocaine-exposed brains, he found, the dendrites grow 30% to 50% longer, and—perhaps to accommodate their length—seem to weave in and around one another. Neurobiologist Hazel Murphy, also of Allegheny, has shown that the longer neurons have more connections to one another. What effect these changes have on cognition is difficult to say, Levitt says, "but clearly the circuitry is not normal" in areas involved in attention and learning.

The change in the D1 receptor may also help explain the anecdotal reports that some children with impaired attention due to drug exposure do not respond as well to stimulants, like Ritalin, that help other children, says Harvard's Kosofsky. Ritalin acts much like the drug amphetamine, increasing the release of dopamine into the gap between brain cells. But if the problems are related to ineffective signaling through that receptor, such a drug would do little to help. Kosofsky is currently testing drugs that stimulate the cellular response to the dopamine receptor to see if he can lessen the behavioral deficits caused by cocaine in mice.

In the meantime, he and others are looking for ways to exploit their findings. Now that scientists know what behaviors to watch for as a result of cocaine exposure in the womb, they can begin to figure out which kids born to cocaine-addicted mothers will need help and what kinds of intervention will work best. For example, he says, "if mom does a little less drugs, is her child less vulnerable? If you intervene postnatally, is the outcome going to be better?" Such studies, he says, may show how to soften the "double whammy from nature and nurture" that these children have received.

—Gretchen Vogel

Additional Reading

P. Levitt et al., "New evidence for neurotransmitter influences on brain development," *Trends in Neuroscience* **20**, 269 (1997).

V. Delaney-Black et al., "Prenatal cocaine and neonatal outcome: Evaluation of dose-response relationship," *Pediatrics* **98**, 735 (1996).

L. Mayes et al., "Information processing and developmental assessments in 3-month-old infants exposed prenatally to cocaine," *Pediatrics* **95**, 539 (1995).

The Critical Question before Drug Treatment: A Summary of A Social Policy symposium.

What Type of Addict Are You?

Erik Banks

Are there different types of addicts? Is the success of treatment dependent on understanding these types? These were among the questions posed at a *Social Policy* conference in November on the current state of addiction treatment. We examined how addicts who are physically, habitually, or socially dependent on a drug, but who can stop at will, seem less grave than addicts for whom the need for the substance overwhelms their centers of judgment and motivation. Although participants agreed that there were more and less serious addictions, they used different typologies to categorize them.

George DeLeon, director of the Center for Therapeutic Community Research, classifies addicts according to their social population. His types are addict-convicts, addicted and mentally ill, adolescents, homeless, and multiple combinations of these types. In addition, DeLeon emphasized that addicts go through "cycles" of more and less severe dependence. Each stage in the cycle of the individual addict is also a different type. DeLeon believes in "community as method," that recovering addicts should be treated in a group setting so that the peer community can have a chance to influence the individual's psychology.

Albert Ellis, founder of the Albert Ellis Institute for Rational Emotive Therapy, distinguishes between the "nice neurotics"—people who medicate their low threshold for frustration—and those with a more severe personality disorder. He believes the number of the latter is quite high—

Erik Banks is a graduate student in philosophy at the Graduate School and University Center, the City University of New York.

From *Social Policy,* Winter 1998, pp. 5-9. © 1999 by Social Policy Corporation. Reprinted by permission.

at least 3 out of every 10 addicted persons. Ellis believes he can make headway with a number of "nice neurotics" who can be argued out of their neurotic frustrations and steered toward a stoical unconditional acceptance of human shortcomings in both themselves and others. Ellis also discussed Jack Trimpy's "voice recognition" technique used in Rational Recovery, a novel approach where addicts listen to recordings of themselves and learn to identify an alien Doppelganger within who is a serious addict.

Lirio Covey, of Columbia University's College of Physicians and Surgeons, described the smoking cessation studies that she and Alexander Glassmann have conducted. Their stunning finding is that a significant number of seriously addicted smokers have a history of recurrent major depression that reemerges when their smoking ceases, making it extremely difficult to quit. Both the depression and the use of smoking to medicate it are traceable to a common cause that is, in part, genetic.

Frank Riessman is in the process of developing an "intensive self-help group" for addiction. This group would be self-determined and rely on recovering addicts who share the secrets of their success, but it would eschew the 12-Step framework, using instead the principles of self-help. The spiritual or values dimension of the group, for example, would not center around the disease model or give the problem over to a higher power.

Keith Humphreys, of the Department of Veterans Affairs, at Stanford University's School of Medicine, submitted a paper but did not attend. He argued that self-help groups like AA could form a "first line of defense" in the battle against addiction, avoiding expensive professional treatment in appropriate cases and making for a better allocation of resources.

A complex addict cannot introspectively tell the difference between natural feelings of joy or sorrow and the highs and lows of rush and withdrawal.

Humphreys' approach suggests a more general question: Why is there no overall "gatekeeper" for steering addicts into the treatment most appropriate for them? With different programs adopting different philosophies and typologies, wouldn't our resources be better allocated if there was a system for sorting them out prior to treatment? Who is to say whether you need Ellis' Rational-Emotive approach, AA, Trimpy's Rational Recovery, or DeLeon's Therapeutic Community? There is no guide to this shopping mall of treatments. All participants at the conference acknowledged that no treatment works for all of the people all of the time, no matter if the goal is abstinence, a reduction in harmful use, or stopping longer cycles of quitting and relapse. On the other hand, there is no telling how much better the various treatments might do on a pre-screened population, not randomized clinical trials. It would be unfortunate if addiction were to go the way of so many social programs, balkanized into mutually exclusive programs competing for funding dollars and fighting off competitors for its own niche. This state of affairs enhances the public's perception that social programs are messy, of dubious efficacy, and a waste of money.

Simple and Complex Addiction

The distinction between addicts with mental illness and those without is an element of typology on which all seem to agree. But after that, the question gets complicated. I agree with Frank Riessman that there is a further distinction to be made among those without mental illness, who can be simple or complex addicts.

A simple addiction is a physical, behavioral, or social dependence on a substance that manifests tolerance and withdrawal symptoms but can be overcome by an act of will. For example, many Vietnam veterans who were addicted to heroin during the war were able to quit when they returned to the US; almost all patients who are given morphine in the hospital are able to endure the withdrawal symptoms and get off the drug; nicotine and alcohol addicts are often able to quit on their own when they perceive a threat to their health, job, or relationships.

Some 90 percent of addicts seem to have the simple form. For the complex addict, however, the need for the substance has merged with his or her emotional structure, judgment, and motivation to such an extreme degree that these cannot be separated. Complex addicts often report a feeling of having their psyches "hijacked."

"Original Existences"

The philosopher David Hume called the motivating passions "original existences." By

---

this he meant that we are motivated by sentiments or feelings that we take only at face value. He added that the customary rationalizations we give are illusory because they presuppose our sentiments.

As long as addicts can introspectively tell the difference between their natural feelings of joy or sorrow and the rush and withdrawal induced by the substance, they remain simple addicts. For example, hospitalized patients who get morphine have had insufficient cause to confuse their natural feelings with the artificial morphine-induced ones because they are constantly reminded by their surroundings that the situation is not normal. In the case of many addicts who quit on their own, their natural impulses remain strong enough to override the substance.

A complex addict, on the other hand, cannot introspectively tell the difference between natural feelings of joy or sorrow and the highs and lows of rush and withdrawal. Indeed, like colors close enough together on the spectrum, there comes a point when these feelings are no longer distinguishable. The author remembers when his cigarette smoking, which started as a tool to fit in with peers, became a complex addiction. When he needed a cigarette and felt depressed, he would interpret the depression as a natural motivation coming from other circumstances that happened to be on his mind—lighting up the cigarette as a mere afterthought. Also, the rush of the cigarette was interpreted as the well-deserved feeling that the problem was solved and "things were going okay."

It is this confusion of original existences that seems to us to be responsible for the complex addiction on top of the simple physical dependence. Of course, the complex predisposition to confuse some feelings for others produced by a drug depends on the type of substance and the feeling it replaces, the emotional profile, social and habit forming factors, and the like—just as color blindness of one type promotes only the confusion of red and green shades. Yet for all the complexity in predisposition, the fundamental distinction must be made introspectively—in the first person—by the addict him or herself, else all external treatment is likely to miss the mark.

Recovered addicts seem to have learned from experience the skill to detect internal differences in feeling. A threat to health or a "wake-up call" may also arouse strong natural motivations that demand to be distinguished. Stages of addiction, then, should be interpreted as stages of development in this skill and the different treatments seen as different means to this end. In any case, some general typology urgently needs to be developed.

Keith Humphreys responded to the question of "types" in the following way:

"There are many defensible ways to subtype alcohol and drug dependent people. As a health policy analyst, I take the pragmatic approach of dividing them into those who can recover using personal (e.g., self-control) and community (e.g., religious organizations, self-help groups) resources, and those who can only recover if they receive professional intervention. This distinction helps us recognize that in the most just and efficient health care system only the latter type of addicted person would receive professional treatment.

Under the collapsed fee-for-service insurance model, those who needed treatment the least tended to get the most of it because they could pay for it. Within the new managed care reimbursement system, there are new incentives to reserve professional treatment for those who actually need it, and let the rest of the substance-abusing population rely on personal and community resources. However, a change in thinking and some advocacy will be required for these incentives to be translated into a better overall approach to the care of addicted people."

ALCOHOLISM:
CHARACTER OR GENETICS?

By Mark Gauvreau Judge

For years, conventional wisdom said alcohol dependence was a character defect. New research points to a genetic basis for it, but not everyone is convinced.

Jim Milam thinks there's a revolution going on. "You can really sense that things are starting to change," he says from his home outside Seattle. "People are really starting to get it."

According to Milam, a clinical psychologist and author of *Under the Influence: A Guide to the Myths and Realities of Alcoholism,* people are gaining a new understanding of what constitutes alcoholism, a disease the federal government claims costs the United States more than $80 billion a year. Milam has dedicated 30 years of his life to the study of alcohol addiction. He has produced a substantial body of scholarly work, including a recent paper titled "The Alcoholism Revolution," and is champion of what he considers a world-changing idea: The causes of alcoholism strictly are biological.

"When people say that someone's environment or mental or emotional problems turned them into an alcoholic, that is like saying loneliness causes syphilis," says Milam. "Environment may increase exposure to alcohol, but the actual process that results in addiction is biochemical and involuntary."

In *Under the Influence* and on his World Wide Web site (aaw.com), Milam cites research indicating that in some people alcohol affects brain-wave patterns, enzymes and metabolism differently than others, and that it is such biological differences—not emotional, environmental or familial problems—that lead to alcoholism. He calls alcoholism "a deteriorative brain syndrome" that over time creates symptoms (depression, confusion, anxiety) that are misdiagnosed as the reason rather than the result of the addiction.

Among many researchers, Milam's theory that alcoholism is biological is regarded as partly valid. While startling developments have occurred during the last several years that lead experts to acknowledge certain genes as responsible for susceptibility to alcoholism, researchers are quick to point out that alcoholism is a complicated disorder and that declaring it solely genetic may be an oversimplification.

"There is no doubt that genetics plays a role in alcoholism," says Enoch Gordis, director of the National Institute on Alcohol Abuse and Alcoholism, or NIAAA, a federal agency in Rockville, Md. "We have twins and adoption studies going back 25 years that prove this. But do we say it's only genetic? Of course not. Social issues, family issues and environment all play out. We know that some people are loaded genetically, but obviously they can't become alcoholic unless they take a drink. The genes are for risk, not for destiny."

According to the NIAAA's most recent *Special Report to Congress on Alcohol and Health,* as many as 80 percent of alcoholics in treatment have "close biological relatives with a history of alcohol-related problems." Gordis estimates that 60 percent of alcoholics acquire their addiction genetically, leaving 40 percent who become alcoholics for psychological, social and environmental reasons.

Whether as a result of genetics, personality or environment, the cost of alcohol abuse and dependence is high. An estimated 15 million Americans have problems with alcohol abuse and dependence; alcohol is involved in half of all fatal car crashes and is directly responsible for 5 percent of all deaths in the United States. The medical consequences add up to more than $6 billion, including more than $1 billion to treat fetal alcohol syndrome. Considering that federally estimated total of $80 billion in total damages, this is just scratching the surface.

While Gordis is not ready to announce that all alcoholism is genetic, he believes the research increasingly is pointing in that direction. He cites the work of Marc Schuckit, a psychiatrist at the University of San Diego, who has conducted studies showing that, from the time they start drinking, some children of alcoholics metabolize alcohol abnormally and exhibit a genetically based higher tolerance for the drug than the general population.

Gordis also points to the work of C. Robert Cloninger, a professor of psychiatry at Washington University in St. Louis. In 1981 Cloninger conducted extensive studies with 2,000 adopted children in Sweden, concluding that children of alcoholic birth parents, raised by nonalcoholics, are at four times the risk of developing the illness as members of the adoptive family. In 1996 Cloninger conducted the same experiment with a different group and achieved "exact replication."

However, it's not "all about genes," Cloninger says. "Right now it's only genetically verifiable in about 60 percent of cases. The other 40 percent can be caused by a variety of factors—environment and personality traits like anxiety and impulsivity."

Yet what if the "impulsivity" and "anxiety" that lead to alcoholism are genetic traits? Henri Begleiter, a psychiatrist at the Health Science Center at the State University of New York, has discovered "deficiencies" in brain waves of many recovering alcoholics. While in many cases these deficiencies cleared up in long-term recovery, Begleiter found that in some cases they were chronic. He then tested the sons of alcoholics and found that many had the same brain-wave deficiencies—even though they had not yet taken their first drink. Begleiter speculates that brain-wave abnormalities could be responsible for anxiety and impulsivity in some people, and that for them alcohol might have a "compensatory" affect on their brains—in short, that they self-medicate. "The most remarkable thing I hear when I ask many alcoholics about their first drink," he says, "is not about how great and wonderful it was, but simply 'it made me feel normal.'"

Some children of alcoholics metabolize alcohol abnormally and exhibit a higher tolerance.

In 1989 Begleiter was made the head of the Collaborative Study on the Genetics of Alcoholism, or COGA, a $60 million project sponsored by the NIAAA that is one of the biggest studies of its kind ever undertaken. Last year, COGA researchers discovered areas on human chromosomes—so-called "hot spots"—they believe are connected to a propensity for alcoholism. "There are four hot spots that they've found on the chromosomes," says Gordis. "It's a real breakthrough, but it's too early to get overly excited. It's like we started out trying to find someone who lived somewhere in the United States, and now we know he's somewhere between Chicago and Cleveland. Now all we have to do is find the house."

For some skeptics, however, both Milam and the NIAAA studies are talking nonsense. "There's no such thing as a genetic cause of alcoholism," announces Stanton Peele, a fellow at the Lindesmith Center in New York, a drug-policy foundation, and author of *The Truth About Addiction and Recovery, Diseasing of America* and other books about addiction. "The best predictors of alcoholism are all psychosocial factors—who you hang out with, whether you have a job. The whole genetic argument is misguided and unjustified." According to Peele, the genetic-based argument makes people victims and gives them an excuse for self-destructive behavior. He believes that moderating drinking is the wave of the future for treatment.

"Stanton Peele is a liar," retorts Milam. "He's in total denial of science and has been completely shut out of the scientific community." Milam believes the genetic model actually makes people more, not less, responsible. "If you know you have a predisposition to this, then there's no excuse to drink. You couldn't blame society or your parents for the problem. It would be your responsibility to deal with." (At least one prominent conservative agrees. William F. Buckley Jr., who has promoted the idea of legalizing drugs, calls Milam's writings "enlightening" and "persuasive.")

Milam claims that controlled-drinking advocates such as Peele have disregarded science to bolster their claims that anyone can learn to drink moderately. As proof, Milam cites one of the most explosive controversies in alcoholism study—the clash between Irving Maltzman and the husband-wife team of Mark and Linda Sobell.

The Maltzman-Sobell war goes back to 1972, when the Sobells, behavioral-therapy researchers, claimed that by using behavioral-modification techniques they had taught alcoholics to drink moderately. The study widely was reported on the mass media. However, Maltzman, a psychiatrist at the University of California at Los Angeles, claims he was tipped off by the staff at the hospital where the research was conducted that those alcoholics the Sobells claimed were drinking moderately in fact had been rehospitalized for alcoholism.

Maltzman conducted his own research and found that "the majority were not functioning well," and many had been rehospitalized. He charged the Sobells with fraud by falsification of data. The Sobells admitted that they had made an "overstatement" about the frequency of their follow-ups but questioned the validity of Maltzman's research and the trustworthiness of the patients he had interviewed. In 1983 Maltzman submitted his findings to *Science* magazine, which then was threatened by the Sobells with a lawsuit if it published. *Science* found Maltzman's paper free of libel and published it, then ran a letter from editor Philip Abelson claiming that the Sobells' attempts to stonewall Maltzman were "unprecedented in my experience of more than 20 years."

Since the controversy, Maltzman has continued to have problems getting his work into behavioral-therapy and alcoholism journals. According to both Maltzman and Milam, the tragic result of what they see as blackballing by the behavioralists is that it pre-

vents scientific evidence about the role of genetics in alcoholism from reaching the media and convinces alcoholics they can drink moderately.

Contacted by **Insight** about the Maltzman charges, the Sobells declined comment. Instead, they sent a paper they authored in 1989 showing they had been investigated both by the Addiction Research Foundation of Toronto and James Jensen, an investigator for the House Science and Technology subcommittee on Investigations. Both groups had found the Sobells conducted their research "in good faith" and were innocent of fraud.

While the Sobells were reluctant to comment on the controversy, others in their field were not. "Irving Maltzman is a mean man," says G. Alan Marlatt, director of the Center for Behavior Studies at the University of Washington in Seattle and a friend of the Sobells. "He's only interested in discrediting moderation drinking as an alternative, and he's very tenacious." Like Peele, Marlatt believes alcoholics can be taught to drink in moderation using behavioral techniques. "Since 1992 there has been a resurgence in controlled drinking as an alternative to abstinence," he says. "And it's now being used successfully."

For his part, Maltzman says he supports neither the purely biological nor behavioral approaches but rather the more complicated NIAAA findings. "Alcoholism is an enormously complicated interaction between biology, genetics and environment," he says. "Both Milam and Marlatt represent two extremes that miss the mark."

Ironically, one of the biggest hindrances to recognition of the genetic models for alcoholism is Alcoholics Anonymous, or AA, the most famous program for treating alcoholism. AA was founded in 1935 and, though it recognizes a physical dependency, much of its philosophy is based on the concept that spiritual problems and "character defects" cause alcoholism. The AA organization was the result of a meeting in Akron, Ohio, between Bill Wilson, a New York stockbroker, and Bob Smith, an Ohio physician. A few months earlier Wilson had been in a New York hospital detoxing from one of his benders when he experienced a religious conversion that changed his life. He concluded that the only way to defeat demon rum was by deflating the ego, which was responsible for the will to drink. Borrowing from religion, he came up with the Twelve Steps, which encourage alcoholics to turn their lives over to God, "make a fearless and searching moral inventory," make "amends" to those they have hurt and live a more conscientious, spiritual life.

While AA is brandished as the best hope for alcoholics, the figures about its success are revealing. Although the constant fluctuation in the number of AA members makes precision difficult, most research reveals that only about 25 percent of those who enter AA manage to achieve sobriety.

And a curiously overlooked chapter in AA history is relevant to arguments about the biochemical nature of alcoholism. During the fifties, AA cofounder Wilson, frustrated that his program was helping so few alcoholics stay sober, late in life became interested in the biochemical nature of alcoholism. He was introduced to research that indicated many alcoholics suffer from hypoglycemia, a low blood-sugar disorder that can cause emotional and physical distress, and that Vitamin B_3, also called niacin, had produced remarkable results in treating the condition. Wilson became so excited he claimed he would be remembered more for this discovery than for cofounding AA.

However, AA didn't want any part of Wilson's medical theories. At a 1967 conference, the organization recommended separation from the controversy, pointing out that Wilson himself had created an AA tradition that advised AA should "have no opinion on

Alcoholics Anonymous is brandished as the best hope for alcoholics, but most research reveals that only 25 percent of those who enter AA manage to achieve sobriety.

outside issues" and therefore never be "drawn into public controversy." In 1971 Wilson published his last paper boosting B_3 and died shortly thereafter.

In light of Wilson's findings and the recent research, AA has become something of a paradox. On one hand, the organization has done more than any other to convince people that alcoholism is an illness. On the other, its literature and philosophy still reflect its Depression-era origins, when people

believed addiction was the result not of biology but of spiritual and psychological problems—or "character defects," in the popular AA jargon.

Genetics booster Milam believes AA should join the fray. "Yes, AA members are alcoholics following a tradition of anonymity and not getting involved in controversies," he says. "But they are also American citizens, and they have the opportunity to do something about a problem that is tearing this country apart."

When AA members are asked about the genetics of alcoholics, the answers vary depending on who's responding. A visit to the AA headquarters in Washington to ask about the role of genetics in alcoholism is met with the terse comment that "AA does not take positions on outside issues." Asked about the medical side of addiction, an AA member in her thirties snaps, "This is a spiritual disease."

Still, with the genetic evidence mounting, some AA members believe it might be time for a compromise. "Our understanding of the disease of alcoholism is different today than in Bill Wilson's time," offers a fiftysomething member of AA who has been sober for eight years. "I know it's controversial, but new things do become known through science and they're often things that enable us to grow."

New pieces filling in addiction puzzle

Research that links specific genes to smoking is helping scientists piece together a biobehavioral model of smoking.

By Beth Azar
Monitor staff

Lou, the oldest of three brothers, smoked from his early 20s until a quadruple bypass in his late 50s forced him to quit. Even then it took him several tries, and even years after quitting, he complained of terrible cravings.

Joe, the middle brother, began smoking in his teens, going through two packs a day at one point. He quit cold turkey in his early 50s when he realized how much money he was spending on cigarettes.

Bob, the youngest, bummed cigarettes off his friends now and then, but never took up the habit.

These three brothers demonstrate the complexity of the smoking addiction puzzle. Their environment—living above their father's smoky bar in an urban neighborhood—gave them plenty of exposure to cigarettes, which, during their formative years in the 1940s and 1950s, were hip and mainstream. Yet each responded differently.

Researchers must account for the experiences of all three brothers if they are to piece together a biobehavioral model of smoking that accounts for environmental as well as genetic factors.

And recent studies have brought them tantalizingly close to having enough pieces of the puzzle: Over the past year, several studies have begun

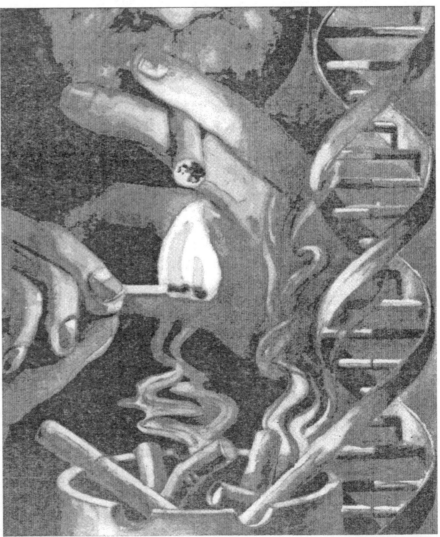

John Michael Yanson

Men cite nicotine, women say social intangibles are behind urge to smoke

Nicotine clearly drives a man's desire to smoke, but it may be less of a catalyst for women, according to research by psychologist Kenneth Perkins, PhD.

That's not to say that nicotine isn't important for women, he says. Rather, he has found that the external pleasures of smoking, such as holding and smelling a cigarette, seem to be more important to them. In contrast, nicotine, more so than external factors, seems to influence men's smoking the most.

These findings may have implications for smoking-cessation programs that hope to help women. Several studies find that female smokers have a harder time quitting than men do, particularly with nicotine replacement therapies, indicating that other techniques may be needed.

"Women appear to be less sensitive to different doses of nicotine than men," says Perkins, professor of psychiatry at the University of Pittsburgh. For example, if he asks smokers to use a nasal spray with varying doses of nicotine or a placebo, women can't tell the difference—even between nicotine and no nicotine. Men, in contrast, can tell the difference even between different doses of nicotine, says Perkins.

This phenomenon, he says, may result from a general inability of women to perceive their own physiological activity, as found in several studies by psychologist James Pennebaker, PhD, of the University of Texas at Austin. In a laboratory environment women are less able than men to perceive physiological changes such as increased blood pressure, heart rate or blood glucose levels, finds Pennebaker.

However, women are just as good as men if asked to observe the same physiological functions in context. For example, if women are exercising or watching a scary movie, they are just as sensitive as men to heart rate fluctuations.

Women appear to be more perceptive to contextual and social cues than to internal cues, says Perkins. So, in terms of smoking, women likely pay more attention to the sight and smell of a cigarette than to the dose of nicotine they're receiving from the cigarette.

In his studies with the nicotine nasal spray, he's stripped the experience of nicotine from the context of smoking. For men, it doesn't matter as much. They feel as comfortable and relaxed in response to nicotine they sprayed into their noses as they do when they're smoking. But for women, these positive effects only occurred when they smoked cigarettes, not when they used the nicotine nasal spray.

"It can't only be the nicotine that women are responding to," says Perkins. "Women to some extent are reacting positively to the way they take nicotine in through smoking."

Perkins isn't saying that women don't become dependent on nicotine, he emphasizes. Both nicotine and non-nicotine factors are related to smoking for men and women. But nicotine appears to be less important for women while non-nicotine factors are more important.

Such a finding is significant for treatment. If nicotine replacement therapy is all people are relying on, women will get short-changed, says Perkins.

—B. Azar

according to studies that show identical twins are far more likely to share a smoking habit than fraternal twins.

In addition, as with most behavioral traits, there are likely many genes that contribute to one's proclivity to smoke. And each gene likely wields a relatively small effect and interacts not only with the other genes but also with the environment, says Swan.

In their search for "smoking genes" researchers are using what they know about how the brain processes nicotine to sift through genes already identified as playing a role in that process.

For example, variations in genes for proteins known to metabolize nicotine might make people react differently to nicotine. And differences in genes known to be involved in the brain's reward system—which is triggered by nicotine—might make people more or less vulnerable to addiction.

Messing with metabolism . . .

Rachel Tyndale, PhD, and her colleagues at the University of Toronto aimed their sights at a gene that encodes the enzyme CYP2A6, which breaks down nicotine when it enters the liver. There are several forms, or alleles, of the CYP2A6 gene, at least one of which produces an inactive form of the enzyme. People who carry this inactive form of the gene, researchers speculate, keep nicotine in their bodies longer than people with the active form of the enzyme. Such a scenario may increase nicotine's adverse effects, making some people less likely to become regular smokers. And in people who do smoke, longer-lasting nicotine would limit the number of cigarettes needed to maintain a preferred nicotine dose.

In fact, Tyndale and her colleagues find that nonsmokers are twice as likely than smokers to have a defective allele for CYP2A6. And smokers who have the defective allele smoke significantly fewer cigarettes than smokers with active forms of the gene. These findings were published

to pinpoint specific genes associated with smoking. The trick now becomes combining that information with what researchers know about the environment.

The ultimate model will not only help researchers better understand addiction, but it will also allow them to design smoking-cessation programs tailored to individual needs. The key to building such a model will be cooperation among psychologists, epidemiologists and geneticists, says Gary Swan, PhD, director of the Center for

Health Sciences at SRI International in Menlo Park, Calif.

Many genes, small effects

Researchers already know that about half the blame for smoking goes to environmental factors, including parents and friends who smoke, society's acceptance of smoking, the availability of cigarettes and the abundance of cigarette advertising. The other half can be blamed on heredity, last year in the journal *Nature* (Vol. 393, p. 750).

Other researchers have yet to replicate the Toronto researchers' findings. But they're intriguing, say some, indicating a possible mechanism that makes some people more or less vulnerable to nicotine addiction.

"Understanding the critical role this enzyme plays in nicotine addiction gives a new target for developing more effective medications to help people stop smoking," said National Institute on Drug Abuse Director Alan Leshner, PhD, when the study was released.

...and wrecking reward

Other researchers are concentrating on the brain's reward system as a potential area for finding genes associated with smoking. In particular, they are looking at genes related to the neurotransmitter dopamine—a major player in the reward system—which may influence people's inclination to smoke, according to the results of several studies.

Most recently, two research teams report in this month's issue of *Health Psychology* (Vol. 18, No. 1) a connection between smoking and the gene for a dopamine transporter—a protein that sweeps up dopamine after it's released by a nerve cell. The studies link the presence of a form of the gene, called the SLC6A3 "9-repeat allele," to whether people smoke and the ease with which smokers can quit. Other studies have linked the 9-repeat allele to increased levels of dopamine, indicating that the transporter the gene encodes is less efficient at clearing out excess dopamine than other forms of the transporter.

In one study comparing 289 smokers with 233 nonsmokers, psychologist Caryn Lerman, PhD, of Georgetown University Medical Center, and her colleagues found that people with the 9-repeat allele were less likely to be smokers than people with other forms of the dopamine transporter gene. This relationship was particularly strong if people also carried another gene related to dopamine—a

form of the D2 dopamine receptor that provides plenty of places for dopamine to "dock" when excess dopamine is left by the inefficient transporter. In fact, people with both genes were half as likely to be smokers as people without the genes, the researchers report.

The National Cancer Institute's (NCI) Sue Sabol, PhD, Dean Hamer, PhD, and their colleagues also found a link between the 9-repeat allele and smoking. In particular, among 1,107 nonsmokers, current smokers and former smokers, former smokers were more likely than current smokers to have the 9-repeat allele, says Hamer. This finding implies that the allele may boost people's ability to quit

How? Perhaps through a connection with the personality trait known as "novelty seeking," says Hamer. He and his colleagues found that people with the 9-repeat allele scored low on novelty seeking, which was also the most significant predictor of whether people quit smoking. The 9-repeat allele, they hypothesize, increases the amount of dopamine in the brain and reduces people's need for novelty and reward through external stimuli such as smoking.

These connections among personality, genes and smoking must be examined carefully in the context of other environmental factors, including cultural and societal views of smoking, says Hamer. It may turn out that a trait that put people at risk for smoking 50 years ago is protective today. For example, during the 1940s and 50s, smoking was related to sociability, extroversion and affability. But to-

day it is "clearly antisocial," says Hamer. So if genes contributing to sociability are related to smoking, they would have the opposite effect today than they had 50 years ago.

Proceed with caution

The overlap between the two dopamine transporter studies "is very encouraging," says Lerman. But it's important to note that it is difficult to draw conclusions from these early studies because they are looking at relatively small groups of people, and ethnic differences within and between study populations may affect the results.

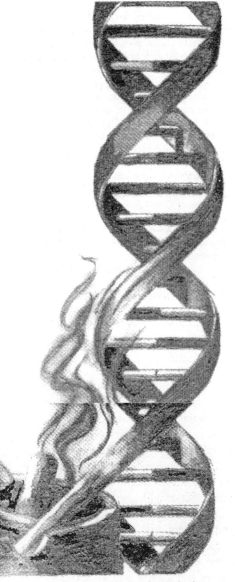

John Michael Yanson

"**The next step is to see how these genetic effects relate to psychological, social and environmental factors and to develop a comprehensive model of addiction. These are the preliminary studies to lay the foundation for those more complex studies.**"

Caryn Lerman
Georgetown University Medical Center

"It may turn out that all of this is wrong," adds NCI researcher Peter Shields, PhD, one of Lerman's coauthors. "But we have good reason to think that it is right. Our data are fairly tight and consistent."

It's also important to note that with any complex behavior, including smoking, the contribution of any single gene is likely to be very small, says Lerman.

For example, researchers know from studies of twins that genes account for at least half the variance in smoking, says Lerman. But within that are multiple genes, each exerting a small effect on smoking and interacting with environmental, cultural and psychological factors.

"The next step is to see how these genetic effects relate to psychological, social and environmental factors and to develop a comprehensive model of addiction," Lerman says. "These are the preliminary studies to lay the foundation for those more complex studies."

The easy part is finding genes, adds Swan. The hard part is sorting through the gene-environment interactions. And that's where behavioral researchers, in tight collaboration with geneticists and biologists, will be critical.

In addition, these multidisciplinary research teams will need to collaborate among themselves, as some have already begun to do, to move the field of smoking susceptibility research forward and avoid the pitfalls of some other areas of research, says Swan.

In the area of obesity, for example, researchers have not cooperated, he says, and they now have many potential genes but no coherent model of how they interact with each other or the environment to cause obesity. The same could easily happen in the area of smoking unless researchers work together to form a coherent and cooperative research program, he says.

"I don't want to be looking back 20 years from now having all the genes and no where to go," Swan says. "The public health imperative of the smoking problem almost demands that we put aside the traditional way of doing things and work in a focused, energetic and supportive environment relatively free of competition among team members."

Television

Taping the horror

**While preparing an anti-drug documentary,
Vancouver's Odd Squad has learned compassion**

BY CHRIS WOOD

Const. Al Arsenault has spent 12 years walking one of the most violent and dispiriting police beats in Canada. Vancouver's Downtown Eastside, roughly a 10-block area adjoining the trendy Gastown tourist district, is seedy enough by day. After dark, it becomes an open-air marketplace of drugs, violence and despair. In alleys, addicts kneel amidst filth, scrabbling through used condoms for crumbs of crack. Outside dollar-a-draft beer halls, the drug dealing barely pauses except when there is a dispute to settle with blows and blood. Almost every day, someone dies with a heroin needle at his or her feet—or still in an arm. But a year after Arsenault and fellow officers began carrying a video camera on patrol, the footage they have gathered is moving for more than its graphic horror. "I have been amazed by the resilience of the human spirit," says the soft-spoken martial-arts and weapons expert. "In all that poverty, it shines through."

If that sounds uncharacteristic of a hard-nosed skid row cop, it is just one of the surprises in store when the Vancouver police officers' amateur video reaches television screens across Canada, likely next year, in a documentary entitled *Through a Blue Lens*. Last month, the National Film Board signed an agreement with Vancouver documentary maker Veronica Alice Mannix to package video footage shot by the members of Odd Squad Productions—all of them past or present Downtown Eastside beat officers—into an hour-long documentary for broadcast, as well as two shorter video packages to be shown in classrooms.

With cameramen in blue still shooting (they hope to wrap up their project in June), many scenes already gathered are gruesome. A few are grimly humorous. But all are tragic—a point the uniformed officers of Odd Squad hope gets through to the group it considers its most important audience: adolescents tempted by the surface glamour and seductive danger of drug use. It should at least get their attention. In Vancouver-area high schools, some of the early footage has struck even snickering, back-of-the-room cynics into shocked silence.

The seeds of the project were sown at a "beat party" thrown early in 1997 by the foot soldiers of the Vancouver Police Department's District 2. Arsenault had been carrying not only a handgun but a still camera on the job for years; he was considered a bit eccentric. But when he showed some of his slides to the party, the powerful scenes immediately grabbed the attention of Arsenault's patrol partner, Toby Hinton. At the time, Hinton had been making presentations about the neighbourhood for five years to audiences of glazed-eyed high-school students, as well as other community groups. Soon, Arsenault's photos began to inject a grim dose of reality into the force's school talks, and Hinton also bought himself a camera. Last March, the two partners and five fellow policemen formed their nonprofit production company, each contributing $400 to buy a broadcast-quality video camera in the belief that what they taped might drive home an anti-drug message even more forcefully.

On shift, policing still comes before taping for the members of the Odd Squad. But when an opportunity arises to capture a vignette of life on the mean streets, the camera comes out. One sequence shows a woman named Carlee, fidgeting in front of a narrow vanity cluttered with drug paraphernalia. Minutes earlier, her boyfriend—who subsequently died—had shot himself in the head. He had turned the gun on himself after being reluctantly talked out of a plan to commit an armed robbery for drug money; Carlee had walked a block to a pay phone to call an ambulance. Now she is doing the shuffle of an addict beginning to need a fix, and halfheartedly spraying disinfectant on a five-inch open wound on her left forearm. "That's the result of picking bugs out of my arm," Carlee explains flatly. Doctors tell her the bugs are hallucinations. She doesn't believe them. "The bugs are in there," Carlee insists. "I don't care what anybody says."

Another woman sums up what has become of her once promising life. The pampered daughter of a wealthy family, Nicola was introduced to cocaine while still a teenager—by

From *Maclean's*, February 22, 1999, pp. 72-73. © 1999 by Maclean Hunter, Ltd. Reprinted by permission.

trainers at the stable where she kept her horse. Estranged from her family by 20, she became a high-end call girl to support her habit. Now 40, she has lost her looks and sleeps most of the time on the street. Crouched in an alcove by a vent for warmth, she describes an addict's existence: "You are a slave. You have no life. Everything you do revolves around getting your next fix."

But the mission the Odd Squad had set out on—to capture the depths of the misery that flows from addiction to alcohol, cocaine and heroin—soon began to open the eyes of the officers behind the cameras. "When I first started out down here," recalls Const. Len Hollingsworth, "I saw the people as junkies or hypes. I had no use for them." But as the group's taping began to focus closely on about a dozen individuals, the stories that emerged transformed his perceptions. "I think one of the biggest things out of this is that we have all learned much more compassion," he says. "This could be your brother, your sister—this *is* somebody's brother or sister."

Documentary maker Mannix found it easy to relate to that perspective. The Vancouver-based producer—whose *Down Here,* an hour-long biography of a poet and ex-addict, aired last month on Vision TV—has had personal experience watching a family member succumb to heroin addiction. And after making several successful sports documentaries with her partner and husband, Emmy Award-winning cameraman Daniel Mannix, she had already sought out more challenging material in Vancouver's Downtown Eastside. *Down Here,* completed in late 1997, is a profile of Bud Osborn, who has become one of the few impassioned voices advocating for the residents of what income statistics rank as the country's poorest urban community. Inevitably, while filming there two summers ago, the Mannixes met the officers—and quickly formed a bond. Daniel Mannix gave them tips on camera work. Veronica became intrigued by the double-edged emotional effects of their undertaking. "It not only humanizes the addicts," she observes, "it humanizes the officers."

The officers' emotional involvement becomes evident when Hinton and Hollingsworth join a *Maclean's* reporter for a Saturday night tour of the alleys and bars on either side of the tenderloin stretch of East Hastings Street. They are watchful but relaxed, greeting many denizens of the street by name. When they encounter Don, an alcoholic who is having trouble standing up, Hollingsworth reminds him that he has two daughters in Ontario who would like to hear from him. Then, Henry—a self-styled "ethical" drug dealer who claims he "won't sell to children, or pregnant women, or people who just started"—expresses his respect. "I never could get along with police," he acknowledges out of their earshot. "These guys, I'd shake their hand." It may help as well that their policy is not to use any of the personal drug use captured on film in a criminal prosecution.

Still, it is not really the people skills, or the discretion, of the Odd Squad cops that has secured the co-operation of most of the addicts and alcoholics who have agreed to have their ruined lives profiled. They also strongly support their goal. Down the block from where Henry has faded into an alley, Lana weaves and bobs on the sidewalk, her skinny frame restless in black leggings and a teal sweatshirt. She is another of the officers' subjects, being filmed and interviewed repeatedly. Why is she bothering? "I wouldn't want anyone else to join my nightmare," she says.

At schools such as Windsor Secondary School in prosperous North Vancouver, the unfiltered footage of life and death on skid row may already be discouraging some youths from just that. When Hollingsworth and another member of the Odd Squad, Dale Weidman, addressed about 40 Grade 11 students one Monday morning last month, their presentation at first prompted an undercurrent of whispered jokes and smart-alec remarks around the back of the second-floor classroom. The subdued tittering continued even after the officers began to show some still images from their slide collection. Then, Hollingsworth flicked on the video player, and introduced the teens to Carlee and her bugs. The peanut gallery fell silent. Afterward, 16-year-old Allison Pehleman shared the opinion of several friends that this was one anti-drug message it would be nearly impossible to ignore. "This is amazing," she said. "You see what can happen. They have very hard lives. It's scary." That is a lesson both the creators and the tragic stars of *Through a Blue Lens* hope to deliver to a much larger audience when the hour-long documentary is broadcast.

Unit 3

Unit Selections

Key Points to Consider

❖ How is it that specific drugs evolve, develop use patterns, and lose or gain popularity over time?

❖ How does the manner in which a drug is ingested help define its respective user population?

❖ How does the manner in which a drug is used influence the severity of consequences related to that drug? Or does it?

❖ Why does the use of certain drugs encourage the use of other drugs?

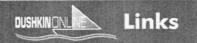 **Links** www.dushkin.com/online/

These sites are annotated on pages 4 and 5.

The following articles discuss those drugs that have prevailed historically as drugs of choice. Although pharmacological modifications emerge periodically to enhance or alter the effects produced by certain drugs or the manner in which various drugs are used, basic pharmacological properties of the drugs remain unchanged. Crack is still cocaine, ice is still methamphetamine, dusters are still phencyclidine (PCP), and black tar is still heroin. In addition, tobacco products all supply the drug nicotine, while alcoholic beverages provide the drug ethyl alcohol. These drugs all influence how we act, think, and feel about ourselves and the world around us. They also produce markedly different effects within the body and within the mind.

To understand why certain drugs remain popular over time, one must be knowledgeable about the effects produced by individual drugs. Why people use drugs is a bigger question than why people use heroin. However, understanding why certain people use heroin, or cocaine, or marijuana, or alcohol is one way to construct a framework from which to tackle the larger question of why people use drugs in general. One of the most complex relationships is the one between Americans and their use of alcohol. Some 76 million Americans have experienced alcoholism in their families. The most recent survey of alcohol use (1998) estimates that 113 million Americans have used the drug in the 30 days prior to the survey. About 33 million are estimated to have engaged in binge drinking (five or more drinks on one occasion), and currently there are 10.5 million drinkers between the ages of 12 and 20. Alcohol prevails as the most popular recreational drug of choice and its use is commonly associated with the use of most illicit drugs. Of the current 11.2 million heavy drinkers, 30 percent (3.3 million people) are illicit drug users. There is also a long-standing and significant relationship between the use of alcohol and the use of tobacco. An estimated 60 million Americans report current cigarette use. The majority consensus is that alcohol is used responsibly by most people who use it even though 10 percent of the American population is believed to be suffering from various stages of alcoholism. The use of alcohol is a powerful force within our national consciousness about drugs.

Misinformation abounds as to the physiological and psychological effects produced by different drugs of abuse. People tend to discuss the subject of drugs generically, often referring to all drugs as narcotics. Narcotics refer to a specific class of drugs, that of opium and its derivatives. Cocaine and LSD, for example, are not narcotics. Understanding the basic differences between different drugs and their properties is significant to understanding how numerous and specific dimensions of drug use are perpetuated.

Understanding why people initially turn to drugs is a huge question that is debated and discussed in a voluminous body of literature. One important reason why the major drugs of use and abuse, such as alcohol, nicotine, cocaine, heroin, marijuana,

and amphetamines, retain their popularity is because they produce certain physical and psychological effects that humans crave. They temporarily restrain our inhibitions; reduce our fears; alleviate mental and physical suffering; produce energy, confidence, and exhilaration; and allow us to relax. They also, albeit artificially, suggest a greater capacity to transcend, redefine, and seek out new levels of consciousness. In addition, they do it upon demand. People initially use a specific drug, or class of drugs, to obtain the desirable effects historically associated with the use of that drug. Heroin and opiate-related drugs produce, in most people, a euphoric, dreamy state of well-being. Cocaine and related stimulant drugs produce euphoria, energy, confidence, and exhilaration. Alcohol produces a loss of inhibitions and a state of well-being. Nicotine and marijuana typically serve as relaxants. Although effects and side effects may vary from user to user, a general pattern of effects is predictable from most major drugs of use. Varying the dosage and altering the manner of ingestion is one way to alter the drug's effects. Some drugs, such as PCP, LSD, and some types of designer drugs, produce effects on the user that are less predictable and more sensitive to variations in dosage level and to the user's physical and psychological makeup.

Although all major drugs of use and abuse have specific reinforcing properties perpetuating their continued use, they also produce undesirable side effects that regular drug users attempt to mitigate. Most often, users attempt to mitigate these effects with the use of other drugs. Cocaine, methamphetamine, heroin, and alcohol have long been used to mitigate each other's side effects. A good example is the classic "speedball" of heroin and cocaine. When they are combined, cocaine accelerates and intensifies the euphoric state of the heroin, while the heroin softens the comedown from cocaine. Most abusers of the major drugs are polydrug users. Additionally, various analogs or chemical cousins known as "designer drugs" replicate the major drugs of use and abuse. These drugs, such as LSD, Ecstasy, GHB, fentenyl, and PCP all lose and gain in popularity over time and typically remain as adjuncts to historically precedented major drugs. Other related drug trends, availability, price, and the public's perception of the drug's safety often influence the degree to which designer drugs remain popular.

Drug abuse in America spans the spectrum of legality. To associate only illegal drugs with abuse and criminality is shortsighted. In terms of drug-related social impacts, any discussion of major drugs could begin and end with the topics of alcohol and nicotine. The pursuit of drugs and the effects they produce may be influenced by, but not bound by, legal status. For the student of drug-related phenomena, an attachment to the concepts of legality or illegality for purposes of comprehensively rationalizing drug-related reality is inappropriate. For example, yearly alcohol-related deaths far outnumber deaths from all illegal drugs combined.

The Major Drugs of Use and Abuse

Resisting Cocaine's Tragic Lure

**Few "recreational" drugs are more dangerous than cocaine.
Here's why people who have used cocaine say, "Stay away!"**

by Jan Farrington

Zack, 19, is a recovering cocaine addict. "That's kind of a shameful thing to have to admit," he says. But admit it he does, because talking to high school students about drugs is a condition of his probation. "I spent four months and 19 days in the county jail in Dallas. I'm on probation until May of the year 2001. I talk to kids [as part of my] probation; I don't know if it does any good. I hope so, because [cocaine is] the most wicked demon I've ever encountered."

Zack knows only too well the price one can pay for giving in to cocaine's tragic lure. "I gave up my best friend for cocaine. I gave up quite a few years of my life. I put my mom through a lot. I stole her car twice. She had to come to Colorado [from Texas] and drive me home. I've been in jail in four different states. I drove all the way to Oregon to get some acid. My high school class graduated without me."

FROM AN EARLY AGE . . .

He was 11 or 12 years old when it started. He was "smoking weed [marijuana] and drinking just about every day—after school, at football games. That's what me and my friends did."

Why he started, he doesn't know. "When I was very young [in Oklahoma], my dad didn't drink much and my parents were together. We lived in an upscale neighborhood. My dad coached all my teams: Little League, basketball, football. My dad told me he'd had some run-ins with cocaine in the early '80s, but by then he'd cleaned up from that. So he'd have a few beers. . . ."

Despite this outward comfort, all was not well. "My friends and I turned into little hoodlums. It [marijuana, mostly]

was pretty easy to get, and it was easy to hide. In all those years, I don't think I was ever caught by my parents or at school. It affected my [school] performance, definitely, but I was never a discipline problem or a troublemaker. I wasn't dealing drugs under the teachers' noses. I was dealing, though—I had to pay for it."

Zack's parents split up when he was 15, and his mother took a job in the affluent town of Plano, just north of Dallas. Zack went with her but couldn't adjust. "I moved back to Oklahoma that summer. My dad was there, but by then he was an alcoholic. He wasn't an authority figure, just one of the guys. I lived with him, my brother, and three other roommates who came and went. I got high with my dad every day that summer."

Zack went back to Plano and his sophomore year in high school. But about mid-year, a new drug came into his life: cocaine.

Again, a parent—this time someone else's—would fail him. "The guy I used to get it from was my best friend's dad. He was about 45 years old, in upper management at one of the telecommunications companies down here," says Zack. "They had a big, nice house, cars and everything. I did a lot of cocaine, because it was doled out to us for free, all day, every day, for about six months. He'd give us his credit cards, and we'd get cash advances at the bank—about $250 every day. We'd drive down south of downtown Dallas and call the dealer, and she'd deliver it to us in the parking lot of a club. We got to be pretty good customers."

But cocaine caught up with his friend's dad. "For cocaine, this guy gave it all up—his family, everything. He put

the house up for auction, and the college degree, the military training, the great job—it was all gone."

Zack understands how it happened because he understands the drug's relentless pull. "I loved doing cocaine. Before I'd ever done it myself, I saw a friend try it. He was sitting in a chair, pale and shaking, and he looked kind of sick. But then he looked up at me, and he was just euphoric."

A DOWNWARD PULL

Soon drugs pulled Zack away from school. "I had good grades, but I just didn't want to be there any more," he remembers. "I'd skip a class to go smoke weed with a friend, and the absences started snowballing. After nine absences I'd lose credit in the class, so then I wouldn't go any more."

He dropped out three times—in 10th, 11th, and 12th grades. He doesn't remember the school counselors ever calling him in to talk about it. But he does remember the drugs: "When I came back on campus the second half of 11th grade, I found a friend. We went around behind the school to smoke weed, and I never made it to even the first class."

In senior year, Zack's girlfriend asked him to stop using cocaine. He says he quit for a while. But within a few months, he and a male friend were looking for drug money. "I didn't have very high moral standards," Zack says bluntly. "I never got to where I was robbing people or anything like that—but I can't say I never stole anything."

Zack and his friend convinced a kid they hardly knew to break into his parents' house. "His folks had kicked him out, and he wanted to go up north to

From *Current Health 2*, February 1999, pp. 6-12. © 1999 by Weekly Reader Corporation. Reprinted by permission.

see his dad. We told him if he went in, we could trade the stuff for drugs, sell them, and give him enough money for a bus ticket. We had it all planned out. He brought us the safe from under the bed, the silverware, stuff like that. And after we did this whole big trade, we never gave the kid any money, just a quarter gram of cocaine."

The boy paid for it, too. "The next day he was arrested," Zack says. "And this is the worst part—he sat in jail for four months before the police put together what happened and came and arrested me and my friend. I was in jail for more than four months."

AN AWAKENING

For the first time, he began to question what he was doing. "My mom brought textbooks and an SAT prep book and got special permission for me to use them in the library. On the fourth day, I asked for a Bible and started reading. . . . And when I came out, things seemed crystal clear to me. I stayed clean for more than a year, until one night—I hate telling this—I smoked weed with an old roommate I'd gone to visit. I've been clean since, though."

Once out of jail, Zack finished high school. "At graduation, they voted me 'Most Improved Student,' and I got a $500 scholarship for that, and another one for $750. Then a friend of my mom sponsored me for $3,000 in college expenses."

Zack's a college freshman now, and he's thinking about studying meteorology or finance—and about playing sports again, something he'd given up during the drug years.

Once or twice, he says, he's gotten the feeling that some teachers don't think he's the right one to talk to their students. He says they think teens will look at him and say, "He's alive, he's got scholarships. Why can't I [fool] around with drugs and then get over it?"

"But I've never had a kid [who uses drugs] ask me that. These kids understand why drugs are dangerous, but it doesn't stop them."

Zack thinks anti-drug workshops that focus on physical dangers are a waste of time. What gets through to teenagers, he says, are "stories like mine."

If you push him, Zack says he's turned away from drugs "because I don't want to go back to jail." But he'll also tell you about the night he thinks the cocaine almost killed him. It's a story he hopes other teens will listen to.

"We did so much cocaine that night," he remembers. "I really kind of felt my brain start to shut down, and I started to feel drunk. That takes a lot of cocaine."

But cocaine's lure is powerful—so powerful, in fact, he nearly let it kill him. "I got dizzy, and my heart was going pretty good. But you know what? I did some more. That was the night I realized it's entirely possible to die from this drug, or to have it just eat up your brain."

Zack's town of Plano has made national news in recent years for multiple teen deaths—first from cocaine and, more recently, from heroin.

"I'm never around drugs any more, and I feel really removed from that life," Zack says. Yet he has never quite shaken the addict's arcane slang, which peppers his conversations. "I know there are a couple of apartment complexes near here where I could go to and find chiva [heroin], no problem."

Still, he stays far away from the drug scene. "My girlfriend will tell you I'm a pretty boring dude," he laughs. "I go to school and work. I work at Blockbuster, so we watch a lot of movies."

As for his male friend, he never sees him. Part of their probation is that they have no contact at all.

And when somebody asks, he tells his story, despite the shame of admitting his past addiction. He hopes it will keep some other kid who's "not afraid of much" from having to fight the same "wicked demon" that nearly wrecked his life.

WHY COCAINE IS DANGEROUS . . .

Cocaine is a white powder that comes from the leaves of the South American coca plant. Usually it is "snorted" into the nasal passages—or, less commonly, injected intravenously. In its altered, smokable form, cocaine is called "crack."

Cocaine belongs to a class of drugs called *stimulants*. Other examples are amphetamines and methamphetamines—including the designer drug "Ecstasy" and "ice," a crystalline form of methamphetamines. The caffeine found in coffee, soft drinks, and many over-the-counter medications is also classified as a stimulant.

Cocaine users report that the drug's "rush" creates strong feelings of pleasure and an illusion of limitless power and energy. On the downswing, cocaine leaves users feeling depressed, edgy, anxious—and craving more of the drug.

Cocaine and crack are highly addictive drugs—and they can kill. They are addictive because they seem to take over the brain's natural "reward circuit"—the mechanism that allows us to experience joy and pleasure. When we have a

pleasurable experience, the brain releases a substance called *dopamine*. What drug abusers find is that cocaine can "fool" the brain into releasing huge amounts of dopamine at one time, producing a rush of pleasure.

That rush comes with a very high price, however. Drug researchers believe that cocaine use permanently alters the brain, reducing its ability to produce dopamine. Users become less and less able to experience any kind of pleasure when they are not high on cocaine.

"Your brain's reward system is depleted," one researcher explained on the PBS special *Close to Home*. "You get no pleasures from anything, except drugs, and even the drugs don't do it anymore."

Cocaine is physically addictive. Brain experts say that with special imaging techniques they can actually see parts of the brain light up with activity as drug addicts report cravings for cocaine.

The drug is psychologically addictive, too. It creates strong "learned" emotional memories that addicts find hard to ignore.

Cocaine is also a killer. Even first-time users can experience fatal seizures or heart attacks, strokes, or shutdowns of their respiratory systems. As Zack knew all too well, cocaine can cause the heart to beat unsteadily or abnormally fast. The drug causes blood vessels to narrow, starving the heart muscle by reducing the flow of blood and oxygen to the heart. At the same time, the cocaine-fueled heart forces more and more blood through the narrowed blood vessels. The resultant rise in blood pressure can cause blood vessels to split or break anywhere in the body, including the heart and brain, causing a heart attack or a stroke. Even super-fit professional athletes have died suddenly of cocaine-induced heart attacks.

Beyond these quick deaths, cocaine and crack have contributed to drownings, car crashes, falls, burns, and suicides. The psychological risks are tremendous: violent, paranoid behavior; hallucinations and "coke bugs"—sensations of insects crawling over the skin; loss of interest in food, sex, friends, family. Some users—like Zack's best friend's father—spend hundreds or thousands of dollars on cocaine or crack each week, and become increasingly willing to commit crimes or put themselves in danger to pay for the drug.

There is no good news about cocaine. But fewer high school and college-age teens are using it—and that's encouraging. In a recent survey of more than 50,000 teens by the University of Michigan, 5 percent of 12th grade students reported having used cocaine powder at least once in the past year. That's down from 17 percent of high

Help
When You Need It

You can phone, fax, or cybersurf your way to help for yourself, a family member, or a friend. Check the local phone book (there's usually a center section with "Helpful Numbers") for community drug hot lines, treatment services/clinics, and other community groups. Here are some places you can call from anywhere in the United States:

Cocaine Help Line: 1-800-COCAINE
National Clearinghouse for Alcohol and Drug Information (NCADI): a one-stop resource for prevention and treatment information. Call **1-800-729-6686 (1-310-468-2600** if

you live in the Washington, D.C., area). Or visit their Web site at **http://www.health.org.**
National Institute on Drug Abuse Help Line: 1-800-662-HELP (4357); their Web site is **http://www.nida.nih.gov.**

---

school seniors in 1985. In the same survey, 10 percent of 12th-graders said they had used some kind of stimulant—from caffeine to methamphetamine—during the same time period.

That surely isn't good news.

In addition to this, heroin has begun to compete with cocaine for the title of Public Drug Enemy #1. After the cocaine heyday of the mid-1980s, the U.S. market for the drug slowly began to shrink. According to *The New York Times*, the number of users declined from more than 6 million a decade ago to 2 million today. So the drug producers in South America developed a replacement product. "Then Colombian cocaine cartels started growing poppies in the Andes," the *Times* reported. From the poppies, they developed a new, purer form of heroin that was easy to transport—and much more profitable than the old form.

And a few teens began to try it.

THE COCAINE-HEROIN CONNECTION

They call it chiva, horse, hammer, junk, smack.

It comes as a white or brown powder, or as something that looks like sticky black tar. And, like cocaine, it can kill you.

"A lot of kids who tried it had no clue they were using heroin," says Nancy Griffin, who heads a Dallas-area group working to educate teens and parents about today's drug dangers. Today's heroin may seem less dangerous because

you don't need a needle. "You can sniff, snort, swallow, or smoke this stuff," says Griffin. And for some teens, heroin has a kind of violent glamour because they associate it with Kurt Cobain, River Phoenix, and the movies *Pulp Fiction, My Own Private Idaho, Trainspotting.*

"Our town was specifically targeted by the drug cartels [producers], especially the Mexican cartel," says Griffin, who lives in Plano, Texas. Most families have a little money to spend—and so do their teenage sons and daughters. Four years ago, Plano drew national attention for a sudden increase in cocaine-related deaths among teens and young adults. But over the past two years, the fatal overdoses making the news in Plano have been caused by heroin.

Nancy Griffin and her family were part of the story, too. Her son Jason, about to graduate from a Plano high school in 1997, had a history of cocaine abuse. Then she found out he was using heroin. "He was arrested in June [1997], and we never bailed him out."

Griffin's tough-love decision set off a public debate about how hard parents had to be to help drug-addicted teens. But, after more than a year, Griffin is sure she did the right thing. "It's the best thing that could have happened to him. It saved his life," she says. "Jason has been in jail or a prison drug program for 16 months—and he's been clean for all that time. The longer you can do that, the better your chance of being able to stay clean."

Griffin worries about what will happen once Jason leaves prison. "I hope he has the strength he needs," she says. She takes heart from her son's words. Jason told me, "I know where [heroin] took me, and I know where it would take me the next time. I'm not doing that again."

Heroin is more addictive and more deadly than ever. Hospital ERs are seeing teens who've mixed cocaine and heroin into "speedballs." These concoctions are thought to help abusers avoid the terrible depression that often follows a brief cocaine high. A doctor at a Plano hospital says it's not unusual for him to deal with three or four heroin overdose victims during a 12-hour shift on the weekend. Similar reports are being heard from other places, including Denver, Colorado; north suburban New Jersey; Orlando, Florida; and Philadelphia, Pennsylvania.

In the wake of recent heroin deaths, families try to handle the grief. One family found their son dead in his bed of a heroin overdose the morning after he'd come home from college for a weekend visit. Another Plano student has been left terribly brain damaged after a heroin-induced seizure. His friends struggle with the guilt of knowing that they failed to stop him from abusing heroin.

"We've had so many kids lost," says Nancy Griffin. "At the funerals, their friends come up to the parents saying, 'I'm so sorry, I'm so sorry.' 'Did you know?' 'Yes.' '*Why* didn't you let us know?' 'I guess I was afraid she'd/he'd

HOW Can I Tell If a Friend Has a Drug Problem?

"Sometimes it's hard to tell," says the National Clearinghouse for Alcohol and Drug Information. But these are clear warning signs:

- *using drugs more and more often, and needing more of the drug(s) to get high*
- *lying about things in general, or the amount of drugs they are using*
- *turning to drugs after confrontations or arguments, or to relieve uncomfortable feelings*
- *giving up activities they used to enjoy (sports, music, dance, etc.)*
- *poor school or work performance*
- *getting into trouble with the law, school suspension, etc.*
- *taking risks, including sexual risks and driving under the influence of drugs*
- *changing to a new group of "friends" who also use drugs*
- *believing they can't have fun without drugs*
- *talking constantly about drugs*
- *pressuring others to use drugs*
- *reporting feeling run-down, hopeless, depressed, or even suicidal*

If you think a friend is using (or see yourself in some of these symptoms), look for help now. Talk things over with an adult you can trust, and decide on some specific actions that will start moving things in a positive direction. Don't wait for a "better time." It will never come. Drug abuse problems change because people start to change their behavior and make better choices—even though their lives are tough.

"I was always looking for the answer to the question 'How can I feel better?'" says a young recovering cocaine addict. "It never occurred to me I could do that on my own [without drugs]."

be mad at me.' Well, being mad at you is one thing. Being dead is another."

Griffin's group, the Starfish Foundation, has high school and college-age members who talk to teens about how important it is to break the "code of silence" surrounding drug use. "Teens grow up with that idea about 'not telling' on their friends, but this is a matter of life and death," says Griffin. "One thing they need to know is that they can get the information to the parents without actually phoning them or going to their front door. You can tell a counselor, a teacher, a principal about a friend who's in trouble—and they will get word to the parents."

Teens who've used heroin sometimes talk about "chasing the dragon"—always trying to recapture the incredible first-time high. "This is one of the reasons you get hooked," a heroin addict said on the recent PBS series, *Close to Home*. "You keep going, trying to find that first time again, and you *never* find it."

That's chasing the dragon—until one day you realize your life is about nothing but your next hit. And then you know the dragon is chasing you.

HOW TO FIGHT THE "LURES"

No guarantees, of course—but counselors say these are some of the best ways for teens to avoid getting lured into drug abuse in the first place:

- **Find an adult mentor** You need somebody (a parent, older sibling, grandparent, neighbor, or teacher) who's lived longer and seen more . . . and who can help you across the rough spots in life without using drugs.
- **Set some goals for your life:** things you want to do this year, four or five years from now, etc. Not just work, college, family—but other things that might bring you a sense of self-worth and joy.

- Stick with a close group of **friends who DO NOT use drugs.** Groups of good friends can create a powerful and safe environment for one another.
- **Keep busy.** Fill your time with good stuff: play a sport, act in the school play, volunteer with a community group.
- **Feed your spirit.** You can live without movies that glamorize drugs, drinking, violence, etc. Try plugging into a more beautiful reality: the natural world, great music, fabulous old movies, good books, or whatever makes you feel better about the world. To some extent, it's true: You "are" what you eat, see, hear, and think about.

Sound corny? Well, look around. If you look hard at the kids in your school who seem to have friends, do pretty well in school, get along with teachers and families—and who **don't** do drugs—you're likely to find them using most or all of these prevention techniques. They can help you, too.

TEENS

Heroin High

It wasn't just 'bad kids.' Cheerleaders, football players and preppies in Plano, Texas, were using heroin—and dying. Inside a three-year drug war.

By T. Trent Gegax and
Sarah Van Boven

DEBBIE MARSTEN CAN TELL YOU exactly how her son became a statistic. On Nov. 12, 1998, she and her husband, Todd, bailed 18-year-old Tyler out of a Plano, Texas, jail after an arrest for heroin possession. The family had tried rehab and they'd tried kicking Tyler out of the house, but after two years of addiction they were out of ideas. So they brought him home. Tyler knew he had missed a lot of schoolwork during his three days in jail, but he didn't realize that his body's tolerance to heroin had dipped. When the goateed senior went to school the next day to pick up some homework, he also picked up a lethal dose of the drug. When he went to bed that night he seemed happy to be home, telling Todd, "Good night, Dad, I love you. My alarm is set." But it was Tyler's dog Skeeter that woke the family at 3 a.m., not an alarm clock. When the barking wouldn't stop, Debbie ran into her son's room. "He was cold. Gone," she remembers. "He wasn't even home 36 hours."

In the last three years, the affluent town of Plano has buried 19 young people because of heroin. The most recent casualty, Tyler Marsten, wasn't like some of the early ones, kids who didn't know what was actually inside the $10 "chiva" capsules they were buying, often from Mexican dealers. He knew he was snorting heroin, with a purity that ran as high as 35 percent. Nor were his parents in denial. Debbie used to cut out of the local papers pictures of kids who had OD'd and use them as a starting point for discussions about the dangers of drugs. But Tyler still died. When leaders of this manicured Dallas suburb realized in 1997 that Plano was in the middle of an epidemic and that not even the "good" kids were safe, they also attacked the problem head on. Elaborate undercover drug stings have led to dozens of arrests. But some kids there are still using

heroin. In recent years there's been a well-publicized national increase in heroin use among middle-class teens. Even in that context, though, Plano remains a mystery. Many of the town's 200,000 residents—the ER doctor, the undercover cop, the preppy 18-year-old who OD'd—can tell you how this tragedy happened. What they can't tell you is when, or if, it will ever be over.

> "If the drugs were becoming prevalent in the schools, then we had to be just as prevalent . . . We had to infiltrate."

"In the beginning I was so against it. I was raised in a real strong Christian home, and I'm strong-willed. But once you're around it every day it becomes pretty ordinary. Then you get curious, and you think it's not a big deal to do it one time." For "Lindsey," heroin stopped being ordinary in July 1996, when she woke up in the emergency room; the Sunday-school teacher and recent East Plano High grad was one of the city's first ODs. Heroin had come to Plano early that year. Though the local schools had their share of burnouts and stoners, they weren't the ones who discovered the drug first. Instead, it was a core group of wealth-

ier cool kids, preppies and jocks, who started sniffing and smoking the brown powder at parties. Older Plano kids, some of whom had gone on to nearby University of Texas at Dallas, threw the parties in their apartments or rented out motel rooms. By the end of the school year, plenty of other teens had taken up the drug, and it was common to hear both girls and guys whisper that they "had a Mexican"—a dealer who could be found at the gas station, or in a church parking lot. Tyler Marsten, for one, was introduced to heroin by his co-workers at a fast-food restaurant. But most of the future addicts were white, middle-class kids with plenty to lose. "Cheerleaders, the football players, the popular group, the pretty girls," Lindsey remembers. "Everyone was at least trying it."

Lindsey was released from the hospital into the custody of her angry parents on July 6. Later the same day, 17-year-old Jason Blair wasn't so lucky—he became one of three city kids who would die a heroin-related death in 1996. He'd thrown up after injecting heroin into his stomach, and he drowned after his friends dumped him in a Jacuzzi to clean him off. Despite those deaths, the city and its parents were still in "big-time denial," says Dr. Larry Alexander, attending physician at the Medical Center of Plano. The hospital saw an estimated 75 ODs between November 1996 and November 1997; under Texas law, administrators couldn't even report the specifics of overdoses to the police. Alexander recalls telling one father that his son had tested positive for opiates, only to have the man throw him up against the wall in the ER and shout, "You g—d—— liar—you don't know what you're talking about!" Even when the boy confessed he was sniffing heroin, Alexander says, the father replied, "No, son. You're just confused about what you're doing."

Matt Shaunfield, 22
Hoped to be a writer; died in Utah 1/2/96

Jason Blair, 17
Altar boy and Boy Scout; died 6/7/96

Victor Garcia, 14
Loved soccer, his 10 siblings; died 4/97

Cathy Sharp, 17
Loved to read and travel; died 4/6/97

Milan Malina, 17
Clean two months before dying 6/8/97

Wes Scott, 19
UT philosophy student; died 6/24/97

Rob Hill, 18
Football player; OD'd 8/20/97

Chad Welsh, 18
Went to a private school; died 10/7/97

Erin Baker, 16
Died at a college party, 11/7/97

Tacha Campbell, 17
The high-school dropout died 2/9/98

Jay Aguanno, 19
Went through rehab twice; died 7/7/98

Tyler Marsten, 18
Had ADD and an IQ of 147; died 11/14/98

By early 1997, A. D. Paul, a burly police sergeant in charge of the city's undercover squad, had become all too familiar with the heroin horror stories: The seventh-grade soccer player whose friends dumped his stiffening body in a church parking lot. The member of the girls' varsity swim team caught trading sex for heroin. The clean-cut young marine home on leave just long enough to OD. Sergeant Paul began speaking at schools, at community groups, even at ladies' coffee klatsches about heroin—"community policing at its rawest," as he remembers it. Sometimes Alexander would go along, delivering a speech on how it feels to die of a heroin overdose so graphic that students would burst into tears or even faint. But Sergeant Paul knew that even as his officers were busting street-corner dealers, a more dramatic step was needed. He got Police Chief Bruce Glasscock to fund a $14,000 undercover sting at Plano East and Plano Senior Highs. Code name: Operation Rockfest.

But Rockfest would take months, and by May 1997, three more Plano teens were dead. The time had come to confront the crisis, so Glasscock, Mayor John Longstreet and state Sen. Florence Shapiro made a brave—and desperate—decision. "I said, 'We're going to significantly increase media presence and take a marketing approach to educating the community'," remembers Glasscock. The task force had decided to voluntarily brand Plano as Heroin City, USA. As the city implemented high-profile drug-prevention programs in the schools and advised parents to search their children's rooms for drugs, the TV news trucks started rolling into town. "The initial negative publicity may have been painful," Longstreet maintains, "but in the long run it was going to save lives." The community campaign reached its climax in November 1997, when more than 1,800 people showed up at a city-wide meeting to mourn their dead and talk about the future. The silence, at least, was over.

The teenagers crying in the audience that November night didn't know that Sergeant Paul's hand-chosen narc was already in their midst. Ashley Lomen (not her real name), 28, was fresh-faced and fresh from the police academy. In the late summer, she had gone "deep undercover," telling everyone but her mother that she had given up police work, and "enrolled" at Plano Senior High. She started wearing an eight-ball necklace and baggy pants, streaking her flowing red hair blond and rarely washing it (which, coupled with heavy makeup, caused some authentically teenage acne). Adopting the persona of a troubled, artistic loner, Ashley sat sullenly at her desk drawing endless psychedelic doodles and made sure her pack of Marlboros was visible peeking out of her purse. Her most precarious moment came when a sociology teacher used an unnervingly accurate analogy for why control groups were necessary in experiments: "She said, 'For example, sometimes the police department will put an undercover officer in the school'," Lomen remembers. " 'What if the police first came up in front of you and said, "Students, I'd like you to meet your undercover cop, Ashley"? You'd change the way you acted in front of her'." None of the heroin-using crowd she had finally infiltrated took the teacher's unwitting advice.

While the November 1997 town meeting had had an immediate effect—just one death in the first three months of 1998 and a sharp increase in kids enrolling in rehab—the undercover officer still had no problem buying heroin. Lomen was scoring chiva, even "freaking out" when a dealer cheated. Halfway through the year she got herself transferred to Plano East, where she kept writing down the names of dealers and users on the soles of her shoes after each transaction. Then, in March of last year—when the Plano death toll stood at 16—the squad cars pulled up at the high schools. Rockfest was a success: in total, 19 students and 19 adults were arrested, including members of the area's largest heroin ring. A more conventional bust in July 1998 netted 29 more suspected dealers. When 16 defendants go before federal court on Feb. 2, prosecutors will ask that the judge consider tacking 15 years onto any eventual sentence, under a little-used law that says dealers can be penalized if a fatal dose can be linked to their drug supply. Senator Shapiro has also sponsored four drug-abuse-prevention bills, one of which would allow hospitals to report ODs to a state agency so epidemics can be identified more quickly.

After three years, heroin is slowly, slowly loosening its grip on Plano, Texas. Will Tyler Marsten be the last casualty? Many of the remaining dealers have moved on to other suburbs. "We displaced the problem, we didn't solve it," admits Chief Glasscock. Maybe kids like Tyler have picked up some of the junkie's street savvy and now know better than to let their friends "sleep off" a potentially fatal OD. But after all the police work and community organization, the real reason drug use is beginning to taper off is depressingly simple. Standing in the parking lot of Plano Senior on a cold January day, spiky-haired softball player Kris Kidwell, 17, tosses off the answer as if it's the most obvious thing in the world: "Nearly everyone knows somebody that's died."

HEROIN AND COCAINE — A GLOBAL THREAT

The huge quantities of heroin and cocaine that are currently being trafficked around the world have resulted in a growing global addiction problem. This has especially affected the developed countries of Western Europe, North America and Australasia, where most of these drugs are consumed. It has, however, also impacted on producer and transit countries, many of which have suffered substantial rises in recent years. The threat posed by global trade in heroin and cocaine covers at least four dimensions.

The criminal threat

First, and most visibly, it contributes to growing social instability by fuelling high rates of crime. This emanates both from users struggling to finance their habit as well as traffickers and distributors striving to gain control of a greater share of the narcotics market. Drug-related arrests in the Chinese province of Guandong have increased nearly 50 times on account of the Southeast Asian heroin trade. It has been estimated that 80 per cent of all crime committed in the southern Chinese provinces are committed by heroin addicts. Figures in the Czech Republic are even more dramatic. In 1997, the country's main anti-drug squad, the Nardoni Proti-Drogovy Central (NPDC), reported a staggering 300 per cent increase in drug-related crime, with street-level violence linked to the heroin trade becoming virtually a daily occurrence in Prague.

In the USA, cocaine and crack sales fuel much of the country's drug violence as gangs compete for lucrative sales territory and addicts steal to feed their habit. In early 1993, a wave of violence exploded over Colombia as a result of inter-factional fighting within the Medellin cartel between Pablo Escobar and a rival group, Pepes. In one month, Pepes killed over 20 Escobar loyalists and carried out 11 dynamite attacks, causing approximately US$8 million worth of damage to properties.

The period since 1990 has seen Russia literally torn apart by a series of highly destabilising drug turf wars, with most bloodletting connected to the attempts by the Mafiya to eliminate new threats from the bespredel'chiki, a younger, newer generation of narcotics criminals. In Australia, it has been estimated that more than A$312 million is raised each year by heroin users and dealers engaging in various forms of property crime, while in 1994, over 2,000 Albanians were being held in Swiss jails on heroin-related offences.

Virtually all countries that have been assailed by cocaine and heroin use in recent years have suffered from similar patterns of endemic crime and violence. In certain inner city ghettos such as those of Peru, Brazil and Mexico, the problem has become so great that any notion of civil society has largely disappeared. As John McFarlane, Special Advisor for the Australian Federal Police (AFP) Office of the Deputy Commissioner, observes, in these instances crime is not only seen as the fast track to success; it is often regarded as the only path to survival. The ensuing instability encourages yet more crime, thus perpetuating the problem.

The medical threat

Heroin use is helping to foster the spread of one of the most lethal diseases of our time, AIDS. This has been particularly evident in Southeast Asia as a result of the intravenous injection of heroin. According to the Office of Narcotics Control Board (ONCB) in Bangkok, Thailand currently has to administer at least 50,000 confirmed heroin addicts, the majority of whom are also HIV positive as a result of sharing needles. Similarly Burma, which was free of AIDS only a few years ago, now has an estimated 200,000 people carrying the HIV virus, 74 per cent of whom are

Reprinted from *Jane's Intelligence Review*, June 1, 1998, p. 14. © 1998 by Jane's Information Group, Ltd.

tested heroin drug users. China (PRC) has been especially hard hit. The Beijing government officially admits that the outbreak of an AIDS epidemic is directly related to drug addicts sharing needles to inject heroin. Ruili, a small border town in Yunnan with one of the highest concentrations of opium addicts in the province, is now in the unenviable position of also being the AIDS capital of China.

The economic threat

The costs associated with trying to control the global cocaine and heroin trade are contributing to a lack of economic performance in source, transit and consumer states. As production and trafficking of these narcotics increase, so more and more resources have to be diverted to treat addicts through detoxification, health and rehabilitation programs, as well as to finance the clinics to treat those afflicted with AIDS on account of their habit. Moreover, the violence, crime and organized illicit activities that have come to surround heroin and cocaine addiction and especially trafficking mean that public resources also have to be channelled into law enforcement, further reducing the availability of funds to stimulate economic productivity.

The true extent of the finances needed to control the drug trade is well exemplified by the USA. In February 1998, President Clinton allocated almost US$16 billion to fund the country's anti-drug effort. Over the last 10 years, the US government has spent, at the federal level, US$110 billion to fight drugs. If one includes monies allocated by state and local governments in addition to out-of-pocket efforts by businesses, communities, schools and private individuals, the total rises to a staggering US$500 billion. Yet this sum does not include the indirect costs of drug use measured in terms of human suffering, increased violence and lost lives. Every year, the US anti-drug effort consumes the overwhelming majority of federal state funds as well as the resources allocated by state, local and private groups. On average, this amounts to more than US$30 billion annually. 1998 looks as though it will be every bit as costly, at least at the US government level.

The democratic threat

Drug money from the illicit trade in cocaine and heroin is playing a key role in weakening and undermining already weak and vulnerable regimes by encouraging involvement by government and military circles. The profit margins involved in the sale of illicit narcotics are truly colossal, and all the more so because they are untaxed. The wholesale price for one kilogram of heroin in Thailand, for instance, is estimated to be US$3,400–US$5,600. It is believed that the same kilogram would cost a British wholesaler up to US$51,000, with the price rising to US$250,000 in the USA. The current cost of a single hit of heroin (less than 1 gram) in London is around Pds10, while the street price for a whole kilogram sold in New York is well over 14 times the purchase price in Yunnan. The potential profits from the cocaine trade are just as dramatic. As the US State Department observes:

"Assuming an average retail price street price of US$100 dollars per gram, a metric ton of pure cocaine has a retail value of US$100 million on the streets of a US city, and two or three times as much if the drug is cut with adulterants. By this measure, the 100 or so metric tons of cocaine that the US government typically seizes each year are theoretically worth as much as US$10 billion to the drug trade, more than the gross domestic product of many countries."

Russia, Mexico, Colombia, Thailand and Italy all provide examples of states where the problem of drug-induced corruption has been especially serious. In Russia, none of the country's main institutions have escaped allegations of links with the Mafiya, including the prime minister's office, the civil service, armed forces, big business, regional authorities and the Duma. The downfall of the former government of Carlos Salinas de Gortari in Mexico was brought about mainly by revelations concerning his administration's links with various cocaine drug lords. In 1996, 43 high-ranking officials in Colombia were detained in a series of narcotics-related investigations, including members of President Samper's Cabinet (Samper, himself, was exonerated of corruption charges by the Colombian Congress); an additional 2,000 policemen suspected of corruption were removed from their positions. In Thailand, numerous members of parliament, including Vatana Asavaname, a former deputy interior minister and deputy leader of Chart Thai, and Narong Wongwan, leader of the prominent Justice and Unity Party, have been fingered by the US government for their involvement in the Golden Triangle's drug trade. In Italy, over 3,000 executives, politicians and government personnel were implicated in a pervasive corruption network that was revealed as part of a major crackdown against the Sicilian Mafia between 1992 and 1993.

The drinking dilemma

By calling abstinence the only cure, we ensure that the nation's $100 billion alcohol problem won't be solved

BY NANCY SHUTE

"Would you like something to drink?" the waitress asks Elisa DeCarlo as she plops into a chair in an Asian restaurant on Manhattan's Upper West Side. DeCarlo, a 37-year-old actress, would *love* something to drink. She has just finished a performance of her one-woman show at an off-off-Broadway theater. Only a dozen people showed up, and they laughed in the wrong places. After a show, when she is thirsty and wound up, is the time she loves a drink most.

"Nothing at the moment, thank you," DeCarlo says, reaching for a water glass and draining it. She drinks two more glasses of water and waits for the food to arrive before ordering a good French pinot blanc. By the end of the night, she's had three glasses of wine; more than her usual two, but still within the limits of Moderation Management, the controlled-drinking self-help program she has followed for the past 16 months. A self-described problem drinker who used to pound down so much booze after a show she felt lousy the next morning, she had checked out Alcoholics Anonymous but was put off by the group's famous first step: "We admitted we were powerless over alcohol—that our lives had become unmanageable."

"If you choose to overdrink, you choose to overdrink and you know it," DeCarlo says. She was happily married; she had published two novels; she toured nationally. She didn't feel that her life was unmanageable, just that alcohol was taking up too much of it. Following Moderation Management guidelines, she quit drinking for 30 days and now takes no more than nine drinks a week, no more than three a day, and *never* drinks and drives. (The guideline's limit for men is 14 drinks a week, four on any given day.) "It's a really nice feeling to know I can have a drink and stop and feel fine the next day," she says. "It's made a tremendous difference. My life is too interesting to mess it up with a drinking problem."

DeCarlo's strategy is, depending on how you look at it, either the best hope for problem drinking in America or the most threatening form of self-delusion. She and other imbibers experimenting with controlled-drinking programs around the country have innocently stumbled into the most hotly contested issue in alcohol treatment: whether cutting back, as opposed to total abstinence, is an option for some people who drink too much.

Narrow path. There are 40 million problem drinkers in the United States—people whose drinking causes economic, physical, or family harm but who are not technically alcoholic (defined as being physiologically dependent on alcohol). But for the past six decades, beginning shortly after Prohibition was repealed in 1933, treatment for drinking problems in this country has focused almost exclusively on alcoholics, has offered abstinence as the sole cure for their problems, and has laid just two paths to that cure: Alcoholics Anonymous, the spiritual self-help group founded in 1935; and a variety of related 12-step programs, originally developed at the Hazelden Foundation and other Minnesota clinics in the 1950s, which combine psychological and peer counseling and AA attendance. (AA is the granddaddy of 12-step programs, but the two approaches are not synonymous. AA is a self-help group aimed at sobriety and spiritual renewal; 12-step alcohol-treatment programs adopt some of AA's tenets but include a wide array of secular treatments, from psychotherapy to acupuncture.)

A *U.S. News* reporter, querying a dozen treatment centers about her options as someone concerned about her drinking, was offered only abstinence-based programs. The Mayo Clinic told her she was welcome to try cutting back on her own and then to come back if she failed. At the Betty Ford Center, a kindly woman answering the phone said, "For people like us, one drink always leads to another. You may be functional now, but it's progressive."

The problem with that advice is that for many people it's not true. For at least the past decade, researchers have known that the majority of people who drink heavily don't become alcoholics; some experts place that number as high as 75 percent. Other drinkers may meet the clinical criteria for alcohol dependence but can sustain controlled drinking for months, even years, before getting into trouble. And the majority of people who cut back or quit drinking do so on their own. Many of those people binge drank in their 20s at college parties, at after-work happy hours, or during Sunday afternoon football games, then got a good job, got married, got busy, and lost interest in getting smashed. In the researchers' lingo, they "matured out."

Moreover, alcoholism cannot be blamed for the majority of social ills linked to drinking in this country. Misuse of alcohol costs the nation dearly—$100 billion a year in quantifiable costs, in addition to untold emotional pain. Yet the bulk of these costs are incurred not by alcoholics but by problem drinkers,

From *U.S. News & World Report*, September 8, 1997, pp. 54-65. © 1997 by U.S. News & World Report. Reprinted by permission.

Is moderation the best hope for problem drinkers or the most threatening form of self-delusion?

who are four times more numerous than alcoholics, are more active in society, and usually reject abstinence as a solution. Alcohol figures in 41 percent of traffic crash fatalities and is a factor in 50 percent of homicides, 30 percent of suicides, and 30 percent of accidental deaths. (Last week, a 20-year-old Louisiana State University student drank himself to death during fraternity pledge week; three other students were hospitalized.) Heavy drinking also increases the risk of cancer, heart disease, and stroke, long before people have to worry about cirrhosis of the liver, brain damage, or other skid-row ailments. A 1990 report by the Institute of Medicine, an arm of the National Academy of Sciences, concluded that the harmful consequences of alcohol could not be reduced significantly unless more options were offered to people with only "mild to moderate" alcohol problems.

Threats and firings. Public-health experts recognized the social costs of alcohol abuse long ago and have responded with programs such as free soft drinks for designated drivers and free taxi rides home on New Year's Eve. But because of deeply held beliefs in the American alcohol-treatment community, this kind of pragmatic, public-health-centered approach has rarely been applied to individuals with drinking problems. Europe, Great Britain, and Australia long ago defined problem drinking as a public-health concern and have established controlled-drinking programs to reduce its physical harm and social costs. Forty-three percent of Canadian treatment programs deem moderate drinking acceptable for some clients.

But in the United States, researchers and counselors who have championed— or even tried to investigate—moderation as a treatment strategy have been threatened, sometimes fired. "We've been accused of murder. That we're all in denial. That we're enablers," says Alan Marlatt, a professor of psychology and moderate-drinking proponent who is director of the University of Washington's Addictive Behaviors Research Center.

A big part of the problem is that it's hard to draw a clear line between alcohol dependency and problem drinking.

According to a 1996 report by the University of Connecticut's Alcohol Research Center, 20 percent of American adults are problem drinkers, compared with 5 percent who are alcohol dependent. The National Institute on Alcohol Abuse and Alcoholism, using much stricter criteria, puts the numbers at 3 percent alcohol abusers, 1.7 percent alcohol dependents, and 2.7 percent drinkers who exhibit characteristics of both. (Discrepancies in alcohol statistics abound.)

Briefly put, problem drinkers are people who have had problems because of drinking (a DUI arrest, marital discord, showing up late to work). But they usually don't drink steadily and don't go through withdrawal when they stop. By contrast, someone who is alcohol dependent (the medically preferred term for alcoholic) exhibits at least three of the following symptoms: tolerance; withdrawal; an inability to cut down; sacrificing work, family, or social events to drink; devoting a lot of time to finding and consuming alcohol; or persistence in drinking despite related health problems.

Even so, the distinctions leave plenty of diagnostic wiggle room. The medical- and alcohol-treatment communities in the United States have dealt with this ambiguity by applying to all drinkers the advice appropriate for the most severely afflicted: abstinence. Any other strategy, they feel, is too risky. "Every alcoholic would like to drink moderately," says Douglas Talbott, a physician and president of the American Society of Addiction Medicine. "Ninety percent have tried. This just feeds into the denial of the alcoholic."

Moderate-drinking proponents concede that some alcoholics will seize upon controlled drinking as an excuse to avoid abstinence. But they say that they explicitly warn that the strategy is not for alcoholics, only for people with less severe drinking problems; that tests (box, "Should you worry?") can evaluate the intensity of difficulties; and that they regularly refer dependent drinkers to AA. Controlled drinking, says Marc Kern, a Los Angeles psychologist, can "reduce harm by reducing alcohol consumption" and can propel people who fail at moderation into abstinence.

Medical or moral? America's ambivalence toward alcohol is long standing. In the early days of the republic, we were a nation of lushes. Per capital consumption of alcohol was three times today's. The first temperance effort, led by Philadelphia physician Benjamin Rush in the 1780s, prescribed moderation: Rush urged people to switch from rum and gin to the more salubrious beer and wine.

Temperance soon moved from the doctor's office to the church. In 1826, the Rev. Lyman Beecher galvanized the movement with his *Six Sermons on Intemperance,* which held that alcohol was a poison and that abstinence was the only answer. "This is the way to death!" Beecher said of the drinking life. Ever since, the nature of alcohol abuse has been debated, the arguments often mixing the medical and the moral. Is it a bad habit, a matter of will, or a disease?

The medical model that has dominated alcohol treatment for more than a half century holds that alcohol dependence is an ailment with biological and genetic roots. Recent research suggests there is a genetic predisposition toward alcoholism; identical twins, for instance, are more apt to share a drinking problem than fraternal twins, and adopted children whose birth parents were alcoholics are four times likelier than children adopted from nonalcoholic homes to become alcohol dependent. This disease approach is challenged by behaviorists, the primary advocates of controlled drinking, who say alcohol abuse is a behavior influenced by psychological, cultural, and environmental forces, not just physiology.

Science has yet to come up with enough information to resolve the disease vs. behavior argument. Odds are that alcohol abuse will prove to be a combination of both, the behavioral factors dominating in problem drinkers and biological factors weighing more heavily in people who are physically addicted. But in the meantime, the disease and behavior camps have been warring as if the evidence were absolute. A 1976 Rand report saying that a very small number of alcoholics successfully mod-

Europe, Britain, and Australia long ago adopted moderate-drinking programs to reduce alcohol's harm.

erate their drinking was fiercely attacked. "It was like desecrating the altar," says Frederick Glaser, a psychiatrist at East Carolina University School of Medicine in Greenville, N.C., who was a researcher at the time. Mark and Linda Sobell, two psychologists who in the 1970s published similar findings, were accused of faking their results and were hauled up before a congressional committee. The Sobells were later vindicated.

Just say whoa! Though most people in the mainstream treatment community hold tightly to the disease concept of alcoholism, the treatment they offer is based on a combination of folklore and personal experience rather than on science. As Robin Room, a Canadian sociologist who is critical of American alcohol treatment, asks: "What kind of field is it that claims [alcoholism is] a disease, but the treatment is nonmedical?" Enoch Gordis, director of the NIAAA, wrote in 1987 of the nation's $3.8 billion alcohol-treatment effort: "In the case of alcoholism, our whole treatment system . . . is founded on hunch, not evidence, and not on science."

A decade later, quality still varies widely, and anyone seeking solid data on what treatments work best is justified in feeling confused. In a comprehensive 1995 review of the effectiveness of treatment programs, New Mexico psychologists Reid Hester and William Miller concluded that, even for people with severe drinking problems, behavioral treatments (such as brief interventions, contracts governing drinkers' conduct, and coping-skills training) worked significantly better than the fare routinely offered by 12-step programs: group psychotherapy, educational lecturers, confrontational counseling, and referral to AA. The gap between those treatments shown to be effective and those that are widely used, they found, "could hardly be larger if one intentionally constructed treatment programs from those approaches with the *least* evidence of efficacy." But the researchers cautioned that their analysis was a "first approximation," because the quality of the studies surveyed was uneven.

Not for everyone. Analyzing the effectiveness of Alcoholics Anonymous is even more difficult because of the nature of the organization. The self-help group keeps no membership records and does not participate in research. "We're not treatment," says Valerie O., an AA member who answered the phone in the group's New York office. "We just sit there and tell our stories to anyone who asks." Only three trials of AA's effectiveness have been performed, and all three used drunk drivers and others forced to attend the program, which violates the group's creed of voluntary membership. None of these trials rated AA as more effective than alternatives. In a 1990 survey, 65 percent of AA members said they had been sober for a year or more; the survey also found that the majority of people who start AA drop out within a year. When AA works, it works extraordinarily well: The testimonies of lives saved by AA are legion. But it's not for everyone.

Because alcohol treatment is so unscientific, some of the most basic and effective standards of care are ignored. Instead of adhering to the stepped-care protocol employed in other areas of medicine—where the least invasive treatment is used first—alcohol treatment starts with its most drastic remedy: lifetime abstinence, meetings, and, until recently, a 28-day residential stay in a substance-abuse clinic. As a result, many people who need help don't seek it. Others try AA but feel it doesn't meet their needs.

That's what happened to Moderation Management founder Audrey Kishline. In her 20s, she was drinking five or six glasses of wine a night, drinking alone, drinking and driving. Diagnosed as an alcoholic, she was sent to detoxification, to residential treatment, and to AA. But Kishline didn't feel she had been alcohol dependent: She had no withdrawal symptoms, and she found it easy to abstain for months. She started researching alcohol treatment, and was outraged to find that alternatives common in Europe were never even mentioned here. "The public's not getting the full story," Kishline says. Now 40, married and raising two children, she occasionally has a glass of wine with dinner. Had she initially been offered less drastic treatment, Kishline believes, she would have

reached this point of temperance years sooner.

Other veterans of the treatment system object to AA's explicitly spiritual focus, a reliance on God or a "higher power" that permeates many 12-step programs as well. Last year, the New York State Court of Appeals ruled the prisoners are constitutionally protected from being forced to participate in AA because of its religious orientation. Similar rulings have been made in California and other states. And several abstinence-based self-help groups, including Rational Recovery, Secular Organizations for Sobriety, and SMART Recovery Self-Help Network, have been founded by people critical either of AA's spiritual focus or of the belief that they are powerless against alcohol.

Changing times. Gradually, however, the alcohol-treatment portfolio is diversifying. After expanding wildly in the 1970s and 1980s, residential 12-step programs are falling on hard times: Insurers and employers, pressed by rising health care costs, find little benefit to justify the programs' considerable expense and are seeking cheaper, less intensive alternatives. Alcohol-treatment research is moving slowly toward a more scientific, empirically based approach. And a national trend away from heavy drinking—alcohol consumption has fallen by 15 percent since 1980, paralleling declines in smoking and illegal drug use—makes it, oddly enough, more acceptable to treat those with only mild alcohol problems, not just *Days of Wine and Roses*-style lushes.

Wisconsin offers a sense of what the future may hold. It is a big drinking state; 25 percent of its residents say they binge drink. "Every little town has a church and a bar," says Michael Fleming, a University of Wisconsin Medical School family physician. "Most of the patients in my practice drinking six drinks a day are not alcoholics. But if we can get them to cut down from six drinks to two, from a public-health perspective you've made a huge impact."

In April, Fleming published the first large U.S. study of brief interventions for problem drinkers in the *Journal of the American Medical Association*. The study, patterned on research over the

Telling drinkers they can cut back "just feeds into the denial of the alcoholic," says Dr. Douglas Talbott.

past 20 years in Great Britain and Sweden, selected 774 problem drinkers from patients at 17 Wisconsin clinics. Half the patients met for two 15-minute sessions, one month apart, with their physicians, discussed their current health behavior and the effects of alcohol, and signed a prescription-like drinking contract. A year later, the men had reduced their alcohol use by 14 percent; the women, by 30 percent. (Women are usu-

ally more successful than men at moderating.) The control group also reduced its drinking, but the brief intervention group was twice as likely to reduce it by 20 percent or more.

Other promising research is coming from Seattle, where University of Washington psychologist Marlatt is working with a notoriously immoderate population—college students. For the past seven years, he has followed 350 stu-

dents who were identified while still in high school as high-risk drinkers. A year after half the students were given a one-hour, one-on-one educational session in their freshman year, 80 percent had reduced binge drinking substantially. Those who didn't were given more education and counseling, with the intensity escalating each year. "It's a harm-reduction approach," Marlatt says, using a phrase more often applied to needle ex-

---

Should you worry? *No questionnaire can tell you for sure if you're a problem drinker. But many alcohol-abuse experts use the following test.*

	0	1	2	3	4	Total
1. How often do you have a drink containing alcohol? (one drink is a beer, glass of wine, or mixed drink)	Never	Monthly or less	2–4 times a month	2–3 times a week	4 or more times a week	
2. How many drinks containing alcohol do you have on a typical day when you are drinking?	1 or 2	3 or 4	5 or 6	7 to 9	10 or more	
3. How often do you have six or more drinks on one occasion?	Never	Less than monthly	Monthly	Weekly	Daily or almost daily	
4. How often during the past year have you been unable to stop drinking once you started?	Never	Less than monthly	Monthly	Weekly	Daily or almost daily	
5. How often during the past year have you failed to do what was normally expected of you because of drinking?	Never	Less than monthly	Monthly	Weekly	Daily or almost daily	
6. How often during the past year have you needed a drink in the morning to get going after a heavy drinking session?	Never	Less than monthly	Monthly	Weekly	Daily or almost daily	
7. How often during the past year have you had a feeling of guilt or remorse after drinking?	Never	Less than monthly	Monthly	Weekly	Daily or almost daily	
8. How often during the past year have you been unable to remember what happened the night before because of drinking?	Never	Less than monthly	Monthly	Weekly	Daily or almost daily	
9. Have you or someone else been injured as a result of your drinking?	No		Yes, but not in the past year		Yes. During the past year	
10. Has a relative, friend, doctor, or other health worker been concerned about your drinking or suggested you cut down?	No		Yes, but not in the past year		Yes. During the past year	

Scoring: *A total score of 8–15 may indicate a problem with alcohol use. You may want to ask your physician about cutting down or becoming abstinent. A total score of 16 or more suggests a more serious problem. You should contact your physician or an alcohol-treatment program for help.* **TOTAL**

Source: Alcohol Use Disorder Inventory Test, World Health Organization, 1987

Getting problem drinkers to cut down from six drinks to two, says Dr. Michael Fleming, has "a huge impact."

changes and other drug-abuse programs. "With young people, if you only offer abstinence, they're not going to sign up."

Another brief intervention program, offered to adults by the University of Michigan Medical Center's DrinkWise program, is patterned on one developed at Toronto's Addiction Research Foundation. DrinkWise offers four one-hour educational counseling sessions, in person or by phone, with three- and nine-month follow-up calls, for $495. East Carolina University will launch its own DrinkWise program later this year.

Many people enter alcohol treatment not by choice but by court order for drunk driving and other offenses. They, too, are beginning to gain a few more options. Last year California ruled that Los Angeles County does not have to require offenders to attend an abstinence-based self-help group, making room for Moderation Management as a legal alternative to AA.

Cutting back

■ *These organizations and people offer help to those who want to reduce their drinking.*

■ **DrinkWise.** Brief intervention in person or by phone. At the University of Michigan Medical Center, 800-222-5145; www.med.umich.edu/drinkwise. At East Carolina University Medical School, 888-816-2736; E-mail: teonon@brody.med.ecu.edu

■ **Moderation Management.** Self-help group with meetings, an Internet discussion group, and Audrey Kishline's book, Moderate Drinking (Crown, $14): 612-512-1484; com-net.org/mm/

■ **Counselors.** New Mexico psychologist Reid Hester's Web page (www.lobo.net/~rhester/software.htm) lists behavioral counselors and links to other resources.

But these groups are still gnats compared to the elephant of AA. Moderation Management has just 50 volunteer-run groups; AA has an estimated 1.2 million members in the nation. Only 8 to 10 people show up for the weekly Manhattan meeting of MM, which Elisa DeCarlo runs. "We're like booze revolutionaries," she says cheerfully.

There's reason to hope today's revolutionaries will get a more open hearing than their predecessors: The NIAAA, along with other federal agencies, is increasing funding for different alcohol treatments. Someday, perhaps, controlled-drinking programs will be as commonplace as Weight Watchers and Smokenders, and problem drinking will be recognized as a $100 billion public-health problem requiring solutions as varied and complex as our long, tempestuous relationship with alcohol.

With Laura Tangley

Generation Wired

Caffeine Is the New Drug of Choice for Kids

by HELEN CORDES

Anyone remember when caffeine was off-limits for children? ("It'll stunt your growth!") These days constraints on caffeine consumption for kids and young teens are nonexistent. Kids are having caffeine early and often—high-octane Mountain Dew is the preferred soda of the under-6 set—and in much bigger doses than before. Caffeine Inc. is raking it in, often targeting teens and younger kids, and while Coca-Cola's polar bears get the attention, studies showing the negative consequences of child caffeination are virtually ignored.

Look at fast-food joints, convenience stores and restaurants, where many kids get up to 40 percent of their meals. It's common to see young children and teens downing "big gulp"-size caffeinated sodas or lining up for seconds and thirds at refillable soda stations. These megadrinks can pack a wallop equal to three cups of strong coffee—all bombarding a body that may be one-half or two-thirds adult size. And kids are eagerly reaching for the aggressively marketed new drinks that are at or near the legal limit for added caffeine (which is 6 milligrams per ounce) such as Coca-Cola's Surge (51 milligrams in twelve ounces), Pepsi-Cola's Josta (58), Jolt (72), the caffeinated herbal drink XTC (70) and others. And kids may get a near double-dose of caffeine if they buy these juiced-up drinks at vending machines, which increasingly offer only twenty-ounce bottles instead of twelve-ounce cans.

Check out school cafeterias—kids are bypassing milk for cans of Coke (45 milligrams), Pepsi (37), Mountain Dew (55) and Sunkist (40), bought at school pop machines or served at the fast-food franchises now at 13 percent of the nation's schools. Glance at family shopping carts: Sodas are the best-selling product at grocery stores—$11.7 billion annually in sales. And four of the five most popular soft drinks in the United States are caffeinated, with number-four Sprite the sole exception.

The most conservative estimates have children and teens guzzling more than sixty-four gallons of soda a year—an amount that has tripled for teens since 1978, doubled for the 6–11 set and increased by a quarter for under-5 tots, according to a 1994 survey by the Agriculture Department. The top drinkers, teen boys, pop open an average of three sodas a day.

And check out the local coffee shop. For tons of teens, and kids as young as elementary school, the local Starbucks or its equivalent has become the favored hangout. Many juvenile customers scorn decaf in the sugary coffee drinks they prefer. (Twelve ounces of a regular Starbucks coffee contains around 190 milligrams of caffeine. Since coffee is naturally caffeinated—sodas have caffeine added to them—it is not regulated for caffeine content.) Caffeine is even showing up on the playing field: Competitive-minded parents are bringing along

Helen Cordes, a freelance writer, is a contributing editor of Utne Reader.

high-caffeine drinks or packets of the new carbo- and caffeine-packed "sports goo" to help give their young athletes a winner's edge.

Why is "Generation Next" (as Pepsi puts it) downing caffeine at rates never seen before'? One likely reason is that most parents are unaware of the health problems associated with caffeine. Solid scientific research has linked caffeine to anxiety, respiratory ailments, possible bone loss and other health worries—although there has been slight coverage of this. But what turned children on to caffeine in the first place? Kids' desire to get wired didn't simply occur as a mass switch in personal preference. The major caffeine suppliers to kids have been throwing millions into advertising and giveaways. Mountain Dew, for example, has distributed half a million free pagers to kids, who can use them to call friends—but only after they read the Mountain Dew promo that automatically pops up.

The soft-drink companies have also spent tens of millions placing their products and ads where youths are a captive audience: schools. Dozens of school districts have been paid up to $11 million each by Coke or Pepsi for the assurance that only that company's products will be sold on school grounds, and for the right to put ads on gym walls and school buses.

The caffeine lobby has apparently borrowed tactics from the nicotine gang, complete with scientists who say there is no cause for concern.

And the soda barons have used dozens of other sly marketing ploys, such as plastering ads and logos on everything from free textbook covers to computer screensavers and mousepads. Children have few places left to look where they are not exposed to a soft-drink product or logo.

The marketing strategy behind the new high-caffeine products is ingeniously suited to a generation confronting more family instability and a less secure job future, and dogged by stress and powerlessness. The names are pulsing with power: Surge, Zapped, Full Speed, Outburst. Josta, laced with both caffeine and the pick-me-up herb guarana, hypes its "raw, primal power." Mountain Dew promises there's "nothing more intense than slammin' a Dew." Caffeine, then, is the perfect antidote for youths facing the pressures of the nineties: It provides a boost of sociability, enhanced performance and energy. Sure, there's the inevitable droop that follows, but that only reinforces the need to . . . have more.

As for kids' rising attraction to coffee, that may be fueled by the proliferation of coffee shops—Starbucks opens another one every business day—and the perennial desire of kids to ape grown-up behavior. "Coffee bars are the only legal places for kids to hang out," says Gerald Celente, author of *Trends 2000*. Direct youth advertising by coffee interests is minimal, but the coffee industry is busy courting younger drinkers, who "love coffee products that are cold and sweet," notes Ted Lingle, executive director of the Specialty Coffee Association of America.

Plenty of coffee parlors are expanding their sweet-drink menus. Starbucks, in partnership with Pepsi, is pushing its bottled creamy coffee drink Frappuccino and test-marketing Power Frappuccino, its coffee and carbo drink aimed at the hot youth-directed "energy drink" category.

All the major caffeine suppliers Insist they're not targeting the under-12 set. "Our core market is the teen and young adult category," says Pepsi spokesman Larry Jabblonsky. "We don't make a concerted effort to reach those under 12." And Chris Gimbl of Starbucks says, "We don't market to teenagers. However, anyone is welcome at our stores." But Terry Barker, whose company makes the caffeinated water Krank$_2$O, notes, "The only market available is to start them out younger and younger." (He hastens to add that Krank$_2$O markets to those 15 and older.)

Barker's remark reflects economic reality. For the market bulge of the century—baby boomers—caffeine is becoming something to avoid. Coffee drinking is on the rise only for those between ages 15 and 24, while java jiving takes a steady dive thereafter. Ditto for soft-drink consumption: Statistics show that teens and young adults slug the most, with soda sipping sinking slowly from there. In Barker's view, caffeine suppliers are following the example of another supplier of an addictive substance: the tobacco companies. "The goal is to perpetuate the market," he says.

Indeed, there's evidence that the caffeine lobby has borrowed a tactic or two from the nicotine gang. Ask industry representatives about the health consequences of children consuming caffeine, and they frequently point to two "nonprofit research organizations"—the International Life Sciences Institute (I.L.S.I.) and the International Food Information Council. Both are funded by major food, beverage and agribusiness multinationals, including Coca-Cola, Pepsi-Cola and major coffee suppliers Kraft and Procter & Gamble. Both refer questions to scientists who maintain that there is absolutely no cause for concern about caffeine and kids.

"The studies are really quite reassuring," says Dr. Peter Dews, an I.L.S.I. board member and a Harvard School of Medicine professor emeritus. "Nothing has been shown to be harmful." Asked about a 6-year-old ingesting the quantum dose of caffeine in a "big gulp," Dr. Richard Adamson, vice president of scientific and technical affairs for the National Soft Drink Association, asserts, "People generally don't drink big gulps all in one sitting." (Kids ration their big gulps?) Asked why caffeine is necessary in sodas, he says, "It's there solely for the taste. Just take a sip of caffeine-free Pepsi and then a sip of regular Pepsi. Try it! You'll be able to tell!" (I did! I can't!) Asked if there is any health value to caffeinated soda, Adamson claims, "They're a good source of water. Kids need lots of water." Reminded that caffeine is a diuretic, which causes water to be excreted more rapidly, Adamson grudgingly agrees.

Despite soothing words from the industry, a few outfits are taking a stand against the rising use of caffeine by children. Last summer, when the Center for Science in the Public Interest petitioned the Food and Drug Administration to require the posting of caffeine amounts on labels, it cited several caffeine-related risks: miscarriage, osteoporosis, insomnia, anxiety, addiction. Children, the group noted, can suffer some of these adverse effects, and they face additional risks: Caffeine may threaten their developing bone mass and, when sodas are substituted for more nutritional food, impede their overall nutrition. (The F.D.A. was scheduled to respond by February but informed the C.S.P.I. it needed more time to investigate concerns and studies cited in the petition.) In 1997 the American Medical Association registered concerns about the new high-caffeine drinks that are "being aggressively advertised" to a youth audience and passed a resolution calling for caffeine labeling.

In perhaps the only public expression of concern from the industry, Havis Dawson, editor of the trade magazine *Beverage World*, called on the industry a year ago to "pronounce clear guidelines for how much caffeine our children should drink." Since then, he's received no response. "If the industry doesn't come up with guidelines," he says, "someone else who's more scared of caffeine could do it, and they might not be ones industry likes."

Guidelines may indeed be necessary. For years, independent scientific researchers have been urging caution. Their concerns fall into two categories: how children react behaviorally to the addictive and stimulant qualities of caffeine, and how caffeine affects children's bodies. Children respond to caffeine as do adults, according to a number of studies. A low dose may aid concentration and task completion, but higher doses typically make children nervous, anxious, fidgety, frustrated and quicker to anger. National Institute of Mental Health child psychiatry researcher Judith Rapoport found the 8-to-13-year-olds who regularly consumed high doses were judged more restless by teachers—in fact, one-third were hyperactive enough to meet the criteria for attention deficit disorder with hyperactivity (ADHD). When low-caffeine-consuming children were given a daily dose equivalent to that of their higher-consuming peers, parents reported that they became more emotional, inattentive and restless. "Children for whom there is a concern about anxiety should not have caffeine," Rapoport says.

Hofstra University psychology associate professor Mitchell Schare studied almost 400 preschoolers from upper-income New York City suburbs in 1994 and 1995. The heavier caffeine consumers among the children, who had the equivalent of three to four cups of coffee daily, had more "uncontrollable energy," Schare notes. He concludes, "I believe the effects of caffeine can potentially mimic ADHD and be misdiagnosed as ADHD." These kids' chief caffeine source was, surprisingly, iced tea, which many parents may not realize contains caffeine.

Like adults, kids who are regular caffeine drinkers suffer ill effects when they don't get a regular shot. In a recent study by Stanford neurobiologist Avram Goldstein, fifth and sixth graders at a suburban Denver school deprived of daily caffeine reported having symptoms including trouble thinking clearly, not feeling energetic and getting angry. Even children who typically consume 28 milligrams a day (less than an average soda) felt symptoms. "Children can in fact become dependent on caffeine," notes Goldstein, who did pioneer research on caffeine and adults in the sixties. And caffeine-dependent children usually have a handicap adults don't: They can't guarantee a daily fix the way adults can, because they don't typically have the money and mobility to get caffeine at will. Johns Hopkins psychiatry professor and caffeine expert Roland Griffiths worries about this on-again, off-again situation. "A lot of kids already have chaotic lives. Do children need a pharmacological destabilizer on top of that?" he asks.

Caffeine can also be harmful to children's growing bodies, since it can cause excess excretion of calcium and magnesium, says Gail Frank, nutrition professor at California State University, Long Beach, and spokeswoman for the American Dietetic Association. She says, "There's a danger that children won't reach sufficient bone mass." Children are less likely now to replace calcium by drinking milk—consumption has plummeted in recent years, largely because kids are downing soft drinks instead. The phosphoric acid in cola beverages may be particularly detrimental to children's health; there is evidence that it can cause bone fractures, notes Cornell University Medical College registered dietitian Barbara Levine. Phosphoric acid can also break down tooth enamel. And common children's ailments like ear infections and respiratory irritations that produce colds, bronchitis and asthma may be exacerbated by caffeinated, carbonated drinks, according to Dr. William Cochran, pediatric gastroenterologist at Penn State's Geisinger Clinic and a member of the American Academy of Pediatrics nutrition committee. Caffeine and carbonated bubbles can trigger "refluxing," in which a sphincter muscle allows the acidy contents of the upper stomach to back up and irritate portions of the respiratory tract, including the throat and ears. In both his research and pediatric practice, Cochran has found that most children with chronic ear infections and respiratory illnesses have refluxing problems.

As kids guzzle caffeinated and other sodas at increasing rates, researchers like Frank worry about potential problems that won't be seen until kids mature. "What will happen when millions of children with much higher rates of caffeine consumption grow up?" Frank asks. "We may see increasing rates of osteoporosis." She also points to caffeine's ability to raise blood pressure: "We just don't know the long-term effects, and we need to find out." Meanwhile, Frank recommends that children and teens stay well under 100 milligrams of caffeine a day, which amounts to one or two cans of soda, depending on the caffeine content.

Many who'd like to see a decline in children's caffeine consumption know the task is not easy. "I think most parents simply don't realize how much caffeine kids get," says C.S.R.I. executive director Michael Jacobson. "Labeling products would at least give them some way to get the information and make some judgments." (For more information on the center's petition to the F.D.A., see C.S.P.I.'s Web site, www.cspinet.org.) The presence of sodas and their marketing in schools is an obvious target. "Schools are selling off students to soda," charges Marianne Manilov of the Center for Commercial-Free Public Education in Oakland, California. "Is this really what we want in public schools?" But efforts to restrict soda sales in school face much opposition from soda conglomerates' lobbying guns as well as from some school officials who like receiving a cut of vending-machine revenues. Last year a West Virginia law prohibiting the sale of sodas in schools during the school day was overturned after "a great deal of effort from the soft-drink lobby," reports an angry Martha Hill, who heads a county school-lunch program and is president-elect of the American School Food Service Association.

For concerned parents, home education—teaching children that caffeine is a drug and should be seen as such—is probably the best option. That's not what the executives at Coke and Pepsi want. But they are pushing a drug on pre-adults, one that may have serious health consequences for a whole generation. And that view—not the glitzy marketing and snazzy ads—is the real thing.

Opium as Cash Crop Is Still Difficult to Beat

By Warren Richey
Staff writer of The Christian Science Monitor

NAM TIT, BURMA

GROWING opium was a family tradition for Zi Zi Fa. His father grew opium, and his father's father.

But the legacy was broken this year when tribal leaders of the Wa ethnic group ordered Mr. Zi and other farmers in this rugged area near the Chinese border to stop planting opium poppies.

It was a decision that dramatically reduced the income of Zi's family of 10. Last year he received the equivalent of $650 for 12.5 pounds of opium-rich sap harvested from three acres of poppies. This year he is planting soybeans instead and expects to earn about 1/10th of his former income.

Three acres of soybeans replacing three acres of opium poppies is viewed by the US Drug Enforcement Administration as progress in the war on drugs.

But Zi sees it differently. "The family is barely surviving," he says.

It is still too early to know how the Zi family will deal with the economic cold turkey into which it has been thrust. But the ordeal illustrates the difficulty of weaning an entire population of farmers and their families away from the only crop that they believe can give them an economic advantage.

It is essentially the same issue faced by coca growers in the South American Andes, poppy farmers in Afghanistan's Hindu Kush, and even marijuana growers in the American Appalachians: How do you break the cycle of financial dependence on an illicit, lucrative cash crop?

Development needed

One-for-one crop substitution doesn't work, experts say. What does work, they say, are regionwide economic-development projects linked with education and law enforcement. "It is widely understood that you cannot find one crop that will replace opium. There is no magic crop that will generate the same income," says Joern Kristensen of the United Nations International Drug Control Program. "The key is to open up the area so local residents get access to the outside world, access to markets. The key is to link them up to development in a country."

There is no doubt that opium is an easy crop for farmers here. It grows on steep, unfertilized slopes above 3,500 feet, where few other crops can survive. The harvested sap does not need to be refrigerated. And the opium buyers—primarily Chinese middlemen—come directly to the farmer, so growers don't have to worry about transportation or the prospect that their crop might be hijacked on the way to market. Some buyers even offer financial services—providing growers advance loans on a future opium crop. It's their way of keeping poppy farmers dependent on the opium trade.

Cultural acceptance of opium

In addition, opium has been an accepted crop in this region for centuries and is still widely used among the older generation as a medicine, in cultural rites such as weddings, as well as a recreational drug. "We have to educate the people that this is very bad for mankind," says Col. Kyaw Thein, Burma's top antinarcotics official.

Some skeptics say it is impossible to break the grip of opium on these farmers. Indeed, the order by the Wa leadership to quit poppy growing applies only to a tiny fraction of Wa farmers in the Nam Tit region. The vast majority of Wa farmers are still heavily involved in the opium trade.

But development specialists and many antidrug experts say there is reason for hope. They point to nearby Thailand and even to China's Yunnan Province as examples of how local governments turned the tide against opium production while facing exactly the same cultural and development issues that now exist in Burma.

Success in Thailand

In 1969, the hill tribes in northern Thailand produced 150 metric tons of opium. By 1997, Thai production had fallen to 10 metric tons.

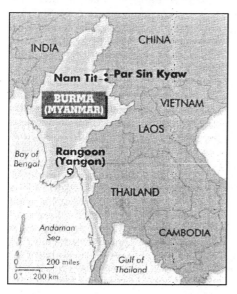

INDIA
CHINA
Nam Tit · Par Sin Kyaw
BURMA (MYANMAR)
VIETNAM
LAOS
Bay of Bengal
Rangoon (Yangon)
THAILAND
Andaman Sea
CAMBODIA
0   200 miles
0   200 km
Gulf of Thailand

STAFF

The conditions in northeastern Burma, where more than half of the world's opium is currently grown, are similar to the conditions that existed in northern Thailand in the late 1960s. There is a lack of roads, which in turn means a lack of access to markets to sell legitimate produce. There is no trucking, no refrigeration, no food processing, and no packaging.

It means that even if a farmer decides on his own to switch to legal crops, he will face an uphill battle trying to find a buyer for his produce.

A former Peace Corps volunteer posted in northern Thailand two decades ago says he remembers former opium-growing hill tribesmen carrying their ripe produce into town to try to sell it. Once in town they were denigrated as hillbillies and offered ridiculous prices for their crops. He says many ended up giving their produce away because there was no developed market, no clearly identified buyers at reliable prices.

He says the same problem exists in Burma today. "No one is reaching out to help them market their produce, they are on their own," he says.

China used a combination of antidrug enforcement and infrastructure development to prevent local farmers in Yunnan province from turning to opium production. Unlike farmers only a few miles away on the Burma side of the border, Chinese farmers have access to roads, trucks, and a central distribution system that creates demand for legitimate produce grown in once-remote mountain areas.

The same crops that are profitable on the Chinese side of the border—rubber, sugarcane, tea, coffee, and mangoes among others—would likely also make money on the Burma side, if roads and other infrastructure existed.

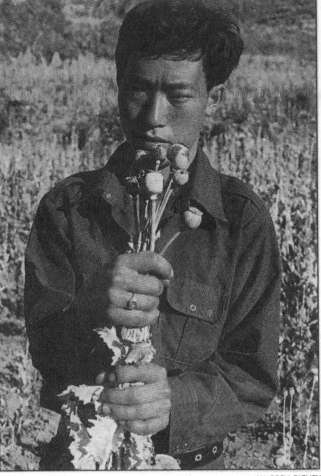

IN THE GOLDEN TRIANGLE: A Burmese soldier holds poppy plants. The government claims it's eradicating opium growing. But Western observers are skeptical.

WARREN RICHEY

'It is a change of lifestyle.'

—UN International Drug Control Program official

"The trick is to find something that grows in the same season as opium," says a Western diplomat. That season runs from October through February.

Japan is supporting a pilot project in northeastern Burma to see if buckwheat might work. The test is whether farmers can harvest three crops a year, including during the prime opium-growing season. Japanese officials promise that all produced buckwheat will be purchased by noodle factories in Japan. But transportation and storage issues must still be worked out.

A United States-backed crop-substitution program sponsored by American veterans who fought here in World War II is introducing farm-management techniques in northeastern Burma. A development project sponsored by the UN is about to start up in a Wa tribal town near the Chinese border. That project will attempt to address the full range of infrastructure problems such as roads, schools, and health clinics, while also teaching local farmers how to become self-sufficient in food production.

Many farmers use opium revenue to buy enough food to feed their families all year. UN project managers say if that food was grown by the farmers themselves, it would be easier to persuade the farmers to grow a second, legal cash crop.

Rubber, sugarcane, and livestock, such as chickens and pigs, are among possible choices, officials say.

"It is a change of lifestyle, introducing other ways of making money," Mr. Kristensen says. As the local infrastructure is developed with better roads, schools, clinics, and market facilities, project managers will begin exploring the creation of support industries, like food packaging and processing plants.

The Buddhist Way To Wean Drug Lords From Opium Trade

By Warren Richey

Staff writer of the Christian Science Monitor

RANGOON, BURMA

REBIRTH is a major theme in Buddhism. But there is a form of "reincarnation" under way in this Buddhist nation that has international drug investigators working overtime.

Burma's ruling junta is trying to prove there is, indeed, life after being a "godfather" in the Golden Triangle.

Just ask Khun Sa and a host of other opium warlords who are benefiting from a government campaign to embrace the region's criminal underworld as legitimate businessmen, provided they invest their narco-money in Burma.

It is a policy that appears rooted in cold pragmatism, perhaps even des-

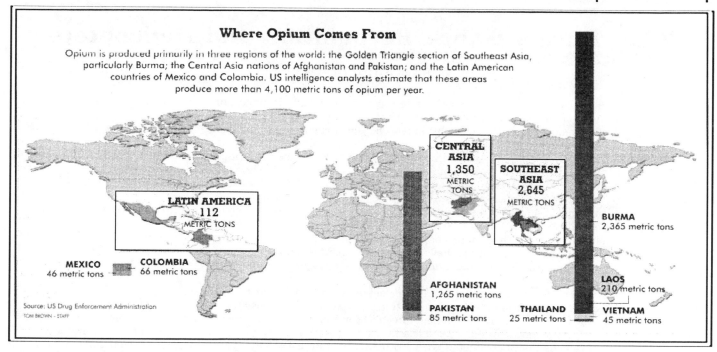

Where Opium Comes From

Opium is produced primarily in three regions of the world: the Golden Triangle section of Southeast Asia, particularly Burma; the Central Asia nations of Afghanistan and Pakistan; and the Latin American countries of Mexico and Colombia. US intelligence analysts estimate that these areas produce more than 4,100 metric tons of opium per year.

CENTRAL ASIA 1,350 METRIC TONS

SOUTHEAST ASIA 2,645 METRIC TONS

LATIN AMERICA 112 METRIC TONS

BURMA 2,365 metric tons

MEXICO 46 metric tons

COLOMBIA 66 metric tons

AFGHANISTAN 1,265 metric tons

PAKISTAN 85 metric tons

THAILAND 25 metric tons

LAOS 210 metric tons

VIETNAM 45 metric tons

Source: US Drug Enforcement Administration
TOM BROWN - STAFF

peration. The governing generals are seeking to prop up their wheezing economy by appealing to drug traffickers—both current and former—to bring their money home.

The key phrase is: No questions asked.

"Opium is the one crop that continues to make money for people here," says a Western diplomat. "How much of the money ultimately comes back here and is invested in the economy, nobody knows."

The policy is raising concerns that the military government may become hooked on drug money.

Given the widening Asian financial crisis, continuing international sanctions against Burma, and less-than-friendly economic conditions inside Burma, the regime has few options for attracting fresh capital.

Narco-investment as rehab?

Government officials defend their policy, justifying it as an attempt to rehabilitate criminals by weaning them away from lives of crime.

But such explanations seem a little convenient to Western diplomats who note that much of the opium and heroin profits are a direct result of lax law enforcement

in the Golden Triangle by Burma's government.

Analysts point to one Rangoon-based business powerhouse with investments in real estate, finance, mining, tourism, and trade. The company is viewed as the commercial arm

From Burma to New York: Opium's Trail to High-Priced Heroin

A farmer in Burma earns **$1,500** for each **15.5 pounds** of raw opium extracted from poppies.

That quantity of opium is refined into a **1.5 pound** brick of heroin and sold from Burma for **$5,600**.

The brick's wholesale price rises as it is sold around the world:

Bangkok $9,100
Hong Kong $15,400
Taipei $42,700
Big US cities $60,000 to $91,000

In New York City, the brick is diluted and distributed in **$10 bags** with a final street value of up to **$140,000**.

Source: US Drug Enforcement Administration
TOM BROWN - STAFF

of the United Wa State Army, a heavily armed militia now considered the largest, most active drug-trafficking group in the Burma sector of the Golden Triangle.

What has some Western analysts in Rangoon concerned is that Burma's drug-money reinvestment policy dovetails with a series of cease-fire agreements reached in 1989 with the same ethnic militias that protect and run the opium and heroin operations.

Under the terms of the cease-fire agreements, the ethnic groups pledged to eventually work toward creation of opium-free zones throughout their regions. Deadlines for an absolute halt to all opium trade have been suggested (some as early as 2000), but it is doubtful they will be honored.

In the meantime, the region's drug trade is enjoying what looks to be a tacit agreement by the government to allow the traffickers to continue their lucrative operations as long as the cease-fires are honored.

Khun Sa's 'surrender'

Among the best-known of Burma's new breed of investors is Khun Sa, also known as Chang Chi-Fu, the flamboyant jungle warlord who "surrendered" to the Burma military in January 1996 and has been living comfortably in Rangoon.

What Burma Wants: Recognition and Helicopters

RANGOON, BURMA

OFFICIALS in Burma complain that they are in the midst of a significant antidrug campaign but that it is being ignored by most of the world, particularly the United States.

The US cut off all aid to Burma, including extensive joint drug-fighting assistance, in 1988 as a result of major human rights violations committed by the ruling junta while crushing antiregime demonstrations.

Now, the military government suggests that the US should reconsider its aid ban in light of recent anti-opium measures undertaken in Burma. The government says it has eradicated 40,000 acres of poppy fields in the past year. Western diplomats in the capital, Rangoon, acknowledge that some eradication has taken place, but the envoys say they are unable to verify how much has been destroyed.

Analysts suggest that if 40,000 acres had been destroyed, as the government claims, opium production for the year would fall substantially. No such fall has been seen, they say.

Government officials counter that there has been a significant decline in opium production, but the US and other nations are ignoring it. "Since 1995, there have been many seizures and we managed to destroy a lot of [clandestine heroin] refineries. I think this is an indication that we are seriously doing our work," says Maj. Gen. Siha Sura Tin Aung, a regional Army commander.

At the core of their request, Burmese officials are seeking equipment from the US that they say will help them to wage a more effective war on drugs. "We are ready to do any kind of suppression to the drug traffickers," says U Hla Thann, a Ministry of Defense official who is also director of a company that seeks to attract new investors to Burma. He says that among its stepped up enforcement efforts, the government would resume an aerial opium-eradication spraying operation that had been conducted with US help prior to the 1988 aid cutoff. In particular, officials say, they need helicopters, surveillance planes, support arms, including rocket launchers, night vision goggles, satellite navigation equipment, and thermal-imaging sensors.

Some Burma analysts say any new equipment would be used to fight insurgent armies seeking autonomy from the central government and to strengthen the junta's grip on power rather than to stop opium traffickers.

At present the full extent of US-Burma cooperation on drug trafficking matters involves the sharing of Drug Enforcement Administration intelligence information with Burmese officials. The US government maintains it will not consider lifting existing sanctions until the ruling generals make significant progress toward achieving democratic rule and recognizing human rights.

—W. R.

At the height of his power, Khun Sa supposedly controlled one-third of the world's opium supplies and commanded 48,000 armed men.

The US government has posted a $2 million bounty on his head. Federal prosecutors in Brooklyn, N.Y., are seeking his capture so he can stand trial on 1994 charges that he smuggled thousands of pounds of heroin into the US over 20 years.

But apparently having Khun Sa as a resident in Rangoon is worth more than $2 million to the Burmese government. The full details of the agreement between Burma and Khun Sa have never been revealed. But officials justify the arrangement, saying his surrender ended a long war.

To coax Khun Sa out of the jungle, Burma's ruling generals offered him safety and the chance to become a tycoon in Rangoon. He was granted a loan by the government to set up a bus and trucking company and was awarded government concessions in jade and gem sales. In addition, he has been offered a lucrative contract to repave the road from Rangoon to Mandalay.

Part of the government's benevolent treatment of Khun Sa may be sincerely rooted in the Buddhist faith and the understanding that good deeds never go unrewarded.

But part is also rooted in his value as a source of intelligence information. "We could just shut him up with one bullet but we are trying to keep him alive because he is a walking encyclopedia," says Lt. Col. Hla Min, deputy director of the Office of Strategic Studies at the Ministry of Defense. "This [opium trade] is a multibillion-dollar business," he adds. "He knows who is involved. And now what he knows, we know."

Some government officials liken the arrangement with Khun Sa to a plea bargain, a common arrangement in the US justice system.

Although his living conditions are said to be comfortable in a guarded military housing compound in a quiet Rangoon neighborhood, he is nonetheless under surveillance. And he still faces the prospect that someone might try to turn him in for the US reward.

"Khun Sa is stuck. He can't move around. If he goes to any third world country, we're going to grab him," says an American official stationed in the region.

HIDDEN DANGERS
of OVER THE
COUNTER DRUGS

By William Ecenbarger

WHEN THE 18-year-old staggered into the emergency room, she was wild-eyed and gasping for air. Her air passages were swelling dramatically. Quick-acting doctors in that Midwestern hospital managed to regulate her breathing with an emergency tracheotomy and intravenous drug treatment. She was admitted to the respiratory intensive-care unit for follow-up treatment and eventually recovered.

The young woman's nearly fatal experience was brought on by an allergic reaction to aspirin. She knew she was allergic to aspirin, but she had taken it inadvertently. How?

At the onset of a headache, she had reached for a common over-the-counter (OTC) drug that she thought contained acetaminophen. It did—but had she bothered to read the label closely, she would have seen the small print that said it also contained aspirin.

A near-death experience with an OTC drug is, thankfully, uncommon. But the young woman's mistake—failure to read the label—is all too common. A survey by the American Pharmaceutical Association last year found that 47 percent of adults did not always read the labels on OTC pain relievers, fewer than 40 percent consulted a pharmacist before taking these products, and 43 percent were unaware of the potential risks associated with taking these remedies along with prescription medicines.

The dangers can be considerable. The remedies we buy for allergy, headache, upset stomach and other common ailments are drugs. And they must be used responsibly. If you are taking prescription medications, be sure to consult your doctor or pharmacist. Consumers who fail to do so or who disregard warnings on the labels and the package inserts before they swallow, spray, sip, inhale, insert or smear one of the 100,000 OTC remedies now on the market are taking a risk.

Here are some of the pitfalls:

Overdosing

THERE IS THE IDEA that if one doesn't work, I'll try two," says Joe Graedon, a pharmacologist and author of *The People's Pharmacy* book series. That is not a good idea.

Earlier this year a 45-year-old truck driver showed up at the Houston Headache Clinic complaining of excruciating headaches. The pain would throb and pulsate, waking him out of a sound sleep and making him nauseated.

It didn't take long to find the problem. The man had been swallowing about 200 Excedrin Migraine tablets weekly for nearly a year. The label warns users not to take more than eight tablets per day and not to use the medication for more than 48 hours. Each tablet contains 250 mg. of acetaminophen, 250 mg. of aspirin and 65 mg. of caffeine.

"This is the classic rebound headache," says Dr. Ninan T. Mathew, clinic director. "As the pain got worse, he took more and more painkiller, thinking this was a safe product. We took him off all daily pain medication, introduced a relaxation and stress-management program and gave him drugs to prevent migraines. He is progressing well."

Overuse of OTC drugs may give you more than a headache.

While no definitive studies have been done, Mathew estimates that between two and three percent of the population—as many as eight million Americans may be overusing OTC headache remedies.

Many OTC products are merely lower-dose versions of drugs that can only be obtained with a prescription. For example, the painkiller Orudis KT is a version of the prescription drug ketoprofen, which can cause ulcers and severe stomach bleeding if taken in high doses or for an extended period.

"Habitual and chronic use of pain relievers that have more than one active ingredient may be risky," warns Dr. William Henrich, chairman of the National Kidney Foundation's public-policy committee. "This could lead to kidney damage and a reduction in kidney function." Some experts, though, say an association between kidney disease and use of combination analgesics has not been proved. In any case, these drugs are considered safe when used as directed.

Interaction

MEDICAL AUTHORITIES urge anyone taking a prescription medicine, especially those with a chronic illness, to consult with a doctor or pharmacist before taking any OTC drug. Millions of Americans, for example, take Tagamet HB, a popular remedy for heartburn, acid indigestion and other minor stomach problems. But if they're also taking the widely prescribed drug Coumadin (used to prevent blood clots), they're at risk. Tagamet HB and Coumadin can interact in a way that, in severe cases, may cause internal hemorrhaging and bleeding from the mouth, nose, rectum and urinary tract. The warning about this interaction is present on the Tagamet label, but the reference is to warfarin, the generic name for Coumadin. (The package insert, though, refers to both the brand and generic names.)

Anti-depressants are now among the most widely used drugs in America. Prozac, for example, is America's fifth most often dispensed drug. "People on medication for depression have to be careful about using cold remedies," notes Grant Shetterly, a fellow at the Center for Proper Medication Use in Philadelphia.

A common ingredient in many cough suppressants, dextromethorphan, may interact with an anti-depressant such as Prozac or Paxil to produce a serious, though infrequently reported, problem called serotonin syndrome. One 51-year-old victim was admitted to the emergency room vomiting blood, sweating, shaking, confused and having trouble breathing. His blood pressure was elevated, and his pulse was 122 beats per minute. The man,

who had a pre-existing vascular disease, recovered after some time in intensive care.

Cold remedies also can interact dangerously with another class of anti-depressants called monoamine oxidase inhibitors (MAOIs). These include Nardil and Parnate. Most OTC cough and cold products, like Sudafed, warn specifically against this reaction.

Cancellation

CONSUMERS NEED to be aware of another potential pitfall: one drug can cancel or reduce the effects of another.

Because it provides relief from high blood pressure, Vasotec is one of the most frequently dispensed drugs in America. It is not unusual for someone with high blood pressure to be taking ordinary aspirin as a preventive against heart attacks. "But aspirin may reduce the effectiveness of Vasotec," says pharmacologist Graedon. The same interaction could potentially occur with other widely prescribed heart and blood-pressure drugs—known as ACE inhibitors—such as Accupril , Prinivil and Monopril. People who take these drugs should not avoid aspirin, especially if it has been prescribed by a physician, but should have their blood pressure carefully monitored.

Many people with high blood pressure also have arthritis. Combining certain prescription drugs for the former and too much of an OTC drug for the latter may reduce the effectiveness of their blood-pressure medication. For example, people on beta blockers such as Inderal, Visken and Lopressor should consult their doctors before taking nonsteroidal, anti-inflammatory painkillers (known as NSAIDs), such as aspirin, Advil, Aleve, Motrin and Nuprin.

Grant Shetterly also cautions that the active ingredients in many antacids, including Rolaids and Tums, can reduce the absorption of certain antibiotics–tetracyclines and fluoroquinolones. In some cases they can totally negate the effects of the antibiotics and inhibit the curing of major infections. People should ask their physicians whether they should take both drugs.

Alcohol

WHEN Antonio Benedi caught the flu from his sons, he relieved his symptoms with Extra-Strength Tylenol, the No. 1 best-selling OTC product. Later, when the ambulance came for him at his suburban Washington home, he was in a coma with liver failure. Benedi's liver was destroyed by a toxic reaction to acetaminophen, Tylenol's main ingredient. His habit of drinking two or three glasses of wine with dinner had made his liver more sensitive to the drug. A last-minute liver transplant saved his life.

A study published in 1997 found that overuse of acetaminophen was the leading cause of admission for acute liver failure at Parkland Memorial Hospital in Dallas, Texas, and that heavy drinkers were especially vulnerable. The American Liver Foundation recommends that regular drinkers use less than the normal dosage of OTC acetaminophen products.

Combining alcohol with many popular OTC pain relievers can be hazardous. Under a new FDA regulation, all pain-relief and fever-reducing products will carry labels warning anyone consuming more than three drinks per day to consult a doctor before taking the product.

Medical and pharmaceutical professionals urge consumers to read the label of every OTC product they buy and to ask a doctor or pharmacist about it. They add these precautions:

▲ *Find out for sure whether taking the medication will affect your ability to drive.*

▲ *Don't assume that all products under a given brand name are the same.* For example, there are at least 11 different OTC products with the name Sudafed. Some contain only pseudoephedrine, and others include acetaminophen, guaifenesin and dextromethorphan. Some contain alcohol; others contain caffeine.

▲ *Read the label every time you purchase an OTC product, not just the first time.* Companies can change the ingredients.

▲ *Be extremely cautious if you crush, chew or break a medication before swallowing it.* Sometimes OTC drugs have a coating that keeps them from dissolving as they pass through the stomach; sometimes these drugs are designed to release medication slowly over time—a goal that can be frustrated by not taking them whole.

Help for consumers is on the way. New FDA rules approved earlier this year will make nonprescription drug labels easier for consumers to read and understand. There will be larger type, more white space, a standard format and simpler language to explain side effects, interactions and when to consult a physician.

Nevertheless, all the warnings in the world won't help if you don't read them.

BIG TOBACCO RIDES EAST

With a squinting cowboy, cute cigarette girls, an American allure, and a poorly funded opposition

BY ROBERT DREYFUSS

Standing in the center of Ho Chi Minh City's wholesale tobacco market, a visitor to Dang Dieu Hy's store can easily count about three dozen different brands of cigarettes, most in low-budget packages produced by Vietnam's state-owned tobacco company.

Yet, throughout the market, two color schemes dominate. Both are from foreign brands: the red-and-white chevron of Philip Morris' Marlboro and the regal gold-on-blue of State Express 555, made by British American Tobacco (BAT). This color coding leads visitors straight down Hoc Lac Street to Hy's store, an entire building painted a blinding red. Inside, as the Marlboro Man squints down from a poster, Hy stands serenely amid the commotion. Stylishly dressed, a cellular phone pressed to one ear, she sends her employees scrambling off to prepare orders. Some of the packages are Marlboros that have been processed and packaged in a factory in Vietnam. Others are contraband, marked with the telltale "Made in U.S.A."

Hy remains unfazed when asked about the smuggled packs and refuses to say how she obtained them. She also says she isn't worried about getting caught. "The police only catch the smugglers at the border," she says. "They have no right to interfere in the market. Besides, we can negotiate with them, once in a while paying bribes." After all, her cash business is bustling (behind the counter she keeps a stack of currency roughly 8 inches high).

For Philip Morris, which designed the shop, painted it, and maintains it, Hy plays a crucial role, providing a center of commerce. Philip Morris and other foreign tobacco companies vehemently deny critics' accusations that they play a role in smuggling the vast quantities of cigarettes making their way across the border. They claim smuggling actually hurts profits, forcing them to compete with themselves. But the contraband also provides Western companies the undeniable benefit of making the product more

visible, which is important because their short-term goal isn't to dominate the Vietnamese cigarette market. They're focused on selling something much more important: their brand. And for Philip Morris, that means selling America.

As Taylor Meloan, professor of marketing at the University of Southern California and author of *International and Global Marketing,* sees it, "[Vietnamese] want the American dream, the American lifestyle, the American way of doing things. We are no longer the ugly Americans," he says. "We are the Americans that live the good life, and when people buy a piece of America they are buying a piece of our lifestyle."

Foreign brands currently constitute only about 15 to 18 percent of Vietnam's cigarette market, according to figures from the U.S. Department of Agriculture. The rest is satisfied by the more than 80 brands produced by the country's own Vinataba tobacco company and several local producers. Domestic cigarettes typically sell for 10 to 50 cents a pack, while the Western brands are priced from 70 cents to just under $1.

Nearly three-quarters of the men in Vietnam smoke, according to a study published in the *Journal of the American Medical Association.* That's the highest rate of male smoking in the world, making the nation, with a population of 75 million, a prized market. According to projections by the World Health Organization (WHO), annual smoking-related deaths will rise worldwide from the current 3.5 million (one-third of them in Third World countries) to 10 million over the next two decades (7 million in the Third World).

Meanwhile, tobacco consumption continues its gradual decline in the United States (from an all-time high of 42.4 percent in 1965 to 24.7 percent in 1995, the most recent year for which data is available). In its search for new consumers, the tobacco industry has pinned its greatest hopes on Asia, which boasts nearly 60 percent of the world's population. As a *Tobacco Reporter* editorial put it: "The future is Asia."

Accordingly, Western brands have swept in with an aggressive marketing campaign based on a simple logic: Even if the people can't afford the higher-priced cigarettes right away, they can start wanting them now.

Over the past decade, Vietnam has tried to build a line of defense against the rising incidence of smoking. Since 1990, the government has tightened its ban on imports of U.S. and foreign cigarettes, prohibited tobacco advertising, and banned smoking in many public places—including hospitals, meeting halls, theaters, and aboard buses and planes. And many local bodies have placed additional restrictions on cigarette promotion, and numerous workplaces, ministries, and local people's committees have forbidden or regulated smoking. Once a year, with the help of Canadian and American health experts and WHO, the government promotes anti-smoking events during a weeklong burst of activity surrounding World No-Tobacco Day on May 31.

The slight, soft-spoken physician with the unwieldy task of directing the country's anti-smoking efforts is Tran Thu Thuy, a government health official who oversees the Vietnam Committee on Smoking and Health (Vinacosh). Over tea, she plainly admits that Vietnam is starting late with its public health campaign against tobacco. "We are not experienced in this kind of work," she says, noting that the country has done little research on the incidence, distribution, and control of tobacco-related diseases in Vietnam, or on the cost to the country in lost productivity and medical expenses. It was this last point that helped turn U.S. political and public opinion against the tobacco industry, particularly after several states launched successful legal battles in 1996 to recoup billions of dollars in Medicaid expenses from tobacco-related illnesses.

Vinacosh is poorly funded—it received just 100 million dong (about $7,000) in government funds for its 1997 activities—making it impossible to launch any type of widespread media effort, or anything resembling a modern television and radio public service announcement. A draft tobacco policy report from the Ministry of Health states gloomily: "Neither government funds or any other financial resources have been available for carrying out comprehensive and systematic information-education-communication activities against smoking."

Vietnam requires only vague warning labels on cigarette packs ("Smoking Is Dangerous to Health"), and while Vietnam's media frequently cite information about tobacco-caused illnesses, the news reports are dry and stale, making them easy to ignore. There are also no restrictions on the sale of cigarettes to children. "Fathers ask their sons to bring cigarettes to them," Thuy says.

Meanwhile, looming over Vietnam's anti-smoking efforts are concerns that ongoing trade talks between the

United States and Vietnam could lead to the repeal of some restrictions. An official at the U.S. embassy in Hanoi, for example, suggests that the cigarette import ban might become a casualty. David Wilson, the spokesman for BAT in Vietnam, says that by 2006, when Vietnam has to be in compliance with the trade rules that govern the Southeast Asian nations bloc, the ban might crumble. And a recent congressional attempt to permanently ban U.S. trade negotiators from representing tobacco interests and prohibit U.S. tobacco companies from marketing to children overseas has failed. Rep. Lloyd Doggett (D-Texas), who wrote the legislation, blames its failures on powerful tobacco industry lobbyists in Washington. "It's probably a bad choice of words, but they are able to choke off any attempts at legislation in committee," he says.

In much of Vietnam, meanwhile, people tend to respond to warnings against smoking with indifference rather than outrage or suspicion. The public's attitude comes across loud and clear at Hanoi's Noi Bai Airport, where two men puff away in the waiting lounge, right underneath the No Smoking signs.

At the Thang Long cigarette factory in Hanoi, heavily damaged by a U.S. air strike in 1967, Nguyen Tien Dung, a Vinataba official and vice director of the plant, explains the company's policy. "We pay attention to the consumer, to his health, with the knowledge that cigarettes are harmful," he says. "But the demand exists and is stable. If we do not supply it locally, then this demand will be filled by [smuggled] foreign cigarettes."

Yet, in compliance with government anti-smoking policy, Vinataba does no advertising or promotion. The price, too, is carefully regulated, and the government increases cigarette taxes whenever the Ministry of Health suggests that demand is too high and tobacco consumption needs to be curtailed.

As in other Asian countries, including China, South Korea, and Thailand, the existence of a state-owned quasi-monopoly can give the government significant leverage against multinationals such as Philip Morris and BAT. Tobacco critics actually view such state-run companies as awkward allies. "I think public health is served by clunky, inefficient national monopolies that keep prices high and don't engage in aggressive marketing techniques," says Neil Collishaw, a scientist and senior staff member at WHO's Tobacco-Free Initiative. "Plus, as a government agency, they are more likely to cooperate with the health ministries in trying to reduce the prevalence of smoking."

Though Vinataba might cooperate with tobacco-control efforts, they are hardly going to encourage tobacco eradication. After all, the tobacco industry is profitable for Vietnam, with tobacco taxes making up 3.2 percent ($110 million) of the national budget as recently as 1994.

That year, however, Vietnam made what health advocates would describe as a Trojan horse-style error. The country entered into production agreements with Philip Morris, Rothmans of Pall Mall, and BAT to produce and sell their premium brands in Vietnam, using Vinataba facilities. Vietnam also launched a joint venture with R.J. Reynolds in Da Nang. In a stroke, Madison Avenue took over Hoc Lac Street.

Too late, Hanoi tried to stem the tide. In late '94, the Vietnamese government strengthened its ban on tobacco print and electronic media ads and billboards, which it has since supplemented with a series of decrees limiting cigarette vendors. With some understatement, the Ministry of Health reported in a strategy paper, "It is likely that the introduction of the transnational tobacco companies in Vietnam through joint ventures promoted smoking via more active and sophisticated forms of marketing techniques.

"Together with increased smuggling of cigarettes, the use of tobacco increased," concluded the report. "The ban on tobacco advertising has not been completely effective, [and] tobacco sponsorship of dances, disco, and the distribution by young women has not been affected."

Despite regulations imposed by Hanoi and local jurisdictions, the foreign tobacco companies are still able to promote themselves. In convenience stores, markets, and cafés, posters and point-of-sale displays trumpet the Marlboro, Dunhill, and 555 brands. They are seemingly everywhere: In Hanoi and Ho Chi Minh City, almost every corner boasts a street vendor with a trolley cart, the bottom half of which carries the logo of one of the premium foreign brands, while on top are stacked carton upon carton of cigarettes. In Ho Chi Minh City alone, according to the *Tobacco Reporter,* there are more than 2,000 such trolleys. Typically, the owner gets the cart free from the company, plus a payment of 100,000 Vietnamese dong per month—about $7 (the World Bank places the annual per capita income at $320)—and a busy network of runners keeps carts supplied with a stock of cigarettes from company warehouses and places like the Hoc Lac market.

Along a single block of Trieu Viet Vuong Street in Hanoi, various cafés, inns, and nightspots sport garish Marlboro colors and, inside, display posters of the Marlboro Man. Many are regularly visited by a minivan—also red and white and bearing the Marlboro name—that disgorges attractive young women wearing red and white, who approach male customers with free packs of cigarettes.

"The Challenge" is one of Marlboro's most successful promotions, whose placards are seen widely in and around Vietnam's major cities. By collecting a certain number of empty Marlboro packages, participants can earn binoculars, watches, radios, knives, backpacks, caps, and T-shirts. Local anti-smoking activists say "The Challenge" is popular with children, who scavenge for discarded cigarette boxes.

Philip Morris denies that it targets children in Vietnam or any other part of Asia. "We don't do that," says Don Harris, vice president for Philip Morris Asia, which is based in Hong Kong. "We have a very extensive youth no-smoking program throughout Asia." These programs in Vietnam, however, are limited to training programs aimed at retailers, Harris says. He also maintains that "The Challenge" is open only to people over 18, who "have to verify their age with some sort of documentation."

But the tobacco policy draft report from Vietnam's Ministry of Health tells another story. At the 1998 Hanoi Tet festival (a national New Year's celebration), it reports, Philip Morris had "a large tent with Marlboro horses to ride on for children, and young, nicely dressed cowboy girls offered single cigarettes free of charge to young boys."

"When it comes to advertising, there are two issues: what's on the statute books and what's actually implemented," says Wilson, the BAT spokesman, speaking in his Ho Chi Minh City office.

BAT has more than a century of experience in Asia, especially in China. There, according to *Ashes to Ashes,* Richard Kluger's Pulitzer Prize-winning history of the tobacco industry, the company used "ruthless pricing practices, dubious legal maneuvers, and purchased political influence" to establish market dominance. In South Vietnam, BAT also had a strong presence until 1975, when the Viet Cong overran Saigon and seized the company's factory there. "A lot of the equipment Vinataba is using is old BAT equipment that they took over in '75," says Wilson matter-of-factly. Today, BAT pays the Vietnamese government for the right to use its more modern production facilities for its State Express 555 brand, manufacturing them at the old Saigon Cigarette Factory—a factory it used to own. A hollow victory, but a victory nonetheless.

But manufacturing cigarettes in Vietnam is not as difficult for BAT as selling them, Wilson says. Throughout the country, regulations vary. "People on one side of the street do one thing, and people on the other side do another," he says. For instance, in some areas of Ho Chi Minh City, BAT believes it is able to use its name on the trolleys that carry its product, while in others it resorts to trolleys that bear only 555's futuristic logo without the product's name.

Philip Morris resorts to a similar strategy. In many urban neighborhoods, the unmistakable, craggy features of the Marlboro Man appear alone, without the Marlboro name but with varying slogans. Under one familiar portrait is the slogan, "The strength of self-confidence." Elsewhere, Philip Morris relies solely on the red-and-white chevron that also adorns the Marlboro package, and displays it on trolleys and umbrellas.

Still, BAT and Philip Morris acknowledge that most Vietnamese cannot afford the premium prices for the 555 and Marlboro makes, opting instead for the lower-priced Vinataba brands.

"The consumer who buys 555 is primarily [from] the rising middle class, perhaps for conspicuous consumption purposes," says Wilson. They might, he explains, be able to afford one or two of the cigarettes a month, buying them for special occasions. "The aspirational elements of the brand are very strong. By the middle of the next decade, we anticipate that the premium segment will double in size."

The high-powered marketing efforts in Vietnam seem significantly out of proportion to the limited number of Marlboros and 555s being sold. So far, high-end cigarettes represent only about 4 to 6 percent of the market, and Marlboro represents only a tiny piece of that small share. That leads critics to suggest that the companies' real intent in promoting so aggressively could be to create a demand for smuggled cigarettes.

Many Vietnamese think foreign-made brands are of a higher quality than domestic ones, though Philip Morris insists that the Marlboros made in Vietnam are manufactured to exacting standards that make them the equivalent of Marlboros anywhere. Still, Philip Morris' Don Harris admits the attractiveness of the smuggled version. "It's an American product," he says. "And there is some cachet in 'Made in the U.S.A.'"

Yet worldwide, the tobacco industry faces criticism for doing little or nothing to prevent smuggling. WHO estimates that 30 percent of all cigarettes (355 billion) in international trade end up being smuggled across borders, from Asia to Latin America to Canada.

According to Judith Mackay, chair of WHO's global anti-tobacco program, the smuggling process begins when tobacco companies sell cigarettes in bulk to middlemen in Hong Kong and Singapore. Some of these distributors maintain ties to or are controlled by triads, powerful organized crime groups in Asia. The triads, in turn, organize the smuggling channels.

The companies deny any connection to the smuggling, although in a widely publicized case in Hong Kong this year, a former BAT official was jailed and later fined after being found guilty of receiving million-dollar bribes from a cigarette distributor in exchange for a supply of duty-free cigarettes, according to the *South China Morning Post*. Ultimately, the judge who presided over the case thought BAT should share the blame, saying, according to the *Post*: "In my view the tobacco companies were clearly putting their commercial interests above whatever moral duty they may have towards our society and to some extent such irresponsible behavior amounted to assisting criminals in transnational crime."

Not only do smuggled cigarettes indirectly funnel sales and profits into the companies' worldwide operations, but smuggling has an additional benefit: It puts tremendous pressure on countries such as Vietnam to relax or eliminate their bans on cigarette imports. An estimated 10 percent of Vietnam's demand for cigarettes is met by smuggled varieties, and they can be found everywhere.

Le The Bao, an official with the Ministry of Trade's vice department, says the country is mobilizing border guards, police, and a special unit of the Trade Ministry to coordinate anti-smuggling efforts, fight corruption, and patrol highly porous land and sea borders.

The smugglers are often Vietnamese hill country and border peasants who carry illegal smokes across from Cambodia and Laos, just as, a generation ago, Viet Cong soldiers and porters hauled rice, arms, and ammunition down the Ho Chi Minh Trail. Bao says the government is hoping to remove the incentive for the cigarette traffic by providing capital and employment opportunities to farmers in the border regions.

Nevertheless, you can find illegal cigarettes everywhere in Vietnam, even at the high-profile cigarette shops that ring Hoan Kiem Lake under the shadow of the Ministry of Trade. Though he refused to disclose details, Bao said his government would announce new restrictions on cigarette retailers by year-end to crack down on the sale of smuggled tobacco.

More than 1,000 miles north of Hoc Lac Street, in the southern district of Hanoi, is Bach Mai, the country's largest hospital. Like much of Vietnam's infrastructure, it is old and crumbling. Flakes of paint peel from the walls, and the tiles underfoot are sooty and cracked. In 1972, American warplanes devastated the hospital in the famous Christmas bombing, and evidence of the destruction still remains. Thirty doctors, nurses, and patients died that day as hundreds more huddled in underground tunnels that now store medical supplies.

Dr. Bui Huy Phu barely escaped death that day at Bach Mai, and now he directs the hospital's respiratory disease center. A gentle man with a wry smile, he has intense, inquiring eyes. When asked if he has the resources he needs to treat the increasing number of patients with tobacco-related illnesses, he looks up at a crack that branches across the ceiling. "Sometimes the ceilings fall down," he says.

"Sixty to 70 percent of the patients here are smokers, most of them men," he continues. "Within the last five years, almost all of the lung cancer patients, 87 percent, have been smokers, and we are seeing more and more of them." Just then, seemingly on cue, a colleague rushes in with an X-ray that reveals a tumor the size of a grapefruit in the right lung of one patient. "A smoker," Phu tells the visitor. "With very early cancers, we send them to the cancer hospital. [Others] with more advanced cancers, we send home. We cannot treat them."

Statistics on cigarette consumption are elusive in Vietnam. But smoking rates are clearly climbing. In 1996, Vietnam produced 30 billion cigarettes, up from 24.6 billion in 1992—and this, of course, does not include the millions of cigarettes smuggled into the country. Several studies have begun, in part to spur the government to stronger action against tobacco. For example, in Can Tho province, nestled along the Mekong Delta southwest of Ho Chi Minh City, a major study of the links between smoking and chronic lung diseases is under way.

There's also the possibility that a grassroots movement against the tobacco industry—like the one in the United States—will catch on. But for now, in a country desperate for international respect and eager to embrace all that is American, such a rebellion seems all the more unlikely.

What grassroots opposition does exist comes from young idealists such as Tran Thu Ha and her colleagues at the Research and Training Center for Community Development (RTCCD), a nonprofit group founded in Hanoi in 1996 and supported by grants from Canada, Holland, and Japan. Ha graduated in 1997 from Hanoi National University, where she studied English and Chinese. She has spent the last year coordinating an anti-tobacco project for the RTCCD. With a budget of just $5,000 to $7,000, the group creates posters and stickers it distributes to schools, hospitals, and government offices.

Earnest, with a civility reminiscent of the early women's temperance movement, the group has produced one sticker that reads: "Be Polite—Don't Smoke!" It's a far cry from U.S. anti-smoking tactics like the ongoing series of spots on Massachusetts television that document a woman dying from emphysema.

Like many in Vietnam, Ha worries that Vietnamese women will take up smoking. "Many Vietnamese women are being attracted by inducements from Western tobacco companies," she says.

In Vietnam, women are the next, potentially huge untapped market. Only 4 percent of women smoke in Vietnam, compared to 73 percent of men. While advertising restrictions make it difficult for tobacco companies to target women, there are other ways to promote a brand while not promoting a product. Ha says she has seen silk purses emblazoned with the Marlboro Man. And Philip Morris, of course, has its army of cigarette girls at cafés and clubs.

Like much of the tobacco marketing, this latest attack has left health experts and anti-smoking activists scratching their heads, wondering what they can do to counter such a campaign. Ha's group has had to resort to such basic, if touchingly naive, approaches as peer pressure: When she and her colleagues see a woman smoking, she says, "We stare at her."

Meredith Nicholson provided additional reporting for this story.

Drug abuse

High in the heartland

DES MOINES, IOWA

THE drug tsar, Barry McCaffrey, is unequivocal: "The worst drug ever to hit America is methamphetamine." He may well be right. Methamphetamine—meth, speed, ice, glass, crank, poor man's cocaine—is a powerful stimulant that affects the body in much the same way as cocaine. But it is cheaper than coke, produces a longer high, and is spreading like wildfire.

Although total drug abuse in America has fallen steadily since the mid-1980s, and cocaine's share is down 75% from its peak in 1985, the number of methamphetamine overdoses and deaths in the United States tripled between 1992 and 1996. It has taken hold especially in rural areas where other drugs are less widely available and "cookers" can manufacture the stuff in clandestine laboratories. When Vice-President Al Gore visited Iowa in January, he spoke about three issues: pigs, Social Security and methamphetamine.

What makes this stuff so nasty? To begin with, a $50 investment at the supermarket can produce $3,000-worth of methamphetamine. The active ingredient is either ephedrine or pseudoephedrine, both of which are found in over-the-counter cold medicines. "Cookers" use products such as drain-cleaner, lithium batteries and engine-starter fluid to transform one of the chemical precursors into a powder that can be smoked, snorted, injected or drunk with a soda. The

recipe is on the Internet. The Iowa Division of Narcotics Enforcement busted 320 meth labs in 1998, up from 63 in 1997.

Meth metabolises slowly, and can stay active in the body for up to 12 hours. The result is a prolonged burst of energy and strength. Many midwestern abusers are workers trying to get through a double shift at the meat-packing plant or a long haul in the lorry. High-school students are a growing market: the girls try meth to lose weight, the boys to enhance their athletic and sexual prowess.

Cooking meth may be cheap and easy, but there is nothing safe about it. A quart of ether (drained from cans of starter fluid) can explode with the force of five sticks of dynamite. According to Mr McCaffrey, one in six meth labs explodes or burns up each year. Those that do not combust are just as dangerous. Every pound of methamphetamine leaves behind five to six pounds of toxic waste. Iowa law-enforcement officials spend roughly $5,000 cleaning up every lab they close down.

Meth addicts become paranoid, delusional and violent. Cookers tend to be heavily armed; their laboratories are sometimes booby-trapped. A recent study in Iowa found that methamphetamine is a contributing factor in 80% of all domestic violence cases. Hospital emergency rooms must deal with overdoses in which the abuser stays psychotic for hours.

Despite the boom in home brewing, Iowa officials estimate that 80% of the

methamphetamine sold in the state is still being smuggled in from Mexico or the south-west, where it is manufactured in giant "superlabs". This trade used to be run by motorcycle gangs, but in the late 1980s Mexican drug rings began moving much larger quantities of meth along existing drug routes.

In an effort to stop it, state and federal authorities have increased the penalties for making, using and selling methamphetamine. Shopkeepers help by limiting sales of cold-medicine or tipping off the authorities when customers make suspicious purchases. One "cooker" was busted in Des Moines after he bought $500-worth of lithium batteries. Iowa is running television commercials warning against the false allure of methamphetamine. "We can't arrest our way out of the problem," says one top drug-enforcement official. The best way is still to stop people before they start.

Perhaps the most worrying part is not where methamphetamine has got to in America, but where it can still go. Outside California, America's big cities have been largely unaffected. In 1998, the Drug Enforcement Administration's office in Springfield, Illinois, made nearly ten times as many amphetamine arrests as the Chicago office. "I'm surprised it hasn't come yet," says Joseph Vanacora, the agent in charge of the Chicago office. It probably will, and the result could be devastating.

Unit Selections

Key Points to Consider

❖ How have the drug use increases of the 1990s suggested valid new worries about drug use by the young?

❖ What factors cause drug-related trends and patterns to change?

❖ How are drug-related patterns and trends related to specific subpopulations of Americans?

❖ How significant is socioeconomic class in influencing drug trends?

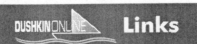 **Links**   **www.dushkin.com/online/**

11. **Marijuana as a Medicine**
    http://mojo.calyx.net/~olsen/MEDICAL/medical.html

These sites are annotated on pages 4 and 5.

Rarely do drug-related patterns and trends lend themselves to precise definition. Identifying, measuring, and predicting the consequences of these trends is an inexact science, to say the least. It is, nevertheless, a very important process.

Some of the most valuable data produced by drug-related trend analysis is the identification of subpopulations whose vulnerability to certain drug phenomena is greater than that of the wider population. These identifications may forewarn of the implications for the general population. Trend analysis may produce specific information that may otherwise be lost or obscured by general statistical indications. For example, tobacco is probably the most prominent of gateway drugs with repeated findings pointing to the correlation between the initial use of tobacco and the use of other drugs. Currently, 4.1 million youths 12 to 17 years of age are users of cigarettes and 10.5 million aged 12 to 20 are users of alcohol. Research suggests that among boys aged 12 to 17 years of age, who have no other problem behaviors, those who report drinking alcohol and/or smoking cigarettes at least once in the previous month are 28 times more likely to use marijuana than those who did not smoke or drink. The relationship is even higher for girls. There are similar findings when researchers study the use of marijuana by youth and its implications for the use of harder drugs. Thus, the analysis of specific trends related to youth smoking is very important, as it provides a threshold from which educators, health care professionals, parents, and young people may respond to significant drug-related health threats and issues.

Historically popular depressant and stimulant drugs, such as alcohol, tobacco, heroin, and cocaine, produce statistics that identify the most visible and sometimes the most constant use patterns. Other drugs such as marijuana, LSD, and Ecstasy often produce patterns widely interpreted to be associated with cultural phenomena such as youth attitudes, popular music trends, and political climate. Still other drugs, such as methamphetamine, suggest potential use patterns of cocaine-like proportions.

Occasionally, sensational drug-related stories, such as those surrounding recent heroin-related deaths of popular rock musicians and stories of drug use by Olympic athletes, serve to promote specific concerns over more general ones. Subsequently, one must weigh carefully the events of today as indicators of overall changing trends. Specific events are sometimes merely "blips on the screen"; sometimes they are tips of an iceberg. Emerging patterns of heroin and particularly methamphetamine use exist as good examples of potentially larger trends currently related to these illegal drugs. The number of persons being admitted to medical facilities for treatment of an overdose and for detoxification services related to the use of these drugs helps affirm our perception of new use patterns. Currently, methamphetamine abuse may pose the greatest threat associated with the use of illegal drugs although its impact has been addressed by a relatively shallow body of research.

Some recent findings are making it easier to speak more confidently about drug use patterns within certain segments of the population. Current research data portrays a good news/bad news illustration of changing drug trends and patterns. Good news is illustrated by a leveling off or, in some cases, a decline in drug use over the past 2 years. Most importantly, teen drug use appears to have leveled off after worrisome increases since 1992. Additionally, there is some new evidence that young people may be associating greater risk with the use of drugs. Still there remains troubling evidence associated with the sheer volume of drug use within society. For example, research attempting to learn when people first use drugs suggests that there are about 3,000 new youth smokers per day and about 5,000 new marijuana users per day. Additionally, the rates of initiation to the use of hallucinogens and heroin by youth have increased alarmingly.

Interestingly, findings continue to suggest a persistent relationship between family structure and drug use by children. For example, one study by the federal government noted that the lowest groups testing positive for drug use are of those juveniles who live with both parents or a parent and a stepparent. The percentage testing positive increases for those juveniles who live with a mother or father only and is highest among those who live with non-parental relatives.

Information concerning drug use patterns and trends obtained from a number of different investigative methods is available from a variety of sources. On the national level, the more prominent sources are the Substance Abuse and Mental Health Services Administration, the National Institute on Drug Abuse, the Drug Abuse Warning Network, the National Centers for Disease Control, the Justice Department, the General Accounting Office, and the Surgeon General. On the state level, various justice departments, including the attorney general's office, the courts, state departments of social services, state universities and colleges, and public health offices maintain data and conduct research. On local levels, criminal justice agencies, social service departments, public hospitals, and health departments provide information. On a private level, various research institutes and universities, professional organizations such as the American Medical Association and the American Cancer Society, hospitals, and treatment centers, as well as private corporations are tracking drug-related trends. Surveys abound, with no apparent lack of available data. As a result, the need for examination of research methods and findings for reliability and accuracy is self-evident.

The articles in unit 4 provide information about some drug-related trends occurring within certain subpopulations of Americans. While reading the articles, it is interesting to contemplate whether the trends and patterns described are confined to specific geographical areas.

Other Trends and Patterns in Drug Use

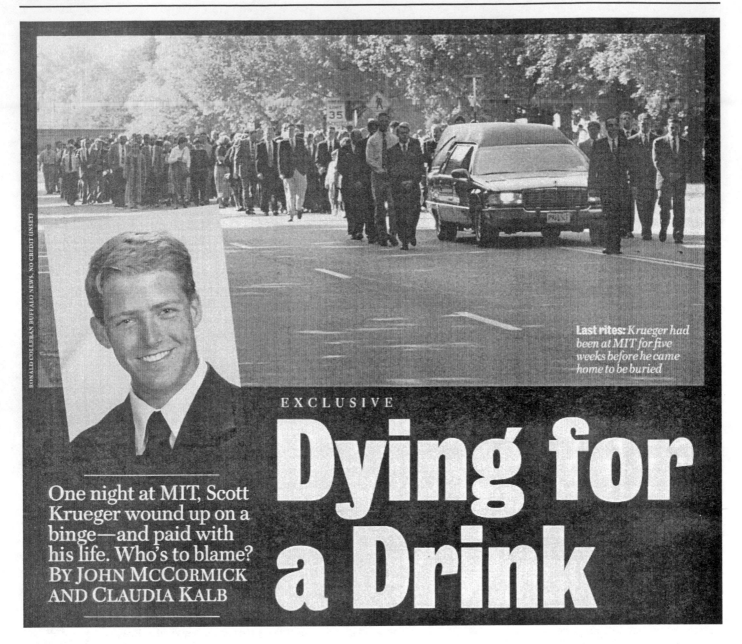

Last rites: *Krueger had been at MIT for five weeks before he came home to be buried*

RONALD COLLERAN BUFFALO NEWS: NO CREDIT (INSET)

EXCLUSIVE

Dying for a Drink

One night at MIT, Scott Krueger wound up on a binge—and paid with his life. Who's to blame?
BY JOHN MCCORMICK AND CLAUDIA KALB

O N THE EVENING OF FRIDAY, Sept. 26, 1997, Katie Krueger spent 37 minutes on the telephone with her twin brother, Scott. Katie, a freshman at Ithaca College in New York, was frustrated by conflicting medical advice she'd received about a knee injury. Scott, speaking from his MIT fraternity house in Boston, tried to soothe her. "Katie, I know you're upset," he said. "Forget about it. Go out and have some fun." In the background, frat brothers told Scott it was time for an event with his pledge class. "If you're upset later," he said, "we'll be here drinking. I won't be able to give you logical answers, but I can listen."

Coming from a kid who hadn't been a big drinker, Scott's words troubled Katie. Be careful, she said. He replied that he would—but, Scott told her, "the class has to drink a collective amount."

The call that every parent fears came seven hours later, at 1 a.m. Saturday, to the upscale Buffalo suburb of Orchard Park. An ER nurse in Boston told Darlene Krueger that her son, MIT Class of '01, was in "very critical condition" with alcohol poisoning. Darlene frantically dialed Conrail trainmasters across New York State. They managed to pull her husband, Bob, off an overnight coal train he was driving to Syracuse. Around

5 a.m. she called Katie and her older daughter, Kelly, also a student in Ithaca: "Your brother is dying in a Boston hospital. Your dad is on the road. He'll pick you up in an hour." At 7:22, Darlene and a friend boarded a US Airways flight east. Maybe, they prayed, it's not so bad. Maybe we'll find a sheepish Scott, sitting up in bed.

Instead they found a boy in a coma, his hair caked with vomit. A ventilator pumped his breaths, and an IV line pushed fluids. Darlene, devastated, caressed her son. "My sweetheart, my baby, I'd have done anything to trade places with him," she recalls. "But you can't do a damn thing except pray, and

After Darlene Krueger's comatose son left his frat in an ambulance, one of the brothers told her, 'You have to understand—this was a *very* big night at our fraternity house.'

hug him, and kiss him, and tell him you just want him to be Scott again." She kept her vigil for 57 hours. On Monday, Scott Steven Krueger died—a victim of "binge drinking."

Who's to blame? For eight months, a grand jury in Boston has quietly investigated the case, the most famous example of a troubling national trend. Binge drinking is medically defined as frequently downing five or more drinks at a time. Alcohol and students have always been a combustible mix. But in a number of cases, from MIT to LSU, the collegiate culture of drinking seems to be moving from keg parties to industrial-strength guzzling. Annual casualties include an estimated 50 deaths and hundreds of alcohol poisonings. For university administrators, this is difficult terrain: there is a limit to what schools can do to control excessive student drinking.

The Krueger case, however, could set an unprecedented standard of accountability for college officials across the country. Legal experts say that the grand jury has four basic options, one of which is to conclude there was no crime. But the length of the probe suggests another outcome. The jury could indict members of the fraternity who were present that night. Or it could settle on more removed targets, like the alumni group that owns the house. The most dramatic possibility is that grand jurors could indict MIT officials, or the university itself, for involuntary manslaughter.

A manslaughter charge could rely less on details of the incident than on whether MIT should have done something to avert it. Unlike most schools, which assign freshmen to dormitories, MIT lets incoming students choose dorms or Greek houses within days of their arrival on campus. (About one third of MIT's undergraduates belong to fraternities or sororities.) Campus critics have long warned that it puts freshmen into a Greek system rife with alcohol

abuses. "MIT dropped Scott into a maze that led him and many others to be living in a dangerous place," says Leo Boyle, the Krueger family's Boston attorney.

MIT denies that its policies put anyone in danger. Students prize their freedom to choose housing, Rosalind Williams, the school's dean of students and undergraduate education, told NEWSWEEK. Freshmen are guaranteed a dorm room if they want one. "We simply do not push students into fraternities," Williams says. MIT trusts students to intelligently take, or leave, Greek life. Students and faculty have rejected proposals to change its housing system, she says, adding that there is no evidence that doing so would prevent a death. In recent years the school has stepped up efforts to educate students about binge drinking, which Williams says is less prevalent at MIT than elsewhere. After this tragedy—the first such death in the school's history—Williams says that MIT has intensified its campaign to curb alcohol abuses.

Behind the legal turmoil lies the human story of Scott Krueger. His family, which has not previously spoken out, agreed to be interviewed for this NEWSWEEK reconstruction of the case. It's the tale of a promising young man's early death—and of his parents' refusal to let the matter rest. One day after a doctor shut off Scott's ventilator, the Kruegers claimed his body in a casketlike cremation box. But they didn't ship him back to Buffalo. He was still a part of the family. They insisted on driving him home, 465 miles, in the rear of their 1988 Buick station wagon. They arrived, exhausted, too late to stop at a funeral home. Darlene didn't want to leave her son alone. So she crawled in the back of the Buick, beside Scott, and spent the rest of the night.

His funeral four days later drew 400 mourners. Midway through, Pastor Dennis Conrad abruptly called for another refrain of the hymn "On Eagle's

Wings." He had just spotted 20 or so of Scott's fraternity brothers, fresh off a bus from Boston, filing into the church. Conrad was stalling, resolute that they hear every word of his sermon. "We are grieving for a brilliant, beautiful, Christ-centered man who was killed by a system," he thundered. "A system that funnels young men fresh away from home into fraternity houses, that builds manhood and brotherhood through alcohol consumption and parties."

Who was Scott Krueger? A young man both breezy and complicated, aware of his uncommon talent but, unlike so many other smart kids, never crippled by it. The Kruegers' four-bedroom colonial, purchased from one of the Buffalo Bills, is on the modest side—fitting for a railroad engineer and his wife, a former math teacher who runs a small computer business. The Kruegers' four kids attended Orchard Park High, a first-tier public school. All were top students, gifted in math and sciences; teachers murmured that it was always good to find a Krueger on next year's class list.

Scott was a star at OPHS. He got into so many advanced courses that friends called him "Skippy." Eager for a special chem class the school didn't offer, he recruited enough kids to justify the course—and then made them promise not to drop it. His writing style was complex, so much so that he was accused of plagiarism. "That would happen the first couple of papers each year," says Jon Wolf, an OPHS guidance counselor. "Then the teachers would realize what they had here." Pressed by one instructor to write conversationally, Scott refused to "dumb down" his work. Wolf and others warned Krueger that his stubbornness was hurting his grades. He wouldn't buckle. Even so, he finished seventh in a class of 339. Grade-point average: 97.644.

In his senior year, Scott hung a list of top engineering schools on his family's refrigerator. He applied to six: Penn, Cornell, Rochester, Rensselaer, Michigan and MIT. As the acceptances rolled in, he narrowed his choices to Cornell, where he'd be near his sisters, and MIT. In April 1997 he rode with a friend, John Bevilacqua III, to see the MIT campus. "He knew MIT was the best," Katie says. "But he worried it was too nerdy." The students were a pleasant surprise. "They weren't all geeks," Bevilacqua says. The boys walked the fabled "Infinite Corridor" and eavesdropped on a class about fracture points in stress analysis. They also accepted an offer from Alpha Tau Omega to spend a night in a frat house. Frat life appealed to Krueger. The older brothers could help him negotiate MIT.

He decided to head to Boston. MIT answered his acceptance with the usual volley of literature, some of it laying out housing options. Soon the frats began recruiting Scott—dozens of phone calls, with tempting offers of trips and parties. The sales pitches were clear: dorms are for girls and dorks, frats are for athletes. Scott, who planned to join the crew and lacrosse teams, studied the housing info during a camping trip to the Adirondacks. Next to the blurbs on each frat, he jotted his impressions in the tight print of an architect: "Not bad," "Kinda dorky," "Doesn't sound like me." Beneath the blurb for Phi Gamma Delta—Fiji, as it's known on campuses nationwide—he wrote, "More than half varsity. Sounds good!"

Summer brought the usual rites: artfully dodging hard labor and partying with friends. Working as a golf-course groundskeeper, he and a friend mounted weed-whacker wars that left his thighs covered with slashes. The parties sometimes included beer-drinking. Scott's parents didn't know about that, but Kelly saw him once when he'd clearly been drinking.

BY ALL ACCOUNTS, THOUGH, HE grew up on the dry side of average. In Orchard Park, "the big drinkers identify themselves in a lot of different ways," says Wolf. In the months since Scott's death, no other kids have confided that Scott drank regularly. Krueger's friends say that's because he didn't. "Scott wasn't prepared for a big drinking experience," Wolf says. Kelly agrees: "He had very little, if any, experience with hard liquor before he went to school." Scott's parents didn't think they needed to warn him about new risks he might encounter. "I didn't go to college," Bob says. "There weren't fraternities at Darlene's state teachers college." Mostly, he trusted his son's judgment. "We'd had *no* trouble with Scott," he says. "My big worry was that he was colorblind—I thought he'd go through a stop sign and hit a tree . . . I wasn't well versed on college life. I didn't think I had to be, with my son going to a place like MIT."

Out of Control: The Bingeing Phenomenon

Many college students, particularly white athletes who join fraternities or sororities, drink heavily. Below, the percentage of students in each category who binge:

Age		Race		Participation in sports	
Under 21	45%	White	48%	Nonparticipant	36%
21–23	48	Hispanic	38	Participant	54
24+	28	Nat. Amer. Nat. Alask.	34	Team leader	58
College residences		Asian/Pacific islander	21	**Attitude**	
Fraternity/sorority	84%	African-American	16	Frequent bingers who think they drink lightly/moderately	
Coed dorm	52	**Gender**			
Off-campus housing	40	Male	50%	Male	91%
Single-sex dorm	38	Female	39	Female	78

SOURCES: HARVARD SCHOOL OF PUBLIC HEALTH, JOURNAL OF AMERICAN COLLEGE HEALTH

Scott's family drove him to MIT on Wednesday, Aug. 20. He wasn't required to report until Thursday, but he wanted extra time to look for housing. Fraternity rush began Friday night. That Sunday, he called home to say he wanted to pledge Fiji. "Whoa! I want to see what this place is like," Darlene told him. Scott said there was no time: "If I don't take the room, someone else will." He quickly moved into the house. When his parents visited him the next weekend, they were surprised that Fiji was a 25-minute walk south of MIT's campus.

Fiji had a reputation as one of the hardest-partying fraternities at MIT. In prior school years, Boston police had been called to quell loud bashes, one of them involving a crowd estimated at up to 2,000. (Williams, the MIT dean, says the school temporarily banned alcohol and social activities at Fiji for those offenses: "It was not a situation that was at all neglected." Bill Martin, executive director of Fiji's national headquarters in Lexington, Ky., says he can't respond to allegations until Fiji can complete its own investigation.) There is no evidence that Scott was unhappy with his choice of MIT or Fiji. "Scott was excited by everything going on at MIT," says Kelly. He told Denise Jewell, a friend at Boston University, that Fiji was "the best fraternity, the best guys."

The Kruegers don't know what, precisely, happened to their son on Sept. 26. His blood-alcohol level was .41—five times the drunken-driving standard in Massachusetts. A reading that high suggests a rapid infusion of alcohol in

toxic quantities that can overwhelm the central nervous system. Richard Schwartzstein, the doctor who oversaw his treatment at Beth Israel Deaconess Medical Center, believes Scott drank beer, Scotch and rum. Attorneys for several fraternity members have declined comment on what happened to Krueger.

Darlene didn't learn much when she called Fiji 90 minutes after the ambulance departed. She says one member told her, "You have to understand—this was a *very* big night at our fraternity house." Another said that Scott fell asleep while drinking and then got sick, so the brothers moved him to a couch in his basement room. "You left my son passed out and throwing up?" she shot back. The young man's answer: "We weren't gone long, Mrs. Krueger. We just went up to have another drink."

According to notes Darlene scribbled during the call, the Fijis returned to find Scott "turning purple." Vomit, including pieces of pizza, blocked his windpipe. At some point, his heart quit beating. The Fijis had called MIT police, who alerted Boston 911. Schwartzstein says ER personnel managed to restart his heart. But an infuriated Darlene couldn't learn how long it might have stopped—a clue to how damaged his brain and organs would be.

When she reached Boston, Darlene got her first briefing in a tiny hospital waiting room. Outside were three Fijis who'd spent the night there. Scott was unchanged. Inhaling his own vomit had seriously damaged his lungs. A CT scan detected swelling of the brain. A neurologist who examined him said little but looked worried. "When will he come out of this?" Darlene asked. The answer: "We don't know if he will." Darlene begged: "Just fix my kid!"

Bob and the couple's three other children—Kelly, Katie and younger brother Jeff—arrived in midafternoon. By Saturday night the Kruegers had been visited by an MIT dean—and by Boston homicide detectives who had learned that Scott might not survive. Sunday brought better news: the doctor was guardedly optimistic. But by midafternoon Scott's pupils had grown large and fixed. His cortex pushed down on his brain stem. More tests confirmed that Scott would not survive. Late Sunday, the Kruegers concluded that their son would die the next day.

Scott's kidneys were shutting down, his face was puffy, his pupils wildly dilated. It was time for his family to make the call. His siblings argued that if he could, Scott would sit up and say, "Get this junk off me." Darlene resisted. She wouldn't relent until everything that would happen after Scott's death—the autopsy, the embalming—had been planned. The last detail was making sure everyone knew the family would be taking Scott home. "He's going in our car," Darlene announced. "No questions asked."

A NURSE WASHED SCOTT'S HAIR. His family gathered around, parents on one side of his bed, siblings on the other. Final tests confirmed no brain-stem function. At 6:40 p.m., Schwartzstein announced, "I'm pronouncing him dead at this time." He detached the ventilator tube from a shorter endotrachial tube sticking out of Scott's mouth, and switched off the respiration, heartbeat and blood-pressure alarms that otherwise would quickly sound. Twenty minutes later, a computer monitor over Scott's bed signaled that his vitals had flat-lined.

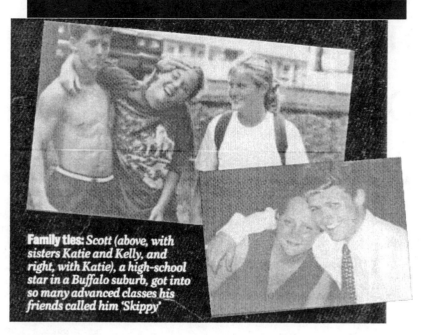

'I wasn't well-versed on college life,'' Scott's father says. 'I didn't think I had to be, with my son going to a place like MIT.'

Family ties: *Scott (above, with sisters Katie and Kelly, and right, with Katie), a high-school star in a Buffalo suburb, got into so many advanced classes his friends called him 'Skippy'*

The next morning, a family friend named Bob Clement took Scott's siblings to the Fiji house. The frat brothers had Scott's belongings boxed and waiting. The Fijis looked chastened—and anxious. A few stepped forward to apologize. They carried the boxes to two cars and helped fend off TV crews.

The Kruegers' chance to help Scott select a college, and a place to live, is long past. But if they could, Darlene says, they would put to use all they've learned. They would visit hospital emergency rooms near campuses. They'd chat up the nurses and ask how often kids arrive with alcohol poisoning. Next stop: the local police, for a fill on what the night shift has to deal with. Then

they'd quiz the admissions office on what is often an afterthought: the details of student housing.

The Kruegers now live amid the relics of Scott's life. His school awards fill a Compaq computer box. In the dining room sits a huge plant from the president of the Fiji house, with a card inscribed, "My warmest and deepest sympathy." The Kruegers keep it as a bitter remembrance. John Bevilacqua remembers Scott talking about why he chose the Massachusetts school. "If I go to Cornell," he told Bevilacqua, "I'll always wonder what would have happened if I'd gone to MIT." Now those who knew Scott Krueger are left to wonder just the opposite.

College students drunk on campus drinking lore, tradition

By Linda Temple
Special for USA TODAY

Spring break's splashy metamorphosis into a week-long public drunk has made it one of the most recognizable of today's college drinking rituals.

Meanwhile, evidence indicates that student drinking is out of control, from the string of agonizing campus deaths that closed out 1997 to the more recent news from Harvard researchers that nearly half of today's college students are binge drinkers.

But while worried adults scramble to dry out the campus, students defend alcohol's ritualized role, handing down their high-octane traditions to the 1 million new freshmen entering U.S. colleges every year.

"The first time I got seriously drunk at college was during Welcome Week," said Brian Kemppainen, a senior at Michigan State University, Lansing. "A street was blocked off, and about 2,000 of us were down there every night, with kegs at every house. It was a really big deal."

On nearly every campus there are rituals to be learned and songs to be sung.

"Fill the steins to dear old Maine" begins the University of Maine's drinking anthem. University of California at Berkeley students sing, "And when the game is over we will buy a keg of booze, and drink to California 'til we wobble in our shoes."

Ivy Leaguers at the University of Pennsylvania toast dear, old Penn with "a highball at nightfall," and even a newly minted rambling wreck from Georgia Tech knows that a hell of an engineer will "drink his whisky clear."

Students say that when they find themselves surrounded by drinkers—85% of those on today's campuses—the warnings they've been pummeled with since childhood become a distant echo.

"Alcohol has been so demonized, of course it's attractive," said University of Colorado at Boulder senior Andrew Simons.

On campus it's as common as ketchup. "During the first month or so you're scared to get caught with it," said Fred Dill, a senior at Ball State University in Indiana, "but pretty soon it's all around you."

They've seen the headlines, but most feel the risks are exaggerated.

"A few freak accidents and all of a sudden it's a big issue," said Michigan State's Kemppainen. "People are going to drink, and nothing's going to change that."

"Most of the people dying are inexperienced freshmen," said Jason Dimberg, 22, a California State Polytechnic University senior. "If I drank then as much as I drink now, I'd have been in the hospital on a daily basis. You throw up and pass out, but eventually your tolerance increases."

Epic acts of alcoholic stupidity form the basis of a rich oral history, and the most legendary excesses are burnished and passed down like treasured heirlooms.

"My sister used to tell us how drunk she got and how people had to carry her home," said Mitchell Whaley, a University of Mississippi senior. "I brought to college the mind-set that the more you're drinking, the more fun you're having."

"During slide shows, the fraternities show you what their parties are like and how crazy they can get," said sophomore Mac Monteith, 19, also of Mississippi. "You think, 'I want to be that crazy. I want to be in some of these pictures next year.'"

Shot glasses and beer mugs stamped with school crests and mascots can be scooped from campus bookstore shelves along with the textbooks and other essentials. "People line them up on their dorm windowsills," said Dianne Reis, 18, a Penn State freshman. "But they're pretty much for show. Everybody drinks out of plastic."

Fake IDs can be snapped up for as little as $20, and although about 60 percent of underage college drinkers said they carry them, many said using them is hardly necessary.

"Most people just go to frat parties or dorms," said Erin Matts, 21, a junior at Colgate University in Hamilton, N.Y. Residence advisers, purportedly the front line in the war on dorm drinking, have always made lousy cops, she said.

"We had parties all the time. Our RA didn't care."

One "bought a keg for us," said Jeff Parker, a senior at Creighton University in Omaha. The RA then disabled an alarm so the beer could be hoisted through a fire escape, he said. "They understand."

Steve Kline, director of public relations and information at Creighton, said: "We require that our students obey laws regarding alcohol use. Illegal or inappropriate use of alcohol is prohibited.

"We do have some resources in place to assist students who might have alcohol problems."

Consequences for getting caught range from written warnings to mandatory alcohol counseling, and while repeat offenders can be ousted from a dorm and even expelled, such cases are reportedly rare.

"If you get caught by somebody who gives a damn, they usually just tell you to pour it out," said Mississippi's Monteith.

Amid the flourishing alcohol task forces and high-profile aversion strategies are many well-entrenched double standards, students said.

"This is supposedly a dry campus, but you see people drinking on the porch of the president's house," said senior Dimberg of Cal Poly. Kegs are toted into the gym for the pre-game parties of alumni, he said. "The rules only apply to some people."

Alumni, whose donations make up as much as a third of some college budgets and total nearly $3 billion nationally, "would go ballistic" if liquor bans were enforced, said University of Mississippi senior Whaley.

Drinking in his school's venerable Grove before football games is a revered alumni tradition, he said. "You can't bite the hand that feeds you."

Alumni aren't the only adults who drink with students. Creighton junior Scott Anderson said he and his 21-and-over classmates went drinking at their professor's invitation last fall. "He's such a cool guy that it didn't surprise me. He used to be in a chapter of my fraternity."

Such customs date to the ancient Greeks, said University of Colorado senior Simons. "Plato used to get drunk with Socrates. It's always been a part of the culture."

More visible Greek traditions are under high-profile attack. Many students feel that the watering down of their fraternity rituals is designed to shield schools from liability, not safeguard students' health.

With things heating up on Greek row, many students are simply drinking elsewhere.

Sports clubs and other social groups are helping fill the breach, and club-sponsored trips on beer-stocked buses to ski resorts and beaches are increasingly popular.

Many universities are promoting alcohol-free events, but students said response has been flat.

"Nobody goes to them, not even nondrinkers," said Bob Wahl, a sophomore at Florida State University, Tallahassee. "People who don't drink want to be where everybody else is. They just go to regular parties and don't drink."

Calls for abstinence have a hypocritical ring, students said, in a society where drinkers make up a nearly two-thirds majority. "Alcohol is a way of life for people in general, not just college students," said Chris Brown, 22, of the University of Colorado.

"Some people feel they need to regulate our morality," said sophomore Michael Zivin of Cornell University in Ithaca, N.Y. "But we're not party animals, just stressed-

Parents urged to open eyes to campus drinking problem

USA TODAY

It is not the problem drinkers but their parents who are in denial.

Nearly half the students surveyed in a recent Harvard study said they frequently binge on alcohol, but fewer than 8 percent of parents believe that their college kids have a drinking problem, another study says.

"It's half imagination and half hope," said David Burns, director of the latter study at Rutgers University in New Jersey and currently head of a health education program for the Association of American Colleges and Universities in Washington, D.C.

"Once parents assure themselves their child is not a problem drinker, they tend not to discuss the issue with them," he said, citing this lack of dialogue at home as a factor in the escalating problem on campus.

Donna Shalala, secretary of Health and Human Services, agreed. "Parents are shocked by what they're seeing, but with nearly 50 percent of our students being binge drinkers, everybody's young person is at risk," she told USA TODAY in an interview Friday.

"Parents need to talk to their young people and ask college officials what's going on," said Shalala, a former college president who was chancellor at the University of Wisconsin at the time of her 1993 appointment to the Cabinet. "Changing the culture of campus drinking is going to take an enormous, com-

prehensive effort, and it has to start now."

Burns, an expert on college drinking, has written a workbook, "College, Alcohol and Choices: An Essential Conversation Guide for Parents and Students" (1996, Wisconsin Clearinghouse for Prevention Resources, 800-322-1468, $24.95) to help families develop a common basis for discussion and to prepare students for what they'll find on campus.

"Whether they drink or not, they still have to negotiate the culture," Burns said. "At home, people aren't throwing up in their bedrooms, but that's exactly what they're about to come in contact with."

The book describes scenarios students may confront in college, options for dealing with them and the skills that will help get them through—topics that are unlikely to be discussed with them once they leave home, he said.

Liability-wary colleges are set up "to avoid entanglement with the problem, not engage with it directly," he said, and it doesn't help that students are the targets of "an unremitting campaign by alcohol manufacturers to get them to drink."

Students will have to solve the college drinking problem for themselves, Burns said. "We have to stop simply making rules and preaching at them and start helping them strengthen their own capacity to manage their lives.

"That is where I believe the solutions are going to come from."

out students who need to unwind on the weekends."

"It would be hard to imagine college without alcohol," said Matts of Colgate. "People think, 'When I get out, I won't be a staggering drunk four nights a week.' But

I'm young, these are my golden years, and I'm going to have as much fun as possible because as soon as I'm out I'll have to bust my tail."—*Contributing: Emily Boling at the University of Mississippi, Oxford, and Heidi Juersivich at Creighton University, Omaha.*

Party Politics

Students stand up for their right to drink.

By Ryan Lizza

Adam Herringa comes from a family of fighters: his great-great-grandfather was a Union cavalryman in the Civil War, and his father volunteered for Korea. So perhaps it is not surprising that Herringa, a 22-year-old recent graduate of Michigan State University, was a principal organizer of one of the largest college demonstrations in recent memory, a 3,000-strong student uprising that convulsed MSU on May 1. And the noble idea behind this act of rebellion? It was a protest against a ban on alcohol at a popular football game tailgating spot. In Herringa's view, tailgaters are being victimized by administrators bent on forcing young people to conform. "They tend to scapegoat alcohol whenever they want to crack down on something," he says. "They use the guise of binge drinking to control issues on campus."

And the outburst at MSU was merely the largest of at least nine alcohol-related disturbances on campuses this spring. At Washington State University this May, a mob of undergraduates, dissatisfied with an alcohol ban at fraternities, assaulted police officers with beer cans and rocks—injuring two dozen officers. In April, students clashed with police over two days at the University of Connecticut, setting fires and vandalizing 27 police cars during an annual weekend of partying. At bucolic Ohio University, in what is becoming a tradition known locally as "the fracas," about 2,000 students took to the streets early on April 5, launching an attack on police to protest the loss of one hour's worth of drinking caused by the shift to daylight saving time.

At some colleges it was the most raucous semester since 1968, and—to hear pro-booze activists like Adam Herringa describe it—it was characterized by the same level of righteousness. Of course the college officials imposing new alcohol rules have a slightly different perspective—informed by the law as well as a well-publicized string of alcohol-related campus deaths. The Massachusetts Institute of Technology or its officials, for example, could face charges of involuntary manslaughter because a drunk student reportedly left alone in a basement by his fraternity brothers passed out, began to vomit, and then choked until his breathing stopped. He died two days later. (MIT says, in a press release, that,

while the student's death was a tragedy, it cannot be held responsible for it. The school also emphasizes that there is "no legal precedent" for bringing criminal charges and that doing so "would be the worst message to send to universities.")

In the last 15 months, according to the Center for Science in the Public Interest, 18 inebriated students have died in alcohol-related mishaps like falling out of windows, falling into rivers, falling down flights of stairs, or simply choking on their own vomit. A 1994 study of almost 18,000 students nationwide, conducted by the Harvard psychologist Henry Wechsler, found that nearly half of the nation's young scholars are binge-drinkers, meaning it's normal for men to chug five or more drinks, and women four or more, in a night. Little wonder that, in survey after survey, college presidents rank drinking as the number one problem on campus.

It wasn't always so. For years universities have been reluctant to take on the extra responsibilities that go along with comprehensive alcohol policies for one reason: liability. Paradoxically, every measure a college adopted to protect a student from the dangers of drinking made the college that much more vulnerable to negligence claims. A string of court decisions reinforced this logic by ruling that colleges were not babysitters and thus were not responsible for controlling private student conduct. (The legal principle of in loco parentis doesn't apply.)

Now schools find themselves in a bind. They're under increasing pressure to crack down on campus drinking, even though doing so would increase their liability. Even the federal government has gotten into the act. In January Donna Shalala, the secretary of health and human services (and former University of Wisconsin chancellor), implored NCAA officials to disassociate themselves from the alcohol industry. Senators Joseph Biden and Robert Byrd, and Representative Joe Kennedy are all sponsoring anti-college-drinking measures on Capitol Hill.

 From *The New Republic*, July 13, 1998, pp. 12-13. © 1998 by The New Republic, Inc. Reprinted by permission.

To Adam Herringa and his companions, this all smacks of overreaction. The issue, Herringa insists, is not drinking per se but rather the fact that colleges set alcohol policy without first consulting students. "We felt alienated," he says, citing a litany of administrative abuses: First, Michigan State shortened the notoriously bacchanalian student orientation period from a week to just a few days. Then, the school banned kegs from tailgate parties at the now infamous Munn Field. ("If they would've just kept kegs," Herringa says with exasperation. "By eliminating one problem they created another.") In hindsight, even the administrators agree that they should have let students in on the decisions. "We're not accepting blame for the riots, but I do believe that communication was definitely a factor," says MSU spokesperson Kristan Tetens.

But the total ban on alcohol did strike at the heart of the student body's most treasured pastime—getting drunk before football games. So, using e-mail, Herringa and a friend organized what they billed as both a "vigil/protest" and "one last party" at Munn Field. For a week the e-mail ricocheted around campus until the entire city of East Lansing was buzzing with anticipation of the Friday night protest. "It just exploded," Herringa says. Soon it wasn't just a party but a revolutionary struggle. By Thursday an op-ed in the school newspaper was calling on students to "stand [and] fight against tyranny" and the "demonizing hegemony."

What occurred was, perhaps, a shade less heroic. A drunken mob gathered until police ordered them off the field. Protesters then decided to march on the university president's home, chanting the MSU fight song and anti-University of Michigan slogans along the way. Then the chief of police stood outside President Peter McPherson's home and addressed the crowd: The president, it turned out, was away for the evening and would not be seeing them. The peaceful vigil descended into a violent riot: Protesters set bonfires and pelted police with bottles and rocks for several hours, until around dawn, when most of the bonfires were extinguished and bursts of tear gas sent the crowds home. Herringa says he was "proud" to be a part of the march, even though he declined to take part in the violence.

Needless to say, older generations of student protesters are not altogether impressed with the self-proclaimed heirs to their tradition. "I think it's pathetic," says Todd Gitlin, the '60s chronicler and former Students for a Democratic Society leader. "There is a certain population who couldn't think of anything more wholesome than fighting for the right to party." In a way, what today's alcohol protests are about is preserving university "traditions" that revolve around booze. (Drinking has always been associated with some college rites of passage. Wechsler likes to point out that in colonial times Harvard University's graduation procession was led by the county sheriff precisely because the University could count on him to control the inebriated graduates.) One of the University of Virginia's quaint customs is the annual Foxfield Races, described by the campus newspaper, The Cavalier Daily, as a "twenty-year tradition of drunken debauchery." Then, there's the "fourth-year fifth," a ritual where seniors down a fifth of a gallon of hard liquor before the start of the last home football game of the year.

Yet today what parents and the media are noticing are the costs of these rites of passage. On any given weekend, about ten UVA revelers seek shelter at the campus emergency room for alcohol-related problems. An average of one to three students die alcohol-related deaths each year. Those sobering statistics and the widely reported death of a student forced UVA to admit there was a problem. "The death of Leslie Baltz"—a student who fell down a flight of stairs after apparently drinking her fourth-year fifth—"was the major impetus for pulling together a[n alcohol] task force," says UVA director of student health, Dr. James Turner.

When fraternities at Virginia were faced with a choice between banning alcohol or pushing the recruitment of new pledges back from the fall to the spring, they chose the latter, despite the huge financial loss it caused. "They chose kegs over money," says Jay Conti, the editor-in-chief of The Cavalier Daily. The fraternity leadership had little choice: Their members threatened a massive protest. It's not just the students whose habits die hard. In May, when an alcohol-policy task force recommended banning booze at tailgate parties, which are technically illegal but have been tolerated by authorities for years, the school's own president, John T. Casteen III, defended the parties as "activities that many here cherish." Alumni also joined in supporting the pre-game bashes. As an old Virginia joke goes, "Whenever two or three UVA students come together, there is bound to be a fifth."

Of course, UVA has not witnessed the kind of rebellions that occurred at schools like Michigan State and Ohio University this year. "It takes a lot to get people riled up and excited at this school," says Jay Conti. "It would take banning alcohol to have a riot here." And UVA's not likely to do that anytime soon. In fact, some universities are licking their wounds and reevaluating their recent crackdowns. At Michigan State, Adam Herringa was invited onto a special "action team" to ensure student participation in future alcohol policymaking. He is triumphant: "If it took a riot to form the action team, then so be it," he says. "I have no regrets."

SOCIETY

The Real Scandal

The greatest threat to international sport isn't payoffs in Salt Lake. It's 'doping,' the use of dangerous performance-enhancing drugs. Do officials turn a blind eye?

BY SHARON BEGLEY AND MARTHA BRANT

IT STARTED TO GO WRONG FOR FRENCH cyclist Erwan Menthéour between Paris and Nice, when race officials tapped him for random drug testing. Just before the 1997 competition, he had taken erythropoietin (EPO), an anemia drug that increases the number of red cells in the blood and thus an athlete's endurance. Menthéour's trainer and doctor swung into action, desperately trying to thin out his blood before he gave a blood sample. They started an IV drip of chilled glucose. They bled him. But still he tested positive. He was thrown off the racing circuit—but not for long. He claimed that his red count seemed high not because he'd taken EPO but because he had had diarrhea and was dehydrated. Menthéour was back on his wheels in two weeks. In fact, his excuses were all a sham: for almost as long as he'd been racing, Menthéour tells NEWSWEEK, he had been taking drugs ("doping") to improve his performance. "For two years I took EPO, growth hormone, anabolic steroids, testosterone, amphetamine," he says. "Just about everything. That was part of the job."

The drumbeat of scandal has filled newscasts and sports pages all year, with revelation after revelation about the Salt Lake City Olympics organizing committee spreading around money and other favors to win the 2002 Games. But a little graft in Utah pales beside what a growing number of coaches, trainers, officials and athletes call the real scandal in sports. The greatest threat to the image, integrity and even the continued existence of elite-level international competi-

tions from the World Cup to the Tour de France to the Olympic Games themselves is the use of illicit performance-enhancing drugs. "Doping" among world-class competitors is rampant, admit many athletes, and the governing bodies of individual sports, as well as the International Olympic Committee, turn a blind eye. "The IOC," charges epidemiologist Charles Yesalis of Pennsylvania State University, an expert on Olympic doping, "has known about the drug epidemic in sport for the last 40 years and has covered it up. There is no difference between the bribery scandal and the drug epidemic in the Olympics. They are intertwined."

Only the most naive sports fan can still be shocked—shocked!—that drugs and athletes go together like socks and sweat. The pressure to win is crushing, the millisecond difference between gold and silver can amount to millions in endorsement contracts and appearance fees and the banning of doping agents in some sports but not others introduces a moral loophole that a trainer can drive a relay team through. Small wonder, then, that one athlete after another is getting nailed for doping. But even more seem to be getting away with it. In part, that reflects the ever more sophisticated ruses trainers and coaches use to elude the IOC's drug-testing system, which has been part of the Games since 1968.

But new evidence emerging in the wake of the Salt Lake City scandal suggests that the IOC and some sport federations, far from being the stalwart defenders of the purity of athleticism, are soft on drugs. Critics con-

tend that the IOC, for instance, has sometimes discarded positive results, fearing they would tarnish the image of the Games. And the IOC continues to use ineffective testing methods that athletes can outwit and challenge. Last week, at the IOC's World Conference on Doping in Sport in Lausanne, Switzerland, this dirty little secret exploded into public view. There, representatives of federations that run such sports as cycling, soccer and track and field failed to reach agreement on a mandatory two-year ban for doping: sports organizations led by soccer and cycling vetoed that as too draconian. Delegates couldn't even agree on how to establish an international anti-doping agency, which was the ostensible purpose of the conference, in large part because European and American sports officials balked at letting the IOC run it. Afterward, Canadian swimmer Mark Tewksbury—three-time Olympic medalist, member of the Canadian Olympic Association and of international swimming's athlete commission—resigned his Olympics posts in protest over "the inability of the IOC to seriously clean its own house." He told NEWSWEEK, "If there's bribery in [selecting] Olympic cities, there's bribery in drug testing."

The IOC flat-out denies that. Since 1967, the IOC's medical code has prohibited doping, which it defines as the use of "substances belonging to prohibited classes of pharmacological agents and/or the use of prohibited methods." Since the 1968 Summer Games in Mexico City, the IOC has been routinely testing competitors for these

---

The pressure to win is crushing; medals can be worth millions of dollars

Mark Tewksbury, Swimmer
The gold medalist quit the Canadian Olympic Association over the IOC's drug stance.

Going for the Gold: Hard Work, Dedication—and Drugs

Some Olympic athletes are turning to a new breed of performance-enhancing substances that are invisible to official tests. The first three described below, human growth hormone, erythropoietin and testosterone, have quickly become the most popular of these drugs. But athletes are still getting caught for more traditional violations such as steroids and stimulants:

Blood testing
The IOC doesn't take blood from its athletes. "I don't think it's going to happen," said one doctor.

Pros Drug concentrations are higher in blood, so drugs are easier to detect.

Cons It's invasive and samples must be refrigerated. Also, there are religious issues.

Urine testing
This is the method that the Olympic committee uses to screen its athletes.

Pros Urine can be easily frozen and there aren't religious objections, as with blood.

Cons Urine samples aren't as concentrated, which makes doping easier to hide.

DRUG	WHAT DOES IT DO?	MASKING/DETECTION	RISKS
Human growth hormone (hGH)	Stimulates the intracellular breakdown of body fat, allowing more to be used for energy.	This is a natural hormone, so added amounts don't show up in blood or urine tests.	Muscle and bone disfigurement—jutting forehead, elongated jaw. Also: heart and metabolic problems.
Erythropoietin (EPO)	Increases the number of red blood cells without having to "dope" using one's own blood.	It's extremely difficult to detect because the extra blood cells are the athlete's own.	Extra cells can make blood the consistency of yogurt. This can lead to a clot, heart attack or stroke.
Testosterone	Used to build muscles. It lets the body recover quickly from strenuous exercise.	Rules allow up to five times the natural body level, giving athletes latitude.	Unnatural levels can cause heart disease, liver cancer and impotence.
Steroids/ androstenedione	Anabolic steroids are incarnations of testosterone; androstenedione is a precursor molecule.	Water-based steroids (most common) are undetectable in urine after several weeks.	Synthetic testosterone carries the same risks as naturally occurring testosterone.
Stimulants	The first category that the IOC tested for. They delay the symptoms of fatigue.	Stimulants such as amphetamines can be detected; diuretics can dilute them in urine.	Fatigue is the body saying "stop"— overriding that message can be dangerous.

agents. An athlete caught doping faces the loss of medals and a suspension from competition. Prince Alexandre de Merode, who has headed the IOC's Medical Commission for all of its 31 years, is unrepentant in the face of criticism of the IOC. "We are not speaking of the past," he said last week. "We have to speak of the future . . . This [conference] is the first time that I hear everybody saying doping is an important problem." He called his critics' charges "coldly insulting."

If doping is, as de Merode noticed, suddenly "an important problem," it is partly because the newest doping agents pose the risk of serious health problems, and even death. But the larger reason is that it is ridiculously easy to dope and not get caught. Doping and detection are like an arms race. First, trainers discover a performance-enhancing drug. Then, sports officials develop a test for it. Trainers retaliate by inventing a way to elude the detectors. So far, doping has stayed a lap ahead. "Undetectable drugs are 90 percent of estimated doping cases," says Hein Verbruggen, head of international cycling.

Czech tennis pro Petr Korda tested positive for the steroid nandrolone after the Wimbledon quarterfinals last May, for instance. (Protesting that he did not know how the chemicals got into his system, he avoided the one-year suspension the International Tennis Association is supposed to impose.) But American pro Jim Courier charged that steroids are far from the worst abuse in tennis. "EPO is the problem," Courier told NEWSWEEK. "I have pretty strong suspicions that guys are using it on the tour. I see guys who are out there week in and week out without taking rests. EPO can help you when it's the fifth set and you've been playing for four-and-a-half hours." Although the endurance-building effects of EPO last for about two weeks, its use can't be detected in urine at all or in blood for more than a day or so after the athlete stops taking it.

EPO is only one weapon in a pharmaceutical arsenal of performance-enhancing substances flowing through sports. Stimulants like amphetamines, ephedrine and caffeine were the first substances to land on the IOC's list of banned agents, and they're still popular. They provide a quick pop of energy, and so are a favorite of sprinters, cyclists and swimmers. They are an ingredient of many

asthma medications. Exercise-induced asthma has inexplicably stricken many Olympians, including 60 percent of the U.S. team in 1994, and medical use of stimulant inhalants is allowed. Are stimulants detectable? Sure, if your trainer's IQ matches his hat size. They clear the urine in hours, so all an athlete has to do is not take them too close to her event. If you've been using too soon before your race, there are always "masking agents." Probenecid, for one, inhibits substances from reaching the urine. And urine tests are all the IOC requires: blood tests, which can detect more substances, are deemed too invasive.

Anabolic steroids, almost all of them derivatives of the hormone testosterone, are the mothers of all doping agents. They build muscles. By most estimates, an athlete can improve strength at least 5 percent by taking steroids either orally or through injection during high-intensity training. Drug-detection machines, such as the high-resolution mass spectrometer used at the Atlanta Games in 1996, can be tuned to detect any synthetic steroid; the Atlanta lab tested for 100 different types. But the Dr. Feelgoods of sport can

Doing Whatever It Takes?

Many are using banned substances, athletes and observers say, but few are busted. Some athletes who've been involved in recent drug-related controversies:

Uta Pippig, Marathon
The three-time Boston Marathon champ was suspended by Germany's track-and-field federation last fall after testing positive for synthetic testosterone. Pippig says birth-control pills caused the high hormone levels.

Michelle Smith, Swimming
She thrilled Ireland and raised questions after soaring from obscurity to win three golds in Atlanta. Last April she was found guilty of tampering with an unannounced drug test and was suspended for four years.

Petr Korda, Tennis
The Czech tested positive for the steroid nandrolone after Wimbledon in May. He claimed he didn't know how it got in his body; citing 'exceptional circumstances,' the International Tennis Foundation didn't suspend him.

Randy Barnes, Track & Field
The 1996 Olympic shot-put champion was banned for life by USA Track and Field last summer for taking androstenedione. Barnes was banned once before, for two years, in 1989 after testing positive for methyltestosterone.

tinker with the molecular structure of common steroids, so they slip through. "There are 72 banned steroids," says one American coach who says he developed drug regimes for athletes in Atlanta, "but the testosterone molecule is changeable in millions of ways. All you have to do is make a steroid not on the list." Or, simply by going cold turkey a few weeks before competition, an athlete can get the muscle-bulking effects without getting caught. If that seems too chancy, athletes can use a diuretic. These drugs, which are also banned, dilute the urine. That makes illicit substances virtually undetectable.

More and more athletes are turning to the source of all steroids: testosterone itself. Natural levels vary, so sports federations and the IOC try to detect doping indirectly. They measure the relative amounts of testosterone and another natural steroid called epitestosterone. In most people, testosterone

levels are no more than twice epi levels. But to allow for individual variation, the IOC set the prohibited level at anything over 6 to 1. That means an athlete can dope himself up to, say, five times his normal testosterone levels, and get away with it. How much of an edge would that provide? A male athlete with a typical testosterone/epitestosterone ratio of 1.3 to 1 could boost that to 6 to 1, stay within the IOC limit and improve his performance at least 10 percent. Women, with a natural ratio of 2.5 to 1, could do even better, since they have less testosterone to begin with and so are more sensitive to added amounts. Testosterone can give women beards, deep voices and tough skin. It can make men's breasts swell and testicles shrivel.

The doping agents of choice today are substances that cannot be detected in urine: EPO and human growth hormone. Even though the performance-enhancing effects of hGH are unproved, many athletes believe it boosts energy. (Athletes dubbed the Atlanta Olympics "The Growth Hormone Games.") hGH can also cause grotesque skeletal deformations by stimulating abnormal bone growth. EPO, by increasing the production of red blood cells up to tenfold, can turn blood the consistency of yogurt, making it too thick to flow freely. The misuse of EPO has apparently killed at least 18 Dutch and Belgian cyclists since 1987.

A handful of other drugs have lower profiles but are popular among athletes looking for any edge. Plain old sodium bicarbonate postpones lactic-acid buildup, for instance, preventing muscle fatigue. Done two or three hours before a race, "soda loading" is especially popular among 400-, 800- and 1,500-meter runners, even though it's banned. Beta blockers, also banned, are cardiac drugs that slow the heart. They are popular among biathletes and archers who need steady hands. Since hands are steadier between beats, the longer the interval, the more time to aim and fire.

Although men do not seem to dope more than women, or vice versa, athletes in some sports dope more than others. "In some sports, such as cycling, it is not possible to compete if you are not using drugs," says Dr. Gabriele Rosa, who advises Kenyan runners. "The culture of doping is spreading to Nordic skiing and especially runners." Yet little is detected. Files collected by the East German secret police document that many of that country's athletes were soaked in anabolic steroids from at least 1969 on. Yet the IOC never once caught a single steroid-popping East German. And in the last decade 27 Chinese swimmers have tested positive, at world meets, for banned substances. The world swimming federation, regarded as tough on drugs, caught them. The IOC didn't.

At the Atlanta Games, several athletes tested positive for Probenecid, the banned masking agent. But the IOC took no action.

Ben Johnson, Track & Field
After testing positive for steroids during the '88 Olympics, the Canadian sprinter was stripped of his world records and later banned for life

Only two Olympians tested positive for steroids. But clinical pharmacologist Donald Catlin, who runs a drug-testing lab at UCLA and oversaw the Atlanta testing, said that other positive samples went unreported. "There were several other steroid positives from around the end of the Games," Catlin told a London newspaper. "I can think of no reason why they [were] not announced." Says one member of the USOC drug committee: "[IOC president Juan Antonio] Samaranch decided the Olympics were over after the last event. There would be no more testing." No confirmation tests were ordered for positive samples. De Merode said he chose not to follow up on positives because he did not trust the new $1 million mass spectrometers. Also, he said, the IOC feared that the results would not withstand legal challenge by an athlete, who could accuse the lab of mixing up or doctoring samples, O. J. Simpson-like.

Sergei Ivanov, Cycling
His Dutch TVM team quit the '98 Tour de France after drugs were found in their hotel; the TVM director and doctor were arrested

But critics suspect other motives may lead the IOC to tacitly allow drugs. "So many Olympic records were made with the help of drugs, and people like to see records broken," says a former American rower. "In some sports, like track and weight lifting, it is considered practically impossible to break records 'clean'." When Canadian sprinter Ben Johnson tested positive for steroids in Seoul in 1988, he was stripped of his gold medal and the Games suffered a black eye. "They will never let something like that be made public again," says Penn State's Yesalis. "The Olympics took such a terrible PR hit that superstars could have drugs oozing out of their eyeballs and the IOC still wouldn't call it." And the Olympics depend on sponsors. "It's very simple," charges John Leonard, executive director of the American

Zhang Yi, Swimming
One of four Chinese swimmers expelled from the 1998 World Championships and suspended for two years after testing positive for a diuretic

Swimming Coaches Association. "The IOC doesn't want sponsors to be unhappy, and sponsors are unhappy any time their brand name is tarnished. That's why the IOC doesn't want the full extent of doping revealed."

The depth of suspicions about the IOC became clear at the anti-doping conference in Lausanne last week. The IOC had called the meeting to establish an agency that would determine how and when to test for performance-enhancing drugs, establish penalties and get the international governing bodies of sports such as FINA (swimming) and IAAF (track and field) to agree to the same rules. The IOC also intended to control the new agency. It didn't work out that way. Politicians and sports officials from Europe and the United States demanded that the IOC keep an arm's length away from the agency. Said Danish Sport Minister Elsebeth Gerner Nielsen, "The IOC has proved that they don't have the power or the will to take care of the fight against doping."

Evidence of its lack of will? Last year the IOC recognized bodybuilding, which is notoriously steroid-soaked, as an official sport. Last July Samaranch called for decreasing the number of drugs on the banned list. Only two days before last week's meeting, de Merode suggested that the IOC reduce penalties against athletes caught using.

And in a performance that stunned many delegates, the IOC threw cold water on what may be the most significant breakthrough in drug testing in years: a test for human growth hormone developed by endocrinologist Peter Sonksen of St. Thomas' Hospital in London. It would use blood drawn from the ear lobe or finger. The IOC said the test needed an additional $5 million worth of work.

There are low-tech strategies to detect doping, however. One is to institute frequent, random, out-of-competition testing, as Canada and a handful of other countries have. Anabolic steroids, for instance, "are training drugs, not something you take the day of the competition," notes Bob Armstrong, chief counsel for a landmark Canadian commission that investigated doping in sport. "At competitions you catch people who are either stupid or careless. You need out-of-competition testing." The IOC doesn't mandate that. In addition, sport federations could freeze all urine samples and subject them to each new detection test that comes along. "If you knew that the undetectable drug you used today might be perfectly detectable a few years from now, and your medals would be taken, and your reputation destroyed, that would make a difference," says American runner Frank Shorter, who won gold at Munich in 1972 and silver in Montreal in 1976.

"You would wait for that knock on your door the rest of your life. That's the deterrence."

Doping has now spread beyond elite sport. "The reason we are involved in this is the 52 million American children," White House drug czar Barry McCaffrey said at the IOC doping conference. That isn't just rhetoric. Since home-run king Mark McGwire admitted to using androstenedione last summer, andro use among kids has soared fivefold, he says. And a study in the journal Pediatrics last year found that 2.7 percent of Massachusetts middle-school athletes were using steroids.

Better drug-detecting strategies and technologies alone won't make sport clean. Athletes themselves have to believe that the IOC and international sport federations will, at least eventually, catch anyone who uses performance-enhancing drugs. They have to believe, in other words, that their competitors aren't getting a free pass. Absent that trust, many athletes will not resist the siren call of swifter, higher, stronger through chemistry. And the luster of the Olympic rings, already so tarnished, will dim even more.

With CRISTOPHER DICKEY *and* KAREN HELMSTAEDT *in Lausanne,* ROD NORDLAND *in Rome,* THOMAS HAYDEN *in New York and bureau reports*

Sex Sells

Viagra Heats Up Market for Sexual Supplements

By Gina Geslewitz

The Baby Boomer Generation who introduced the concept of Free Love in the 60s (enhanced with liberal amounts of drugs), and then as they matured, Safe Sex in the 80s, are now combining the best of both worlds. They are back to their Sex 'N Drugs phase. Only in this case, the drug of choice is not marijuana, but Viagra—successfully combining the previous two phases: it's a drug and it's safe, or at least legal.

When Pfizer introduced Viagra™ — their little blue miracle pill that treats impotence—in March there was a mad rush for prescriptions. Doctors were writing about 300,000 prescriptions a week making Viagra the most successful launch in the history of prescription drugs.

There are reportedly 20 to 30 million American men suffering from chronic impotence in the United States. Add to that, a whole bunch more who merely would like to have stronger and longer-lasting erections and you've got a huge market for the new potency pill.

But Pfizer didn't just introduce a new drug, they opened the door to new expectations and a new willingness among men and women to experiment with products that enhance the sexual act.

While Viagra is effective in about 70 percent of patients, that still leaves 30 percent dissatisfied. It works best for men with milder forms of impotence and is not recommended for those with heart disease. And there are side effects, the most common being blue-tinged blurred vision and light-sensitivity, headaches, skin flushing, and indigestion. And there have been 69 deaths reported among those taking Viagra (although it has not been determined if Viagra was the cause).

Another negative: it's expensive. "The number one side effect of taking Viagra

is poverty," declared Stephen Holt, MD, author of *The Sexual Revolution: Natural and Healthy Alternatives to Viagra.* "At $10 per dose it can be very costly."

James Balch, MD, author of *Prescriptions for Healthy Living,* is even more adamant. "It is suddenly becoming the latest 'cult drug' of millions of Generation X Americans seeking a thrill," he writes in his newsletter. "Men as young as 20 with no sexual problems are buying Viagra illicitly. Then they're taking it like candy in order to achieve multiple erections in one night."

He also warns that Viagra can create a "powerful dependency. If you were having some trouble maintaining an erection before taking Viagra, just wait until you start taking this drug and then have to stop."

Now that Viagra has raised fears among many men (and women), doctors are becoming more cautious, cutting down on the number of prescriptions they write.

Is There a Better Solution?

Many medical and nutritional experts say there is. Not only saying, but betting the house on it.

"Viagra has been described as a lifestyle drug," says Holt. "But the answer to a lifestyle problem is not a drug, but a change in lifestyle."

"No one single agent alone can solve everyone's sexual problems," he stated. "Sexual intercourse involves a response cycle that involves other events than just the erection of the male penis." Holt says the ability to enjoy sex is based on an individual's total health and psychological outlook.

Nevertheless, there are many natural products out there that purport to promote sexual function. And while there

have always been herbs and supplement formulas available for "male potency" and "virility," the pace of new introductions has taken a rather sudden upwards spike since Viagra hit the market. And many of them are openly or less openly taking on the pharmaceutical giant.

Sexual enhancement products can be divided into two categories: Those that work immediately, much like Viagra does (two pills and 30 to 60 minutes later, you're ready); and those that, like most supplement programs, require the user to take them on a daily and long-term basis.

Viagra Competitors

The following products belong in the former category:

Viri-Stat™ . Dr. Holt who is also founder of BioTherapies, Inc., Fairfield, NJ, recently introduced his own patented formula Viri-Stat, which comes in male and female formulas. The male version addresses erectile dysfunction while the female version addresses psychological and menopausal related problems that impact on sexual performance.

Both contain herbs and niacin which has been shown to improve circulation to the lower limbs, where the arterial blood vessels are blocked by arteriosclerosis. It is recommended, like Viagra, to be taken one to two hours before sexual intercourse.

Viri-Stat, said Holt, is currently being tested in seven clinical practices.

Veromax™ . Another brand new product is Veromax, formulated by Melvin J. Duckett, MD, a board certified urologist with the Maryland Urology Group. At the same time that Pfizer was developing Viagra, Dr. Duckett and his researchers were likewise developing Veromax, according to a company paper.

From *Health Foods Business,* December 1998, pp. 36-39. © 1998 by Health Products Business Magazine. Reprinted by permission.

Veromax, like Viagra, increases nitric oxide into the bloodstream, which is a key factor in male erections and also helps women become stimulated. The patent for Veromax was filed in early 1998.

Veromax contains saw palmetto, Siberian ginseng, L-Arginine, L-alanine, glutamic acid, L-lysine and ginkgo biloba. A product brochure said that it is for both men and women who wish to preserve, restore or enhance their sexual functions. It is also compared to Viagra and is said to be superior in terms of increasing the cyclic GMP (guanosine monophosphate) levels. Like Viagra the recommended dosage is two tablets prior to sexual intercourse.

The Maryland Urology Group has conducted clinical research with Veromax using the same International Index used by Pfizer in its clinical trials of Viagra. "After three months of taking Veromax, 75 percent of the 100 customers in our study reported significant satisfaction and stated they would continue to use the product," said Larry Park, vice president, sales and marketing.

Herbal V. Another new Viagra alternative already on some store shelves is Herbal V from Lane Labs. Herbal V, which contains yohimbe, damiana, saw palmetto, panex ginseng, royal jelly and vitamins A and E, zinc and selenium, is said to support genital blood flow for sexual function.

David Miller, new product development manager, said they have just completed a focus group study using 24 single men and five couples. According to their study, 67 percent reported improvement in sex drive and 87 percent said they were satisfied with the product.

Like Viagra, Herbal V is recommended to be taken two hours before sex.

Miller explained that this product is not being marketed as a "sex product," but as a way to help people with sexual dysfunctions. "There definitely is a big market for it," he said.

Wait and See

Many of the older products on the market as well as some new ones, however, take a more gradual approach to sexual enhancement. This group of supplements are designed to be taken over a longer period of time before the consumer will notice a difference.

NutriMan TNT™, from NutriCare, Intl, a Springfield, MO-based company, is one such product. Unlike Viagra which rushes blood to the penis, allowing an erection, TNT, which contains a blend of herbs, is said to "strengthen, tone and increase the muscle mass of the genital area and the male reproductive system,"

and to increase the libido. The product was formulated by Steve Margolis, MD, of Troy, MI, a medical director at AlternaCare P.C.

The product is sold in a 30-day supply, says Daphne Dulle, vice president. She says that for men over 55 it takes about three weeks to build to a steady level in the system, while younger men can see benefits in as little as five to seven days.

Dulle said they offer a money back guarantee and that of the thousands of bottles sold, only one customer has asked for a refund. The company also has a formula for women, NutriFem, which is designed to handle difficulties from PMS to menopause.

Just introduced in the United States is Vigoril, a homeopathic product used to promote sexual function. Manufactured by ELS/Homeocare the product has been used by doctors for their patients in France. (A double blind study is currently underway, reports Edith Scheiner, president.)

"We've received lots of calls for alternatives to Viagra," she said. "We've had a slightly different product for sexual function in private label for a year and a half and it's doing well. While no one product works for 100 percent of people, Vigoril will cover most genital problems of men and works for urinary incontinence as well."

Another homeopathic company that has products that address male potency causes is King Bio. Dr. Frank King, ND, DC, has three formulas that address the issue of male potency. Sometimes a formula named for a specific symptom will actually cure another symptom that is only related by a root cause, points out Scott Blanchard, marketing director. Male Power addresses impotency caused by emotional issues or alcohol or drug abuse; ProstaPower addresses symptoms associated with prostate dysfunction; Muscle Maximizer enhances physical strength in general.

NuMan from Interceuticals, Inc., is based on Traditional Chinese Medicine and is said to "work naturally in the system stabilizing sexual activity by getting to the root of the problem rather than reducing the symptoms for a quick fix," according to a company press release.

Most of the ingredients in the natural sex enhancers sold in health food stores are herbs and vitamins that are sold singly as well. These individual herbs continue to sell well. Among these are: yohimbe, tribulus terrestis, avena sativa, damiana, ginkgo, panax or siberian ginseng, muira puama, saw palmetto and ashwagandha. Supplements for sex include: L-arginine, niacin, zinc and essential fatty acids.

Yohimbe

Before Viagra, yohimbine the active component of the Yohimbe bark, was the only FDA approved drug for impotence. "Like Viagra, Yohimbine heightens potency and maintains erections by increasing blood flow to the penis, writes Rob Ivker, DO in *Natural Health,* Sept.–Oct. 1998. "But unlike Viagra, it does so by increasing the body's production of the adrenal hormone norepinephrine, which is essential for erections."

Yohimbe bark is one of the most popular aphrodisiac herbs available.

Muira Puama (potent wood)

Native to Brazil this herb has been used to increase libido and sexual function. In a French study, presented at The First International Congress on Ethnopharmcology in Strasbourg, France, June, 1990, more than one half (62 percent) of a group of 262 patients receiving muira puama extract claimed that libido was enhanced; more than 50 percent of the individuals who had failures of penile erection reported a benefit from the administration of this herb.

Tribulus terrestis (puncture vine)

Tribulus has been shown to have a pronounced effect on sexual performance and has been clinically shown to boost levels of the male hormone testosterone. In Ayurvedic medicine, Tribulus has been used to treat disorders of the prostate, penis and urinary tract, writes Holt. Tribulus appears to raise the testosterone production via the activation of leutinizing hormone secretion from the pituitary gland.

L-Arginine

L-arginine is an amino acid that is converted in the body into nitric oxide, the same active agent that mediates the sexual response. In the book, *Better Sex Through Chemistry,* authors John Morgenthaler and Dan Joy write, "By facilitating blood flow to the erectile tissue of the penis, nitric oxide produced from L-arginine can give men erections that are bigger, harder and more frequent. Some men also report that L-arginine gives them greater endurance."

Not All Solutions Come in a Pill

Taking an entirely different, more feminine approach, to improving sex is Erotikava, from Pacific Sensuals, West

Los Angeles. Called the "drink of love" and "romance in a bottle" Erotikava is a unique blend of rare Asian herbs chief among them being kava. Kava is known to decrease anxiety and has grown in popularity as a single herb.

Erotikava got a head start on some of the other products mentioned above, coming out in 1996. Just five months later the fledgling company received a major publicity boost when it was featured on the TV newsmagazine "Hard Copy." "It has since been rerun 16 times," said Corina Harmon, director of marketing, "and each time sales go up."

Monique Caulfield, founder of Pacific Sensuals, makes clear that Erotikava is not an herbal Viagra. "A lot of men's impotence is anxiety based. Our product helps people calm down. Most aphrodisiacs are pills that people pop like medicine. They don't improve romance." Women, said Caulfield, are their primary customers.

Eroktikava is designed to be taken by both men and women and the packaging suggests that it be shared in a romantic tea ritual. The producers advise lovers to "complement the experience with candles, music, massage oil and anything your imagination can conjure. . . ." In fact, Pacific Sensuals will soon have available a gift basket with massage oil and an aromatherapy candle.

Another natural product, National Arousal™ for men and Natural Sensation™ for women from Natural Pleasures takes a hands-on approach to delivering sexual satisfaction. Like many of the other products mentioned, they work by increasing blood flow to the genital area. Both contain L-arginine in a cream base and are to be applied topically.

Natural Arousal has been tested by several urologists and general practitioners, according to the company, and preliminary reports showed that nine of eleven patients with self-declared impotence reported restoration of erectile function.

Beginning to Grow

In an informal poll of several retailers throughout the United States, HFB learned that while there is some interest in natural sex enhancers they aren't yet shaking the earth. "We have not had a boon in people asking for Viagra," reports Cynthia Tice of Center Foods in Philadelphia. "Some men are interested in yohimbe, but there hasn't been a significant increase."

John Kay, manager of Health Emporium in Corona Del Mar, CA, said that things are starting to pick up. "We have been getting questions."

Capitol Drugs, with two locations in Southern California, is a pharmacy with a large natural supplement section, and sells both Viagra and its alternatives. Said co-owner Bruce Senesac: "Viagra has been doing great. It's been flying out of here. We haven't heard any complaints (about side effects)," he said. "The only complaint we hear is that some people can't get their doctor to prescribe it."

"The craze has begun to die down. Doctors are being more particular about who they give it to," he added. "People who weren't able to get Viagra are adamant about trying Herbal V. We've reordered it four times." Capitol Drugs sells Herbal V from a display on the counter next to the register in three locations. The pharmacy, the natural section and the sports section.

Senesac noted that it sells best in the sports section.

However, pills are not the only thing customers are sniffing out in connection with sexual activities. Aromatherapy can also be effective in the bedroom. Senesac said that his store offers a number of custom blended private label aromatherapy products. And the most popular blend? Aphrodisiac.

While Senesac didn't say which essential oils were in this stimulating fragrance, Dr. Holt in his book notes that jasmine is considered to promote a "sexy mood". Other romance promoting essential oils include: sandalwood, patchouli and ylang-ylang. Of course, it doesn't hurt that these scents are often applied via a massage which in itself promotes warmth and pleasure.

If you looked around your store, there are probably lots of products that can be used to promote romance and a healthy sex life. With Valentine's Day just around the corner you may want to investigate some of the new sexual enhancement products and provide your customers with a selection of provocative choices.

Pain breakers

Stress from work. Aches from workouts. No wonder we've become a nation of pill poppers.

By David Barton
Bee Staff Writer

Jason Wilson is nothing like his dad. Just ask him.

"My dad was 56 when he died," he says, standing outside City Bicycle Works on K Street in midtown Sacramento. "Fifty pounds overweight, bad diet, never exercised."

He pauses, and glances at the ground.

"It killed him," he adds, a trace of bitterness in his voice. "Heart attack. Which is why I do what I do."

Wilson, a 41-year-old software marketer from Folsom, is doing everything he can—mountain biking, weight lifting, running, volleyball, hiking—anything to forestall the fate that befell his father.

And it's working: Wilson is fit, lean and muscular, and looks as much as 10 years younger than he is. Whatever gets him, it's unlikely to be caused by being fat and out of shape.

Bummer about the knees, though. And that thing with his lower back. . . .

"Yeah, I hurt," he admits, a mixture of concern and pride in his voice. "I beat myself up pretty regularly. Thank God for ibuprofen. I eat that stuff like candy."

Ibuprofen, along with acetaminophen, ketoprofen, naproxen sodium and good old aspirin, are the drugs of choice for millions of people, including members of the exercise-crazy baby boom generation. And some experts say the generation most associated with excessive illegal drug use in the '60s and '70s may be overdoing it with these more benign drugs.

Dale Ogar is editor of the UC Berkeley Wellness Letter, published by the School for Public Health. She says: "People are looking to nonprescription drugs more than they ever did. The increase in the numbers of people exercising, especially older people and people in midlife, has taken the market up enormously."

"The People's Pharmacy," the '70s-era (and recently updated) consumer guide to the benefits and dangers of OTC (over-the-counter) drugs, says that the use of OTC painkillers has skyrocketed. Sales rose a remarkable 60 percent between 1986 and 1996—with no slowdown in sight.

The reason, says Dr. Ron Sockolov, one of the two team physicians for California State University, Sacramento, is that people like Wilson are beating themselves up at a

---

> "We're seeing a lot of overuse type of injuries. People are playing hard, and the body is not used to that . . . . They're working on cumulative trauma."
>
> Dr. Ron Sockolov

---

higher rate than in the past.

"We're seeing a lot of overuse type of injuries," he says. "People are playing hard, and the body is not used to that. The average person in their 30s and 40s hasn't maintained the conditioning they had in their 20s.

"And they're working on cumulative trauma," he adds. "We're seeing classic wear and tear, chronic tendonitis and even arthritis, often in people younger than we'd expect. Our recommendation for people in their 40s and 50s is that they stay in the best shape they can, so that they can go and participate, instead of just going out and playing without getting in shape first."

When such folks go out and hurt themselves, many seem to pop pain relievers until they feel better, without much awareness that they're taking serious drugs. That's a mistake, says Dr. Peter Koo, a pain management specialist at the University of California, San Francisco, Medical Center.

"One of the problems is that people think (over-the-counter) stuff is safe, and that's a myth," he says. "Those drugs are just as active as any other drug, but the OTC dose is lower."

Like any drugs, even these more common remedies can be dangerous if used in excess, says Dr. Scott Fishman, chief of the Division of Pain Medicine at the UC Davis Medical Center.

"They are great drugs, and they really work," says Fishman. "And we can get them over-the-counter. If we don't take more than the directions say, we probably won't have side effects. But in excess, they can be life-threatening.

"The problem with the drugs we have is that there are side effects over time," he says. "These drugs can cause stomach ulcers or kidney problems, and those can be life-threatening. Acetaminophen can cause liver damage. You can overdose on Tylenol (acetaminophen); it is only safe if taken for short periods of time and in the proper doses."

These are powerful drugs, Fishman says.

"Sometimes in the hospital, if someone's in bad pain, we might give them morphine," he says. "And if that doesn't do it, sometimes ibuprofen will. It's a powerful drug."

"People say that if aspirin were a new drug, it wouldn't be available over the counter, because of all the side effects," he adds. "It does the worst in terms of bleeding—if someone has a bleeding ulcer, it takes a while to declare itself, and people can even die if they don't get treatment early."

Still, he adds: "People shouldn't be afraid to take a couple of ibuprofen, or aspirin. It's a great treatment, it's mind-boggling how good these drugs are."

Nevertheless, Koo points out that "the number of deaths caused by drugs every year is in the hundreds of thousands," and the Food and Drug Administration has published estimates that 10,000 to 20,000 of those deaths can be attributed to the use of nonsteroidal anti-inflammatory drugs (NSAIDs). Some 80,000 people a year are hospitalized for complications from the use of acetaminophen and NSAIDs.

The major difference between benefit and disaster is dosage, and doses vary widely. In fact, dosage is

---

In the name of pain

Most of the brand-name, over-the-counter pain relievers—Excedrin, Tylenol, Advil, Aleve, et al.—fall into one of two generic categories: acetaminophen and the NSAID group (non-steroidal anti-inflammatory drugs). The NSAID group includes aspirin, naproxen sodium, ibuprofen and ketoprofen. Here is a list of the five most commonly used pain relievers, along with their brand names, their uses and effects.

GENERIC TYPE	BRAND NAME	USES	EFFECTS AND CAUTIONS
Acetaminophen	Tylenol, Panadol, Anacin-3	Aches, pains, fever	Does not cause gastrointestinal bleeding. Will not reduce inflammation or prevent blood clotting. Should not be used with alcohol or for a hangover.
Aspirin	Excedrin, Bayer, Bufferin, Anacin, others	Aches, pains, fever	Researchers are exploring its preventive effects on conditions such as blood clots and cancer. Can cause stomach irritation, internal bleeding or ulcers.
Ibuprofen	Advil, Motrin, Nuprin, Mediprin	Pain, fever, inflammation	Less gastrointestinal distress than aspirin, but could cause stomach bleeding in some people. Best for menstrual cramps.
Ketoprofen	Orudis KT, Actron	Pain, fever, inflammation	May cause gastrointestinal, kidney or other problems. Not a significant improvement on other over-the-counter painkillers.
Naproxen sodium	Aleve	Pain, fever, inflammation	Less likely to cause gastrointestinal distress than aspirin or ibuprofen. Longer-lasting effects. Not recommended for heavy drinkers or those with ulcers or kidney disease.

—David Barton

Source: "The U.C. Berkeley Wellness Self-Care Handbook" by Dr. John Edward Swartsberg and Dr. Sheldon Margen also the difference between many over-the-counter, brand-name drugs. Extra Strength Excedrin and Excedrin Migraine (or Extra Strength Tylenol and Tylenol Arthritis), marketed as different drugs, are really the same. The difference is merely a matter of a hundred milligrams here and there.

Also, these doctors point out, the difference between brand names is minimal, as long as you're in the same drug category.

"Motrin, Nuprin, Advil, they're all the same," says Sockolov. "They're all ibuprofen. The generics work just as well as the brand names." The same is true of the different aspirins, which are often made different by what they're blended with—Excedrin adds caffeine to aid absorption, Excedrin PM adds an agent to promote sleep. But they're all aspirin.

For that reason, when shopping for these drugs, you are better off with the generics—acetaminophen as opposed to Tylenol, ibuprofen as opposed to Motrin—which are just as reliable as the brand names, and often considerably cheaper. Some are even made with the same ingredients, and in the very same factories, as the more expensive brand names.

Better yet, try forgoing the use of these drugs, at least for a while. For most people with occasional aches and pains from overuse, or from over-indulging, it may be a good idea to back off of the pain relievers and get to the root of the problem.

"First of all, know your body," says Koo. "Know the problem. Educate yourself about yourself. You have to know what you have, then figure out what to do about it."

One thing Koo suggests is that any potential users of even something as simple as ibuprofen read the company literature that comes with the drug. And do not exceed the recommended doses.

"It's also important to note the age of the patient," says Koo. "The older you are, the more susceptible you are to kidney damage. The non-steroidal anti-inflammatory drugs can decrease kidney function, and the older you are, the more likely that is. And people on high-blood-pressure medicines have to be careful about NSAIDs."

This has been a problem with the relatively new drug, Aleve (naproxen sodium), a major selling point of which is the longer duration its effects last (12 hours rather than four). You also need only take one pill, rather than the two that is often recommended for the other drugs.

But people are in the habit of taking two pain relievers, which can actually be dangerous, leading to potential side effects such as stomach bleeding. And just because you don't note any side effects from taking too-high doses doesn't mean that your stomach is not suffering some damage that you may not discover until years later.

For these and other reasons, these doctors say it is often best to simply avoid these drugs and go with a more benign treatment. Sockolov recommends ice.

"I try to keep it simple with the medications," he says. "I like to use ice, I think it works very well to take down the inflammation, which is what we're talking about with these drugs. So ice would be my first recommendation."

"Then, if there's significant inflammation, I'd go to the anti-inflammatories. But you've gotta be careful. If you take it on a regular basis, let your doctor know, and have a blood test. I want a blood test checking their liver every 6–12 months."

As for taking a big dose of Tylenol or Advil to cure a hangover headache, Koo says, forget it.

"Taking acetaminophen for a hangover is the worst thing you can do, because your liver is already stressed, and you're adding a second stress," he says. "For a hangover, take one of the NSAIDs if you have to, but they could easily irritate your stomach lining, just as alcohol does. There's no happy solution.

"The best cure for a hangover is not to drink so much."

That said, Fishman thinks that most people don't abuse these drugs because, when it gets right down to it, they don't need to.

"Typically, people don't take them unless they feel they have to," he says. "Most of us heal within a day or two if we strain ourselves. You'll feel better in a couple of days whether you take Advil or not."

New date-rape drug emerges

Metro parents worry legal product touted by health stores, Internet threatens teens

By Jodi S. Cohen / The Detroit News

Poison-control experts fear that yet another easily available date-rape drug—promoted as a legal replacement for similar drugs that have been banned—is headed for Metro Detroit. The latest products touted on the Internet and in some health food stores and body-building magazines contain 1,4 butanediol (BD), a chemical that can be dangerous—even deadly, according to the U.S. Food and Drug Administration.

On the Internet, it's called a party drug; in the magazines it's hailed as a growth-hormone stimulant; health food stores claim it's a sleep aid.

But it's really another cousin of GHB (gamma hydroxybutyrate), a banned substance known as a date-rape drug because it can render women helpless in fending off sexual attacks, warns the Food and Drug Administration.

The GHB-related drugs have parents and their teens worried, especially during a time when high school students are celebrating at proms and graduation parties.

"Students are party-hopping from house to house because there are so many parties from the end of May until the end of June," said Sheree Hicks of Rockwood, who has two daughters. "Everybody serves open bottles of pop and punch. I would never have thought of that last year when I had a graduation party for my daughter, but I sure think of it now."

'We knew this was coming'

A 15-year-old Rockwood girl died last January after she was slipped a dose of GHB and a related substance, GBL (gamma butyrolactone). Three teens face charges of poisoning the girl by putting the odorless, colorless drug into her Mountain Dew soft drink at a Grosse Ile party.

Manufacturers have designed various substitutes for the banned drugs to boost their sales, authorities say.

"We knew this was coming, so we have been looking out for it," said Dr. Susan Smolinske of the Regional Poison Control Center in Detroit. "As the FDA cracked down on GBL, we knew that there would be other substitutes. The companies are still wanting to make money, so they are relabeling and repackaging it."

But 1,4 butanediol has advantages if used properly, suppliers say.

"If you take it according to directions, it can be wonderful. But there are some people who want to mix it with alcohol—and that's a huge mistake," said Maria Gomez, who owns a dietary-supplement company in Pennsylvania and sells products that contain BD on the Internet.

The latest substitute for GHB—BD—is often called legal GHB or herbal GHB. Drug experts say it quickly converts into GHB inside the body, making it just as dangerous.

This is not the first time this year that authorities have warned about this type of product. In January, the FDA released a warning about products containing GBL, which was manufacturers' first sneaky substitute for GHB. After the FDA threatened court proceedings against makers of GBL, most companies pulled their products.

Authorities believe many of these companies are now substituting BD for GBL and renaming the products. For example, Renewtrient (GBL) is now being called SomatoPro (BD). One Internet company brags that five caps of SomatoPro will convert to 2 grams of GHB.

All three substances—GHB, GBL and BD—can slow breathing and lead to unconsciousness, vomiting, seizures and death. They also increase the effects of alcohol. Products containing BD are sold with benign names such as Revitalize Plus, Serenity, Enliven, SomatoPro, Thunder Nectar and Weight Belt Cleaner.

Recipes on Internet

The chemicals by themselves are not illegal. They're found in floor-strippers, paint-thinners and in the production of plastics. Manufacturers and suppliers contend that when mixed and taken correctly, they can build muscle, reduce fat and improve sleep.

But the difference between a small, euphoria-inducing amount and a higher, fatal dose can be minimal, experts warn. Recipes to mix the chemicals can be found on the Internet, and authorities warn that a person could unknowingly mix a fatal concoction.

Although the drug may have less serious consequences when taken correctly, that's not what is occurring among some college and high school students.

"College kids have no clue how dangerous it can be. A girl in my class was talking about how she works at a bar and said they see it all the time," said Lisa Crawford, 19, a freshman at Macomb County Community College. "Instead of just giving lectures on marijuana and alcohol, high schools and colleges need to include this."

GHB and similar drugs began to surface in greater frequencies in Metro Detroit in late 1997. Since then, area rape-crisis centers have reported cases in which men slipped it into the drinks of women with the hope of rendering them helpless. Young adults also have been using the drugs at parties, especially in the underground rave scene, as a non-fattening way to get a buzz without alcohol.

New law seen as answer

Many hope that efforts in Lansing and around the nation will get the drugs off shelves and Internet sites and onto the list of dangerous, medically useless drugs such as cocaine and heroin. Law enforcement officials say they have had trouble confiscating drugs related to GHB because they are technically not illegal in Michigan and most other states.

But a bill introduced to Congress in March—the Date-rape Prevention Act of 1999—would add GHB and its precursors, like GBL and BD, to the list of Schedule III substances, making possession of the drug a crime punishable by five years in prison and a $250,000 fine.

"Isn't it funny that we started out with GHB and then there was heat put on GHB, so now there is GBL. And now, when there is heat on GBL, we are finding BD," said Grosse Ile police Sgt. G. Mark Faistenhammer, assigned to the Michigan State Police narcotics division. "How does the Legislature or law enforcement keep up with that? We haven't even made a law on the first one yet."

Symptoms and safeguards

There are common signs that someone has ingested a date-rape drug. There are also ways to prevent becoming a victim:

• Symptoms: Slow breathing, sudden vomiting, seizures and coma. Showing signs of intoxication without drinking alcohol.

• Safeguards: Open your own beverages and keep your eye on your glass. Also, watch friends' behavior for signs of trouble.

• Where to call for help: Regional Poison Control Center at (800) POISON1 or Firststep, a rape-crisis center, at (888) 453-5900.

New threat

Authorities fear that 1,4 butanediol and other relatives of the date-rape drug GHB easily can be slipped into women's drinks. Parents and students worry the substances will be present at upcoming graduation parties and other festivities.

• Name: BD (1,4 butanediol)

• Advertised as: Sleep aid, energy inducer, muscle builder and fat reducer.

• What it is: A chemical that can cause slow breathing, unconsciousness, vomiting, seizures and death. It also increases the effects of alcohol.

• Found in: Revitalize Plus, Serenity, SomatoPro, Enliven, Thunder Nectar, Weight Belt Cleaner.

Incidents grow

Here are the 1999 incidents of date-rape drug abuse reported to the Regional Poison Control Center in Detroit through May 19.

• 35 cases, ages 15–40

Previous years

• 1998: 57 cases
• 1997: 23 cases
• 1996: 15 cases

Unit 5

Key Points to Consider

❖ What role do the media play in influencing drug-related crime?

❖ Explain why you believe drug-related crime is either overrepresented or underrepresented.

❖ Survey your class to determine what percentage have been victims of crime. Determine what percentage of those were victims of drug-related crime.

❖ Consider the costs of drug-related crime on the criminal justice, health care, and educational systems in your community.

❖ How is the fear of crime continuing to change the way we live?

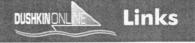 **Links** **www.dushkin.com/online/**

These sites are annotated on pages 4 and 5.

Crime is intrinsic to the world of illegal drugs. The relationship is strong and enduring. The type of crime associated with this world varies according to the type of drugs involved and certain environmental factors associated with them. For example, patterns of violent crime consistently accompany the trafficking of both cocaine and methamphetamine. The lucrative nature of the market, the fierce competition it generates, and the tendency for street dealers to be users of the product all serve to perpetuate violence. The repeated use of cocaine and methamphetamine produces a loss of judgment, paranoia, and psychosis in the user, promoting aggressive and irrational behavior. This behavior is associated with an increased risk of becoming a victim or perpetrator of crime and being present at a place where crime is occurring. Many illicit drugs fall into similar categories due to their associated black market economy or their pharmacology.

The use and abuse of legal drugs, although not as publicly sensational, also produces a significant relationship with crime. The most notable one is alcohol, which studies repeatedly connect to crimes ranging in severity from shoplifting to rape, homicide, and child abuse. The high percentage of perpetrators as well as victims using alcohol before and during the offense is a long-established criminological phenomenon. One study reported that violence was ten times more likely to occur during the commission of a crime if the offender had been drinking. Another recent study suggested that alcohol-related deaths of young people occur at rates 6.5 times higher than those caused by all illegal drugs combined. The best evidence suggests that the relationship between drugs and crime is developmental rather than causal and varies by the nature and intensity of drug use.

Ample evidence exists supporting the strong relationship between drug use, criminal activity, and being arrested. Over half of the crime in this country occurs by persons under the influence of drugs. Research suggests that 80 percent of men and women behind bars in the United States are seriously involved with alcohol and other drugs. Crime increases as drug use increases. Criminal activity is reported to be two to three times higher among frequent users of heroin and cocaine as compared to the criminal activity of irregular users. In most cities surveyed, over 68 percent of arrestees reported recently using drugs. Three out of four arrestees reported drug use in their lifetime. Two out of three state prison inmates reported using drugs once a week or more before their arrest and incarceration.

Juvenile crime related to drugs continues to be a major concern for students, parents, school districts, and the nation. In the aftermath of the tragic Columbine High School shootings, new controversies arose from the concerns of many mental health professionals about the tremendous numbers of school-age youth (approximately 6 million) taking prescribed psychotropic medication for mental disorders. Some are questioning the possible connection between these drugs and violence. Eric Harris, one of the shooters in the Columbine murders, was under the influence of Luvox, an antidepressant prescribed for obsessive-compulsive disorder. In another shooting in Conyers, Georgia, 15-year-old T. J. Solomon was being treated with Ritalin when he fired on and wounded six classmates. In another example, Kip Kinkel, a 15-year-old high school student in Springfield, Oregon, murdered his parents and then proceeded to school where he shot 22 classmates. Kinkel, too, was being treated with Ritalin and also Prozac. The DEA reports that the United States buys and uses 90 percent of the world's Ritalin. The International Control Board, an agency of the United Nations, reported in 1995 that "10 to 12 percent of American boys between the ages of 6 and 14 had been treated with Ritalin." Some point out that Ritalin has pharmacological properties similar to cocaine, long believed responsible for promoting aggressive behavior in the user.

Another different but remarkable dimension of the drugs/crime relationship concerns the relationship between drug use, drug trafficking, and violent crime. Certain legal and illegal drugs such as alcohol, cocaine, and the amphetamines produce profound physiological and psychological influences in the user. These influences, often visible in the form of aggressive, irrational, paranoid, and psychotic behavior, have long been associated with an increased potential for violence. Those arrested for violent crime typically test positive for illegal drugs at rates of 60 to 80 percent. In jurisdictions in the West where methamphetamine is prevalent, rates are even higher.

Currently, no discussion of large-scale drug-related crime and trafficking is possible without recognizing the emergence of powerful Mexican cartels. In addition to purchasing cocaine and heroin directly from Colombian traffickers for sale in the United States, Mexican traffickers now manage the largest-scale methamphetamine manufacturing and distribution network in the hemisphere. According to the Drug Enforcement Administration, Mexican syndicates now control 80 to 90 percent of the methamphetamine distribution in the United States, 33 percent of the cocaine distribution, and 20 percent of the heroin distribution.

Additionally, it is an error to limit the discussion of drug use and violent crime to suspects and perpetrators. Domestic violence and child abuse research consistently express relationships between these crimes and the abuse of drugs. It is important to be sensitive to and aware of the often disproportionate toll of certain drugs on specific populations of Americans.

The articles in unit 5 help illustrate the wide range of criminal activity associated with the manufacture, trafficking, and use of some illicit drugs. As you read, consider the significance of drugs as they relate to the most pervasive fear in this country—the fear of crime.

Drugs and Crime

Border Trafficking

Where the U.S. and Mexico meet, the drug smugglers are riding high

By John Ward Anderson and William Branigin
Washington Post Foreign Service

McALLEN, Tex.

Border patrol agent Joel Martinez and his dog Brutus were on routine patrol eight months ago in Combes, Tex.—checking freight trains for illegal aliens— when the dog started whimpering, barking and chewing the corner of a boxcar. Martinez looked inside. It was empty. But using crowbars and a blowtorch, agents discovered the source of Brutus's unflagging agitation: more than two tons of marijuana stashed behind false walls.

"I damn near kissed that dog on the mouth," Martinez says.

The incident was but one recent example of how the U.S.-Mexican border is under siege by Mexican drug trafficking organizations. The traffickers have virtually unlimited funds to build the most elaborate secret compartments, to buy the best counter-surveillance technology and transport vehicles available, and to corrupt law enforcement officials on both sides of the frontier.

The Southwest border is being attacked from all angles, with traffickers tunneling under it, flying over it, walking and driving across it and boating around it.

Based on the rule of thumb, often cited by law enforcement officials, that only 10 percent to 15 percent of the drug flow is discovered and seized, traffickers are delivering between five and seven tons of cocaine, marijuana, methamphetamine and heroin from Mexico to the United States every day of the year.

That traffic is contributing to drug abuse and crime in the United States; corrupting the Mexican economy, judicial system and government; and poisoning relations between the United States and Mexico. But more immediately, it is wreaking havoc all along the 2,000-mile border between the two countries, distorting and destroying the lives of ranchers, policemen, federal and local officials, and people living in scores of Southwestern towns and cities.

"Texas is now where Florida was 15 years ago, and we need all the help we can get," says Capt. Enrique Espinoza, head of the Texas Department of Public Safety's narcotics unit in McAllen. "We're getting overrun by it."

The flood of drugs is being orchestrated primarily by two major Mexican drug cartels—one based in Tijuana and headed by the Arellano Felix family and the second operating out of Ciudad Juarez on the Texas border and led by Amado Carrillo Fuentes until his death. At least three other smaller but powerful organizations also traffic drugs across the border: the remnants of the Gulf cartel on Mexico's Gulf Coast; the Caro Quintero family's organization based in Sonora along the Arizona border; and the Amezcua family, with a global methamphetamine smuggling business headquartered in the central city of Guadalajara.

The Mexican cartels, which have replaced Colombian-based mafias as the primary traffickers of cocaine, marijuana and other drugs in many parts of the United States, have become so big, so powerful and such a dominant factor in the drug trade that U.S. law enforcement officials now speak of them in almost apocalyptic terms.

"I am not exaggerating when I say that the Mexican drug syndicates are the premier law enforcement threat facing the United States today," U.S. Drug Enforcement Administration Chief Thomas A. Constantine told Congress last year.

What makes the Mexican drug organizations more menacing than those of Colombia or Burma or Nigeria is the proximity—and the porousness—of the border, a thinly guarded strip surrounded by a rapidly growing region populated by tens of millions of Mexicans and Americans. This series of articles about the border will show that:

■ U.S. and Mexican authorities are overwhelmed by the quantities of drugs being smuggled into the United States, and

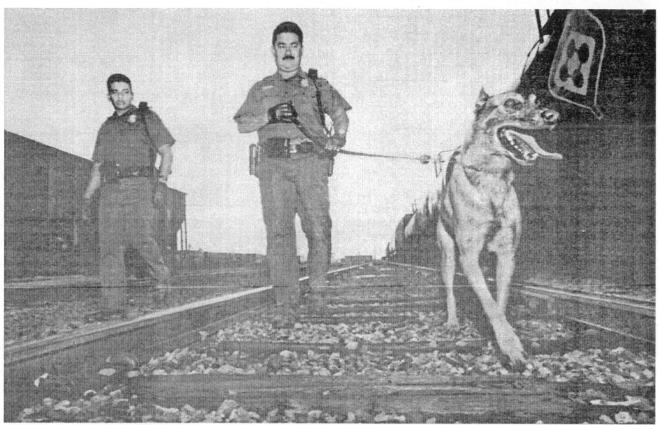

Border Patrol agent Joel Martinez and his dog Brutus discovered two tons of marijuana in a railroad car in Texas. At left is agent Jesse Ramos.

acknowledge that geography, technology, economic trends and the odds overwhelmingly favor the traffickers.

■ Mexican traffickers pay off corrupt police and officials both in Mexico and the United States to allow drugs to cross the border. While corruption in the United States is believed to be episodic rather than systemic, officials are worried that it appears to be increasing.

■ Drug-related crime and violence have made their way across the border as well, with Mexican traffickers enlisting street gang members in U.S. cities as foot soldiers. Cities like San Diego and Phoenix are seeing a vicious new style of murder, while smaller communities along the border have experienced a rash of drug-related kidnappings.

■ Although the United States and Mexico—close allies and free-trade partners—have pledged at the highest levels of government to work together in the fight against drug trafficking, the reality on the border is quite different. Cross-border relations among authorities are more often characterized by suspicion and resentment than by cooperation.

■ The Mexican drug gangs, as their influence reaches deeper into the U.S. heartland, seek to escape notice by immersing themselves in the fast-growing Mexican American communities of the nation's large cities.

Some analysts worry that Mexican immigrants and Mexican Americans might be stigmatized by the drug gangs, much as Italian Americans were stigmatized for years by the Mafia.

THE BORDER IS MORE THAN A battleground in the drug war. It is also a distinctive and complex region where a growing assimilation of peoples, cultures and economies is in some senses making the line between the two countries gradually disappear.

Much of the border region is hot, dusty and poor. There are long stretches of arid ranch land, rugged hill country and desert wilderness, with some of the 38 official border crossings separated by hundreds of miles.

But this desolate expanse is punctuated by bustling cities, sun-baked barrios and vibrant boom towns that face each other across the border in pairs—San Diego and Tijuana; Calexico, Calif., and Mexicali; Douglas, Ariz., and Agua Prieta; El Paso and Ciudad Juarez; McAllen, Tex., and Reynosa; Brownsville, Tex., and Matamoros.

Free trade between the United States and Mexico has drawn migrants from other parts of Mexico north to the border, where small factories and assembly plants have sprouted like desert wildflowers after a sudden rain. People, money and goods move back and forth across the frontier in such profusion that the two sides are more tightly linked—more interdependent, both economically and socially—than ever before.

This melding, for all its beneficial effects, makes halting the flow of drugs across the border all but impossible. Drug smuggling thrives amid a tradition of smuggling that goes back generations; cross-border family ties; high levels of poverty, illiteracy and unemployment; interlocking economies; daily commuting by students, shoppers and workers; and a unique Southwest border culture and language. And thrown into the mix are a lot of money, a little creativity and raw intimidation.

"They are just limited by their imagination," says a U.S. official who closely monitors Mexican trafficking groups. "Money is no obstacle at all."

Trafficking schemes run the gamut from the mundane to the Byzantine. In recent years, drug mafias have bought commercial jetliners and built a fleet of two-man submarines to move drugs to the United States. They have secreted loads in propane tanks and containers of hazardous materials, in small cans of tuna fish and five-gallon drums of jalapeno peppers. One trafficking group fashioned a special mold that was used successfully to ship cocaine from Mexico through the United States and into Canada completely sealed inside the walls of porcelain toilets.

The groups are using satellite-linked navigation and positioning aids to coordinate airplane drops to boats waiting in the Caribbean and to trucks in the Arizona and Texas deserts. They are using small planes equipped with ordinary car radar detectors to probe radar coverage along the border, then slipping other drug-laden aircraft through the gaps before U.S. officials can react. They are racing hauls of drugs up the coast in 22-foot-long powerboats with massive engines, digging holes in the Gulf beaches of Texas and burying their loads like hidden treasure for pickup at a later date.

THE WASHINGTON POST

They are outfitted with automatic weapons, night-vision goggles and the latest high-tech communications devices. In one case, after a wiretap went dead, DEA officials discovered that the traffickers were calling each other on a videophone and holding up written messages.

In another case, 16 people were indicted in Connecticut in June for allegedly selling devices that intercept cellular phone conversations to Mexican traffickers; the traffickers were believed to be using the devices, which are illegal for private citizens to own, to eavesdrop on law enforcement officials and other traffickers. Traffickers also "clone" cellular phones, stealing and using phone numbers that belong to unsuspecting legitimate users.

❏

AMONG THE MORE AMBITIOUS DRUG-SMUGGLING methods in recent years was the construction of tunnels under the border at Douglas, Ariz., and Otay Mesa, Calif. According to the DEA, the former was built by the Jóaquin Guzman Loera organization and was used to smuggle tons of cocaine into the United States until it was shut down following a tip from an informant. It started in a private home in Agua Prieta, Mexico, where the opening was concealed under a section of floor

covered by a pool table and operated by hydraulic lifts. From there, the tunnel went under a chain-link fence marking the border and came up in a lumber warehouse behind a Douglas hardware store.

The tunnel at Otay Mesa ran 60 feet below ground through half a mile of solid rock, U.S. officials say. It was intended to come up near the Otay Mesa port of entry for commercial cargo, but was discovered before it could be used.

California anti-drug officials were first tipped to the growing sophistication of traffickers more than five years ago after noticing tire tracks emerging from a train tunnel that straddles the border near Campo, Calif., about 35 miles east of San Diego.

As Border Patrol agents watched late one night, Mexican drug scouts disabled electronic sensors along the train tracks. The traffickers then ran a pickup truck through the 300-foot-long tunnel, while at the same time jamming the Border Patrol's radios from a hillside in Mexico with a Russian-made device that sent out a staccato clicking sound over every wave band. When the truck hit two "stinger strips" of spikes designed to flatten tires, its special "run flat" tires were unaffected by the puncture holes and it raced down the tracks three-quarters of a mile and up onto a highway.

The Border Patrol gave chase for about 12 miles until the truck sped back into Mexico through the Tecate border crossing, where it was abandoned with about 900 pounds of cocaine in the back. No one was arrested.

"A lot is hidden in plain sight," says one U.S. official, noting that much of the massive drug supply—up to 2,500 tons each year, according to estimates—smuggled from Mexico to the United States gets intermingled and lost in the crush of legitimate commerce and people crossing the world's busiest international border. In 1996, 75 million cars, 3.5 million trucks and railroad boxcars, and 254 million people entered the United States from Mexico. At some of the 38 official border crossings, fewer than 5 percent of the cars and trucks were searched for contraband.

U.S. anti-drug officials say that one of their biggest concerns is the use of legitimate railroad cargo to conceal illegal drug shipments—in the same way that legitimate maritime trade is used. A case in point was the 4,659 pounds of marijuana, worth about $3 million, found in Combes, Tex., in May by agent Martinez and his colleague Brutus, a 5-year-old Belgian Malinois shepherd dog.

The boxcar and marijuana—200 packages double-wrapped with Saran wrap, duct tape and a thick layer of transmission fluid to disguise the smell—apparently had come from the central Mexico city of Guadalajara.

"The whole front of the boxcar was found to be a secret compartment. They'd taken a sheet of metal and welded it over the compartment, then they'd painted it and rammed it with a forklift so it looked old," says Joe Garza, the Border Patrol chief in McAllen, Tex. "We'd never seen anything this sophisticated. I often wonder, how long was this going on? How many got away from us?"

✜

THIS NEEDLE-IN-A-HAYSTACK ASPECT OF THE SEARCH for illegal drug shipments is likely to worsen: Legitimate imports from Mexico have doubled from about $40 billion in 1993, the year before the North American Free Trade Agreement (NAFTA) took effect, to a projected $81 billion last year.

Traffickers often hide drugs in shipments of food, such as fish or produce, that would spoil if they were stopped and thoroughly searched. "Much of the time you're dealing with perishables, and unless we have specific information [that drugs are in the load], the priority is business and trade," says a federal official who, like many others, complains that NAFTA's mandate of unfettered commerce has hampered drug interdiction efforts.

Especially at crowded crossings, where U.S. businesspeople and tourists can swelter in traffic for more than an hour waiting to return to the United States, U.S. border guards often find drugs neatly stacked in car trunks with no effort to conceal the contraband.

"In El Paso in 1996, we had 4,545,657 pedestrian crossings [into the United States], 594,434 commercial vehicles and 16,247,097 private vehicles, for a total of 46,881,381 people," says Tom Kennedy, head of the DEA there. "With that kind of volume, forget corruption. Simple math shows that if you run enough across, the odds are in your favor."

Sometimes, if stopped for a search, so-called "port runners" will simply slam their foot on the accelerator, race through a gate and try to outrun police in high-speed chases.

Drug dealers also ship small packages of drugs to the United States via express courier services or the regular mail. In another favored method, traffickers divide large drug shipments into 50-pound loads that are floated across the Rio Grande and carried in backpacks across remote desert areas by groups of people known as mules. In some stretches, as much as 250 miles of arid wilderness separates the ports of entry.

"It's a very long border, covering thousands of miles of the most remote country you will find anywhere, and to smuggle drugs across it could be as easy as getting a tire and floating across the river," says Leonard Lindheim, the head of Customs Service investigations for southwest Texas.

"It just takes a little ingenuity," says a former DEA official from the border region. "You need a safe house in Mexico where you can store the drugs and take your time.... Wait until it's 115 degrees in Laredo and there are 150 trucks lined up and just pop in line, or until you have a huge train, and build the load into the walls of a boxcar. You can't put a dog

on a train because it's so hot it would kill him, and you need to open it for hours to let it cool down. It's just so damn easy."

Customs and DEA officials say their greatest success comes from cases in which they have informants give specific information about drug shipments. At the border crossings, officials say that their best weapon is a drug-sniffing dog, which can smell a single marijuana cigarette wrapped in plastic and hidden in a dashboard even through thick exhaust. Traffickers, though, have begun acquiring their own drug sniffing dogs so they can evaluate their packaging methods.

Authorities have tried to respond with countermeasures. At many crossings, for example, barriers have been erected to prevent cars and trucks from switching lanes, and to send them into a series of turns when leaving the gates to hinder port running.

More than 5,300 additional inspectors and patrollers have been added to the border force since 1992. The border force is also supplemented by the National Guard. The U.S. military conducted border surveillance for a while, but that program was suspended after a Marine killed a young man who was tending a herd of goats in May, mistaking him for a drug-runner.

"The idea is to be unpredictable, with more hands and more eyes," says Leticia Moran, Customs director at Laredo, Tex., the busiest commercial port on the border in 1996, clearing $20.7 billion in goods from Mexico.

Border officials are trying to counter the increasing technology and ingenuity of drug traffickers with equal doses of their own. At one crossing that is often watched for drug dealers, U.S. officials have begun filming their surveyors with a long-range lens and recently spotted two Mexican police officers helping to coordinate lane shifts by a vehicle loaded with drugs.

Inspectors also use a small gadget called a "buster" to measure the density of materials and a hand-held laser that measures distances down to the fraction of an inch, both of which can help detect hidden compartments. Some crossings are being equipped with giant X-ray machines to let agents inspect cargoes. And most crossings have computers listing licenses of cars and trucks that previously have been used in illegal activities.

✜

IN ADDITION TO THEIR INNOVATIVE SMUGGLING techniques, the Mexican cartels maintain their advantage by adapting quickly and ruthlessly when their organizations are compromised. They have kidnapped and killed informants and their families, and they change their trafficking techniques and profiles at a moment's notice to stay ahead of the law.

The Mexican drug groups also have learned valuable lessons from their Italian Mafia and Colombian cartel counterparts on how to thwart law enforcement. The Mexican groups usually are organized around family ties to prevent infiltration by informants, and they are compartmentalized to protect the leaders and to ensure that if one cell of their group is dismantled, the entire business is not destroyed.

The Southwest border is being attacked from all angles, with traffickers tunneling under it, flying over it, walking and driving across it and boating around it.

"There are many levels between the guy calling the shots in Mexico and the people we arrest here," says a DEA agent on the border. "Often with trucks, the drivers wait around an area near the border and a guy comes and says, 'I need a driver,' and he's told to take a truck from point A to point B in the United States, leave the keys under the floor mat and walk away. If he's caught driving a load, he can legitimately say, 'I was simply hired this morning and don't know anything about the people on either end.' Even if he wanted to cooperate, there's nothing he can say."

And when a driver does have information, he rarely shares it with U.S. police for fear of reprisals against his family in Mexico, investigators say.

Once in the United States, people working for the drug smugglers watch as the smaller loads are subjected to a series of drops and transfers to thwart police surveillance attempts. Finally, the loads are taken to a "stash house" in the border region and reassembled into a larger load, then taken to cities close to the border for shipment to the interior of the United States.

In December 1996, Tucson police found about six tons of neatly packaged cocaine worth about $100 million stacked in a downtown warehouse. And early last year, police found more than 10,000 pounds of marijuana in an empty house in downtown McAllen, then less than a week later discovered another 2,400 pounds in a house just three blocks from the local office of the Texas Department of Public Safety (DPS), the state's main anti-drug agency.

Drug dealers also are quick to adapt to perceived threats and new anti-drug initiatives. Often, what DEA believes is a new trafficking trend is in fact months old, and by the time it has been detected, the drug dealers have moved on to a new technique.

"All drug work is done based on profiles, and the smugglers can adapt to changes quicker than we can adapt to the new profiles," says Robert B. Nestoroff, an airplane smuggling expert with the Texas DPS. A telling example, he says, is the current disagreement among U.S. investigators over how much cross-border smuggling is being done with small planes.

❑

AT THE HEIGHT OF AIRPLANE SMUGGLING IN THE 1970s and '80s, hundreds of planes were used to smuggle drugs into Florida and to hop shipments over the border. But now, Nestoroff says, intelligence experts suggest there is very little plane activity.

"It could be we've lulled ourselves into a false sense of security and are not prioritizing it," he says. "They've adapted to our profile and they know our seams, and we're not recognizing it because we [are] not teaching it anymore. This is the swing of the pendulum."

Others argue that there is no longer a typical profile for drug dealers.

"When I started with the Border Patrol [28 years ago] in Laredo, you'd look for a young person crossing late at night. That was suspicious. We'd catch marijuana in cars, and it would be wide open—you'd look in the back seat or the back of a truck, and there it was," says Garza, the Border Patrol chief in McAllen.

"Now, you sit at the checkpoint and you can't profile anybody," he says. "It could be someone who looks like a grandmother, a lady with children sleeping on the drugs; it could be a bus driver or people in an official vehicle. We find it in drive shafts, in car bumpers, in beer coolers where they put it under ice and beer, in butane tanks, gas tanks, in air conditioner vents, in the pistons of cars being towed. They'll try anything. They carry it on their bodies, in the diapers of their children, on their person anywhere you can imagine."

"The border is absolutely overwhelmed with numbers—people, vehicles, modes of transportation," says a DEA intelligence analyst. Even though conventional wisdom says it is the riskiest choke point in the hemispheric drug pipeline, he says, "it may be that the border is the easiest part of the whole business."

Some of the Bad Guys Wear Badges

EL PASO

A Border Patrol agent in Douglas, Ariz., is convicted on drug-trafficking charges for his role in guiding across the border a vehicle loaded with more than half a ton of cocaine. In Laredo, Tex., two sheriff's officers are arrested for stealing more than a ton of marijuana from police custody and selling it back to drug dealers.

In Calexico, Calif., four current or former Customs and immigration inspectors are jailed for their part in two rings that smuggled more than 11 tons of cocaine, worth at least $165 million, into the United States over five years.

With increasing frequency along the 2,000-mile frontier between the United States and Mexico—a region of remote desert and hard-baked farmland, with a few booming cities and a generations-long tradition of smuggling—U.S. officers entrusted with defending the border have been caught surrendering it to drug traffickers.

These federal, state and local officials have been recruited by Mexican trafficking groups that for years have relied on corruption as their favored method for doing business south of the border. They are offered huge bribes and profits, and run little risk of getting caught. Authorities have had their greatest successes in discovering corruption through sheer luck—leading them to conclude that much is going undetected.

"Unfortunately, both the violence and the corruption that are attendant to the drug trade in Mexico are spilling across the border into the United States," Drug Enforcement Administration (DEA) chief Thomas A. Constantine said in recent Senate testimony. "These criminals will not hesitate to offer U.S. law enforcement officers millions of dollars to look the other way or provide them with information."

PROFITS AND BRIBES

Corruptibility of officials on both sides of the border helps drug traffickers. While official corruption reaches into the highest levels of the Mexican government, corruption on the U.S. side is more random. But the high demand of American consumers, border agents' low wages, the poverty of the border region and the high bribes paid for facilitating or turning a blind eye to the transport of drugs make it that much harder to stanch the flow of cocaine, heroin and other drugs. The profit motive for traffickers is enormous because the price of drugs paid by an American consumer is about 25 times that in a producing country, such as Bolivia.

The number of law enforcement workers along the southwest border has almost doubled in the past five years, but the flood of drugs continues:

(Includes INS inspectors and support, INS Border Patrol, DEA, FBI and U.S. attorneys. In thousands)

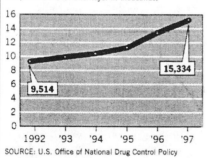

9,514 — 15,334

1992 '93 '94 '95 '96 '97

SOURCE: U.S. Office of National Drug Control Policy

Poverty in many counties in the border area is far above the U.S. average—15.1 percent for 1993—making residents and officials there more vulnerable to easy money offered by drug traffickers.

County	Percentage of population in poverty, 1993
Starr, Tex.	51.0%
Maverick, Tex.	45.3
Zavala, Tex.	45.3
Willacy, Tex.	41.6
Dimmit, Tex.	41.0
Hidalgo, Tex.	40.9
Brooks, Tex.	38.7
Presidio, Tex.	38.6
Cameron, Tex.	38.1
La Salle, Tex.	37.7
Webb, Tex.	36.7
Frio, Tex.	35.8
Zapata, Tex.	35.2
Luna, N.M.	34.9
Duval, Tex.	34.8

SOURCE: U.S. Census Bureau

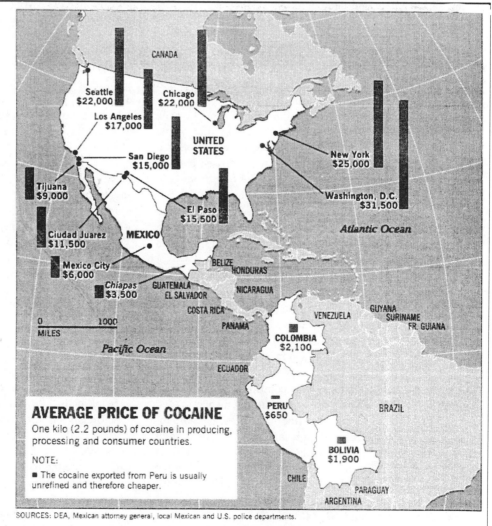

AVERAGE PRICE OF COCAINE

One kilo (2.2 pounds) of cocaine in producing, processing and consumer countries.

NOTE:

■ The cocaine exported from Peru is usually unrefined and therefore cheaper.

SOURCES: DEA, Mexican attorney general, local Mexican and U.S. police departments.

THE WASHINGTON POST

Many senior U.S. officials say that the problem of corruption on the American side of the border is limited to "a few bad apples," to cite a commonly used phrase. They say there is no proof that drug corruption in the United States is widespread or systemic, with entire border crossings or units or agencies conspiring in illegal activities. That level of graft, they say, still is confined to Mexico, where bribes are often kicked rung by rung up the ladder to the highest reaches of government, with every official along the way taking a cut.

🔲

BUT ANECDOTAL EVIDENCE SUGGESTS THAT THE problem in the United States is more extensive than generally acknowledged, particularly in local police agencies along the border. There appears to be no coordinated federal response to border corruption, however, and detecting these crimes is often a matter of chance.

Meanwhile, according to estimates based on official figures, between five and seven tons of illegal drugs are smuggled across the border every day.

"These quantities of coke and marijuana just couldn't be moved across the border if there wasn't some sort of a problem with law enforcement and detection," says Michael F. McCormick, head of the U.S. attorney's office in McAllen, Tex. "You just have to read between the lines."

Echoing that theme, a senior Mexican anti-drug official says, "How am I supposed to believe that there's no corruption in [U.S. law enforcement] when there are rivers of drugs and money corrupting it? It defies common sense."

According to a drug smuggler from Texas who says he worked for a major Mexican kingpin for about four years, every significant shipment he was involved in was protected by Mexican federal police—and, he was told, crossed into the United States at a border checkpoint with the help from U.S. officials who had been bribed. The drug dealer, who was interviewed in a Mexican jail on condition that he not be quoted by name, says he has been involved in the shipment of between 30 and 50 tons of cocaine and more than 100 tons of marijuana since 1993, earning for himself about $1 million.

"They [U.S. officials] give you a time, and you tell them the vehicle, and it's money in their pockets, without taxes," he says. "If you were working for immigration and I told you, 'We're going to cross 500 kilos and we'll give you $50,000 now and $50,000 after it's across,' would you take it or not? It's something to think about. Nobody makes $100,000 in a day."

Officials cite various factors that contribute to corruption, including low morale among many law enforcement workers; sophisticated surveillance of front-line inspectors; possible intimidation of border guards and their families; the cross-border family ties that some border guards have; and the difficulty of detecting corruption, much less proving it in court. But in the end, officials say, greed is the strongest motive for local police officers who make as little as $15,000 a year and federal border agents who start at around $25,000.

"Bribes were once $5,000, but now $30,000 to $60,000 is being offered," says Wayne Beaman, head of the McAllen

branch of the Justice Department's Office of the Inspector General. "The sky is the limit. And these organizations do their homework. . . . They have the resources in money and personnel to match any offensive we can throw at them."

🔲

ALTHOUGH THERE IS CONSIDERABLE DISAGREEMENT about the extent of corruption among U.S. border guards, virtually no one disputes that Mexican law enforcement and army officials play a fundamental role in ensuring that drugs are safely shipped through Mexico up to the border and stock-piled there until a crossing is arranged.

"It's a huge syndicate, so it's better to pay everyone off, because if you don't, someone gets [angry] and holds up the load," says a recently retired DEA official who spent nearly two decades along the border. "Everybody gets their cut—the governor, the military, high-ranking police."

Authorities say they frequently hear traffickers boast of having help on the U.S. side of the border as well—especially from U.S. Customs Service inspectors and Border Patrol guards.

Says one top federal anti-drug official in Texas: "I did a lot of undercover work, and there were hundreds of times traffickers would say, 'We've got the deal set, but not tonight, the right inspector is not in the gate.' But the next night, we had our dope."

According to McCormick, head of the U.S. attorney's office in McAllen, "People who cooperate with the government [on drug cases] give statements saying that they were told to drive a load car to point X, but not to cross until a certain time on a particular day." These informants have no direct knowledge of who was involved, he says, but it is clear the organizations have paid officials to let their drug loads through. That type of corruption "is the most lethal type of corruption you have," says a former DEA official with extensive experience on the border. But investigations of it "are not going well," he says.

"That to me is where the traffickers have made inroads. They don't need a lot of people," the former DEA official says. "They don't need anything sophisticated to happen except to know when the individual is on the line and to make sure he knows when they're going to cross. It's an absence of activity that's involved with him. He simply lets the car or truck or camper pass without a secondary search. It's just that split second."

The federal anti-drug official in Texas estimates that 10 percent to 25 percent of the drugs smuggled into the United States from Mexico each year cross the border with help from corrupt U.S. officials.

Officials say they believe, however, that by far the greater portion of the illegal drug supply that comes across the border does so without the help of corrupt U.S. agents. As evidence, officials cite the increasingly sophisticated techniques Mexican gangs are using to smuggle their loads, as well as the logic of pure arithmetic.

Given that more than 46 million people and 16 million vehicles crossed the border at El Paso in 1996, says Tom Kennedy, the head of the DEA there, "Why would anyone want to pay extra money to come through the gate . . . when all they have to do is hide the coke in a concealed compartment on a semi-trailer with a legitimate load and a legitimate driver who's not even aware of what's going on? The odds are in their favor."

❂

THE VARIOUS FEDERAL AGENCIES CHARGED WITH stopping drugs at the border have begun sniping at one another—although few officials are willing to attach their names to their complaints—over how well they are policing themselves against corruption. Some of the bitter grousing has ethnic overtones.

"The Customs and Border Patrol recruit along the [Rio Grande] river, and many are great kids," says a high-ranking anti-drug official in Texas who asked not to be identified. "The fatal mistake is sending them right back to their home town, because a percentage have family ties to people who are corrupt. When a brother-in-law comes through his lane, what's he going to do—search him? They wave him through. Some are corrupt, and some are unknowingly corrupted. They are manipulated."

Many border officials say they find such suspicions insulting and demeaning to Hispanics, who account for as much as 90 percent of the population in some border counties. In fact, they say, people hired locally often are better at detecting smugglers.

"I think it's an insult to insinuate home [local] people are susceptible to corruption," says Ramon Juarez, the Laredo port director for the Immigration and Naturalization Service (INS). "The inspectors who are most successful at detecting violators are from here. They know the people, the culture, the area. They have a sixth sense about what's going on.

"When I have seen corruption, it's because the system allowed it," he says. "The guys trying to get things across are desperate. They'll do anything. And they have intelligence systems. They'll study us and identify our weak links, and you'll never know why someone is going to be corrupted. But it doesn't mean everybody is corrupt."

Some U.S. agents are lured into corruption gradually by traffickers in a process akin to the recruitment of foreign spies by intelligence agencies. Such was apparently the case with a convicted federal law enforcement official who is completing a prison sentence for conspiracy to smuggle narcotics. The man testified at a recent Senate hearing, using the alias Joe Daedalus.

Wearing a hood and speaking into a microphone that disguised his voice, the Vietnam veteran with 15 years of government service testified that he was slowly "sucked in" by a trafficking ring through Mexican members who befriended him during the course of his duties.

"I did not know at the time that these people were traffickers, but they knew who I was," he testified. He visited them at their homes on special occasions, such as birthdays and baptisms. He received unsolicited gifts, such as baseball tickets, and on one occasion, after mentioning that he wanted to do some landscaping. he returned home to find a couple of

With increasing frequency along the 2,000-mile frontier between the United States and Mexico—a region of remote desert and hard-baked farmland, with a few booming cities and a generations-long tradition of smuggling—U.S. officers entrusted with defending the border have been caught surrendering it to drug traffickers.

fully grown palm trees planted in his lawn. "Before I realized it, they had their hooks into me," he said.

When the pitch to help them smuggle drugs finally came, he said, he was "vulnerable" because of his agency's "lack of recognition" for his hard work and because of "problems with some of my superiors." He said he took payoffs totaling $50,000 for helping the smugglers on about a dozen occasions.

Officials say that vulnerable federal employees—for instance, people who are over their heads in debt—are particularly susceptible to the bribes offered by drug dealers. The risk of federal employees falling prey to drug money can be lowered with regular employee background checks of the sort that are done when they are first hired, but the agencies have not regularly rechecked longtime employees. An effort is now being made, however, to submit inspectors to more frequent and thorough checks, including reviews of their personal finances.

In a September 1995 review of the Border Patrol, the Justice Department's Office of the Inspector General "found that one-third of the Border Patrol was overdue for reinvestigation," according to May Senate testimony by Michael R. Bromwich, head of the office. "INS's neglect of reinvestigations is historic, as had been true of the department generally."

Thorough background checks and periodic monitoring are particularly important given the rapid hiring of federal law enforcement personnel in recent years along the border, officials say. Since 1992, the Border Patrol and its parent agency, the INS, have increased their border staffing by more than 80 percent, from 5,863 employees to 10,746 this year.

Better background checking might have warned officials to watch for potential problems with Thomas Bair, 26. The Border Patrol agent was discovered by two other agents three months ago close to a border fence in a rugged area of eastern

San Diego County with 11 duffel bags in and near his patrol van stuffed with 602 pounds of marijuana worth $300,000.

An investigation of the incident revealed that Bair had declared bankruptcy in 1995 and was working at a paint and body shop in San Diego County when hired by the Border Patrol, says Assistant U.S. Attorney Michael Wheat.

But soon after joining the service, he bought a new Mustang with $100 bills, made $12,000 in payments on another vehicle and paid off $10,000 worth of credit card debt. At the time of his Aug. 5 arrest, he was about to make a $64,000 down payment on a $193,000 house—all on a salary of $29,000 a year, Wheat says. Bair also was found to be residing in the United States only one night a week, spending the rest of his time across the border in Tecate with his Mexican girlfriend. He pleaded not guilty, claiming he had seized his drugs on his own to become the "hero" of his unit, and is being held without bail pending trial, which is expected early this year.

In May, Jorge Luis Mancha, 43, a Border Patrol agent in Douglas, Ariz., was convicted on drug smuggling charges stemming from the September 1995 seizure of a vehicle containing 1,200 pounds of cocaine and 28 pounds of marijuana, a load the Border Patrol says was worth $38.4 million.

Mancha's corruption was discovered after two Border Patrol agents in Douglas intercepted a teenager with a scanner in his car. The youth, a suspected scout for a drug trafficking gang, was allowed to go—but only after one of the agents examined the scanner and wrote down its frequencies. Agents then started monitoring the channels and eventually heard Mancha trying to guide a drug load across the border from Mexico. Later that night, a couple of agents came upon Mancha as he was riding a bicycle along the border and noticed that he was wearing a headset transmitter that he tried to conceal. When agents later found the drug-laden vehicle, there were bicycle tracks all around it, a federal court in Tucson was told.

Evidence presented at his trial showed that Mancha had been involved in drug trafficking for at least three years, amassing more than $444,000 in payoffs.

Some investigations have revealed broader conspiracies. In El Paso, six Customs and INS inspectors have been jailed since 1992 for waving drug loads through their gates. One cocaine-smuggling ring used a system of beepers to tell couriers what time to come and which lane to drive through.

Customs inspector Eduardo V. Ontiveros, 46, was sentenced in 1996 to 24 years in prison in the case. He had provided the ring with confidential information from a Customs computer system and recruited another inspector, Jose de Jesus Ramos, 41, to accept a $1 million bribe to allow a vehicle carrying 2,200 pounds of cocaine to enter the United States, prosecutors said. The April 1995 crossing turned out to be a sting. Ramos, who pleaded guilty and testified against Ontiveros, received a reduced sentence of 7 ½ years in prison.

❏

ANOTHER CONSPIRACY WAS BROKEN UP IN 1995 AFTER a drug courier, a young Mexican, apparently drove through the wrong inspection lane at the Calexico, Calif., port

of entry, and an INS inspector discovered 823 pounds of cocaine stacked unconcealed in her car's trunk and more than $47,000 stashed under the driver's seat.

The woman immediately confessed her role in one of two overlapping Mexican drug trafficking rings that together involved at least four current or former INS and Customs officials. The officials had helped smuggle more than 11 tons of cocaine, worth at least $165 million, into the United States between 1990 and 1995. Investigators seized $1.2 million in cash, most of it from Ernest Garcia, 42, a former INS employee who directed couriers for one of the rings. Garcia and his three accomplices—including his brother, who worked as an INS inspector in Calexico from 1988 to 1995 and was involved in both rings, and another former INS inspector de-

Thorough background checks and periodic monitoring are particularly important given the rapid hiring of federal law enforcement personnel in recent years along the border, officials say. Since 1992, the Border Patrol and its parent agency, the INS, have increased their border staffing by more than 80 percent, from 5,863 employees to 10,746 this year.

scribed by the government as a "narcotics broker" in Calexico—were sentenced in 1996 and 1997 to prison terms ranging from 10 years to life without parole. Six Mexican nationals also were convicted in the case.

Federal officials are deeply divided about how to prevent such rings from developing, but the solution favored by many law enforcement and corruption experts is a regular rotation of personnel—which severs potentially corrupting cross-border ties—along with regular polygraph examinations.

Many Customs and immigration officials strenuously oppose rotation as too disruptive of agents' personal lives, however, and the Customs employees' union also opposes such a policy. Moreover, it is particularly difficult to recruit people from other parts of the United States to work in the hot, dusty, impoverished border area, officials say, adding that border communities offer the biggest pool of bilingual workers. In Senate testimony last year, former Customs commissioner George Weise estimated that staff rotation would cost a prohibitive $60 million a year.

Border officials are trying to foil corruption and defeat surveillance by being as unpredictable as possible—not publishing work assignments in advance, prohibiting inspectors from making calls during their shifts, switching inspectors from booth to booth at a moment's notice, ordering an entire lane of 20 cars to open their trunks or to undergo a more intense secondary inspection.

Local law enforcement officials, while not involved in guarding the border, still can use their police authority to help smugglers move their loads. The extent of that problem became clear in 1994 and 1995 through a series of high-profile local corruption cases along a 300-mile stretch of border in southern Texas. A county judge, a county clerk, the sheriffs of three counties, a local district attorney and a county jail administrator all were convicted of drug crimes. The situation has not improved in recent years, state and federal officials say, making them reluctant to work drug cases with their local counterparts. A case in Webb County illustrates why.

◻

FEDERAL OFFICIALS USUALLY DECLINE TO prosecute small drug cases—generally those involving less than 150 pounds of marijuana—and instead turn them over to state and local officials for adjudication. When that happens, local police take custody of the drugs from federal authorities to use as evidence.

But instead of taking marijuana seized by federal authorities to the local evidence room, Reynaldo Ortegon, 46, the head of the Webb County sheriff's narcotics unit and internal affairs division, and his deputy, Alfredo Tijerina, 35, replaced them with fake bricks made of soap and alfalfa hay, and sold the real stuff back to drug dealers. The deputy also used the captain's official police cruiser to drive a load of cocaine past a Border Patrol checkpoint in what turned out to be a sting.

Court documents show that the pair, who have been sentenced to four years in jail each, employed the scheme on 40 occasions over two years, stealing more than a ton of marijuana.

And on Sept. 23, five former police officers—including two chiefs—from the small south Texas town of Donna were indicted for distributing marijuana, money laundering and official corruption after using police cruisers to escort more than 1,700 pounds of marijuana to delivery points near their town in 1995 and 1996.

"We clearly have seen corruption of sheriffs, Customs Department inspectors and others," White House drug policy director Barry R. McCaffrey said during a recent tour of the Southwest border.

"The drug trade produces billions of dollars which have a corrupting influence on democratic institutions on both sides of the border. . . . The question isn't whether there'll be corruption. The question is, what are we going to do about it?"

—*William Branigin and John Ward Anderson*

Raising the stakes in U.S.–Mexico drug wars

$2.2 million reward for a nobody

BY LINDA ROBINSON IN MEXICO CITY

After seven years of chasing drug traffickers, Richard Fass was no novice when it came to dangerous undercover work. His easy charm and fluent Spanish made him one of the Drug Enforcement Administration's most effective agents. From his Phoenix base, Fass saw methamphetamine, a synthetic drug cooked in rural Mexican and American labs, pouring into the city. Meth was becoming the new scourge of the '90s, and Phoenix one of the top three markets for the white crystals.

On June 30, 1994, Fass was on his last day at work undercover. He was being transferred to a desk job in Mexico, and his wife and four children were waiting for him to go shopping for the move to Monterrey. But Fass had one more drug gang to bust, a job that turned out to be his last.

It has been four years now, and the gang leader allegedly responsible for the killing of Fass, a Mexican named Agustín Vásquez Mendoza, is still a free man. This week the U.S. government is posting a reward of up to $2.2 million in an all-out effort to catch Vásquez. One of the few means to deter traffickers who kill agents is the certainty that they will be hunted down and caught. If that doesn't happen, agents say, it will be open season on them.

Targeting agents. Enforcing the rule has become more critical than ever because the DEA has embarked on a high-stakes effort to dismantle the Mexican trafficking rings that now feed most of the U.S. market. Nine joint U.S.-Mexican teams have been formed to go after the traffickers, and officials fear they will be targeted.

Capturing Vásquez is the DEA's top priority. The only accused killer of an agent still at large, he was put on the FBI's Ten Most Wanted list last year. Now Washington is upping the reward in hopes of smoking him out.

Fass could have kicked back and taken it easy on that last day at work, but he had set up a drug sting, posing as a meth buyer who would pay $160,000 for 10 kilos [22 pounds] of the drug from a tough who called himself Aniceto. About 6:10 p.m., Fass and agent Tony Pelonero drove into the parking lot of a strip mall in Glendale. Leaving Pelonero there with a gym bag full of cash, Fass entered the auto-repair shop where the two dealers were waiting. One of them, Juan Vásquez Rubio, 24, went out to the truck with Fass for the prearranged "flash" of money to prove the buyers' bona fides. Then they went back inside and Vásquez telephoned Aniceto, who was to bring the drugs.

But the elaborate sting suddenly took a deadly turn: Vásquez and his brother-in-law, Rafael Rubio Méndez, 20, pulled their guns and forced Fass into the back office and onto the floor along with two garage employees who were cooperating with the DEA. Whipping out a pair of handcuffs, Rubio clamped Fass's left wrist and told him he was a dead man. Fass yanked his 9-mm Glock pistol with his free hand and shot Rubio through the right breast. Rubio fired back with a lucky shot that knocked the trigger off Fass's pistol.

As Fass and the garage employees begged for their lives, Juan Vásquez aimed his .45-caliber pistol at the DEA agent's head and fired three times. A fourth shot pierced his chest. The other two men were saved when Vásquez accidentally flipped on the safety. Thinking his gun had jammed, he ran for it. The wounded Rubio jumped into a car and fled before Pelonero could get a shot off. The two were caught within minutes by DEA backup teams. But it was too late for Fass, who at age 37 had become the 34th DEA agent killed in the line of duty.

Still free. Four years later, Rubio and Juan Vásquez are serving life in prison, but the man who allegedly set up the deal, Aniceto, Agustín Vásquez Mendoza, remains free. Driving up moments after the shooting, he saw the backup agents and kept going. "Aniceto" was the head of a family gang that specialized in drug-dealer rip-offs. Roaming the West, they would pretend to have drugs, set up deals, then rob and often kill unsuspecting buyers.

Agustín Vásquez first fled to a safe house, then to Mexico, where he burrowed deep: From Sonora to Baja California, then to the state of Michoacán, where the Vásquez clan has lived for generations.

This spring DEA Administrator Thomas Constantine decided to make an

From *U.S. News & World Report*, October 5, 1998, pp. 35–36. © 1998 by U.S. News & World Report. Visit us at our Web site at www.usnews.com for additional information.

all-out push for Vásquez's arrest to send a signal to Mexican traffickers whose business flourishes while the U.S. and Mexican governments squabble. The frictions date to the 1985 torture killing of DEA agent Enrique Camarena.

The quarrel between the two governments intensified this spring after U.S. Customs conducted a massive money-laundering sting, in part on Mexican soil, without letting Mexican officials know. That came on the heels of an uproar last year when Mexico's top antidrug official, Gen. Jess Gutirrez Rebollo, was arrested for taking millions from the biggest Mexican drug lord.

The problems continue. Members of Mexico's new antidrug force are suspended and under investigation for collaborating with traffickers. The brother of a former president of Mexico is accused by the Swiss government of taking $500 million in drug bribes.

Mexico responded with anger this month after the House of Representatives passed a bill aimed at coercing Mexico to let DEA agents carry guns for self-defense in its territory—a matter of bitter dispute for two years.

Last week, Mexico balked at jointly announcing the new U.S. reward for Vásquez. Mike Garland, head of the 45-agent DEA office in Mexico, said: "I wish they had a greater appreciation of how important this is to us."

Catching Agustín Vásquez would not seem that tall an order, even for Mexico, since he's small fry compared with the big-time traffickers. But Mike Huerta's hair has gone gray in the four years that he has been leading the hunt. He spends half his time in Mexico and follows up every lead with the help of 14 agents and a half-dozen state and federal agencies all over the United States. Their zealous pursuit has led to 40 U.S. arrests of suspects wanted for other crimes.

"We get calls from everywhere in the U.S.," said Huerta. But the best intelligence indicates that Vásquez is in his Mexican hideout.

Serious obstacles impede Vásquez's capture. One is foot dragging by a peeved Mexican government that says the manhunt is not its top priority. The other is the very real danger of penetrating the mountains where growing marijuana and opium poppies, cooking meth,

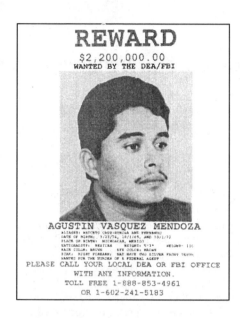

REWARD
$2,200,000.00
WANTED BY THE DEA/FBI

AGUSTIN VASQUEZ MENDOZA
ALIASES: AGUSTO CRUZ-ZUNIGA AND FERNANDO
DATE OF BIRTH: 5/23/74, 10/1/69, AND 10/1/71
PLACE OF BIRTH: MICHOACAN, MEXICO
NATIONALITY: MEXICAN   HEIGHT: 5'3"   WEIGHT: 110
HAIR COLOR: BROWN   EYE COLOR: BROWN
SCAR: RIGHT FOREARM; MAY HAVE TWO SILVER FRONT TEETH
WANTED FOR THE MURDER OF A FEDERAL AGENT
PLEASE CALL YOUR LOCAL DEA OR FBI OFFICE
WITH ANY INFORMATION.
TOLL FREE 1-888-853-4961
OR 1-602-241-5183

Big bounty on small-time rip-off artist

and engaging in violence are a way of life. In a drug raid there in the 1970s, seven Mexican federal policemen were stranded when a helicopter broke down. The next day they were found dead, buried alive. "Everybody up there has a criminal enterprise going," said one senior U.S. official.

Vásquez is hunkered down in a tiny village of 40 people living in wooden shacks with no electricity or telephones.

The long arm of the law, with all its sophisticated technology, is no help here; billion-dollar satellites that record phone calls and photograph license plates have nothing to pick up. "It was easier to catch Pablo Escobar," says Tom Raffanello, the DEA agent in charge of the Phoenix office, referring to the violent Colombian drug lord whose retinue of cars and bodyguards with cell phones aided his capture.

Huerta and other agents doggedly sniff the trail into Michoacán, but any stranger showing up in Vásquez's lair would be an immediate target. It's up to the Mexicans to penetrate the mountains or lie in wait for him in nearby Apatzingán, where he comes down periodically to drink. Last month, after prodding by the DEA, Mexican police agreed to make the trek to follow up a reported sighting of Vásquez, but all they got was one of his relatives. They had to send a force of 300 men, yet failed to seal off escape routes.

Rosa Fass still grieves for her son as if he died yesterday. Richard Fass was the first Fass to go to college; an altar boy till age 18, he almost became a priest but decided to work with juveniles, then joined the DEA. The living room of the family's modest home is lined with Richard's plaques and medals and a framed quotation of Raymond Chandler: "Down these mean streets a man must go who is not himself mean, who is neither tarnished nor afraid. He is the hero. . . ."

Rosa Fass's eyes brim with tears. "I feel that they did not do enough to protect him," she said. "We still have so many unanswered questions." An agent who joined the DEA because he liked and admired Richard Fass said, "That's why I went on the task force. I hope they'll believe [in us] when we find Vásquez."

The Charm City blues

For Baltimore, homicide has become a real-life horror story

BY ANGIE CANNON

In the wee hours of the morning, just four days before Christmas, detectives dug up the battered body of 41-year-old Rufus Washington from a patch of woods in southwest Baltimore. The motive, police said, was the same as for hundreds of other murders they've seen: drugs. But in one way, Washington's death was unlike the others. He was No. 300, the murder that turned Baltimore's crusade to avoid that number into a failure.

In Charm City, life is—sadly—imitating art. Its glitzy Inner Harbor showplace notwithstanding, Baltimore is essentially still the gritty, blue-collar town so familiar to TV viewers as the perfect setting for NBC's police drama *Homicide: Life on the Street.* Ever since 1990, the city has claimed the grim distinction of more than 300 homicides annually, keeping it among the nation's murder capitals even though the number of violent crimes, and notably murders, has precipitously fallen nationwide. No one really knows for sure why places like New York are making such remarkable progress while Baltimore lags. But the answer may lie in the nature of a city's drug trade and the workings of its police culture. For criminologists, Baltimore may be the exception that proves the rule.

The brass was so determined to keep 1998's total below 300 that last month Police Commissioner Thomas C. Frazier ordered an extra 60 to 100 deskbound officers to hit the streets. But the bodies continued to pile up, hitting 313 as the New Year approached.

Assassins. Baltimore's persistent killings are especially puzzling because the number of other kinds of violent crime, such as rapes and aggravated assaults, has declined there over the last few years. But a recent study of shootings turned up a disturbing trend: Many appeared to be premeditated gangland executions. Gunmen were using higher-caliber weapons. They were firing more shots, usually at their victims' heads and at close range. These killings "are assassinations," said Peter Beilenson, commissioner of Baltimore's Health Department.

That sort of MO usually means only one thing: drugs. And in Baltimore, the drug of choice is heroin. A recent University of Maryland study showed that in Baltimore a higher percentage of people arrested tested positive for heroin than in any other U.S. city. Baltimore also has an astonishingly high number of drug addicts—59,000 in a city of 675,000. "What's unique about Baltimore is this addiction problem," said Chuck Wexler, head of the national Police Executive Research Forum. "This is larger than a police problem."

Frazier also believes that crack cocaine came to Baltimore a little later than it did to other cities. Most big cities first saw crack in the mid-1980s but have since seen the violence recede as a younger generation has turned off crack and gang disputes over crack-selling territory have settled out. In cities like Baltimore and Indianapolis, gang clashes may still be raging. Health Department head Beilenson notes the possibility that New York's crime crackdown has sent some drug dealers to Baltimore. "New York has done a good job of zero tolerance, and they have pushed the drug dealers elsewhere," he speculated.

But the fact that tough policing has curtailed the drug trade in other cities raises questions about tensions within the Baltimore police department. Frazier arrived in 1994 from San Jose, Calif., and has made big changes. Frazier says he has put in place strategies that have worked in New York and other cities. For instance, one morning a week, the department's top officers meet to discuss crime patterns and enforcement. Officers are focusing on the city's crime "hot spots."

Cop grumbles. Last year, police blanketed the tough East and West sides, where the streets are jumping with the furtive glances and sly signals of drug dealing. The officers have been shutting down open-air drug markets as well as stopping cars for traffic infractions—as a way to look for guns and drugs. But the new commissioner also reorganized

IS IT SAFE YET?
The incredible shrinking crime rate

For Americans long accustomed to deadbolt locks and blood-soaked bodies on the nightly news, the numbers are nothing short of stunning: Crime across the United States is in a free fall, and no one is sure when the good news will end. In a late Christmas present, the Justice Department's National Crime Victimization Survey revealed last week that Americans suffered less at the hands of criminals in 1997 than they have at any time since the poll was first taken in 1973. Another new Justice Department study found that the nation's 1997 murder rate was the lowest in three decades. And the early word from police departments across the country suggests that things only got better in 1998. The late December total of 414 homicides in Los Angeles for 1998 represented a 27 percent drop from just the previous year, and the lowest tally since 1970. At last count, Chicago tallied 697 homicides in 1998 compared with 760 in 1997. And New York, which had 2,262 murders as recently as 1990, recorded just over 600 last year—fewer than in 1964.

Experts claim there is no single explanation for the decline, but many say the waning crack epidemic in many parts of the country is a major factor. Another cited by criminologists like Northeastern University's James Alan Fox is a significant demographic shift—specifically, a recent drop in the numbers of young people who have traditionally committed a disproportionate number of crimes. Still other factors include tougher prison sentences, stricter gun laws, smarter police strategies—and more police.

Many of those strategies began in New York, where Mayor Rudolph Giuliani and his first police commissioner, William Bratton, re-engineered New York's department, first by embracing the so-called "broken windows" theory that leaving small infractions unpunished would inevitably lead to more serious crime. The NYPD has thus cracked down on nuisance crimes like public urination and blaring boom boxes. The department has also revolutionized crime-fighting by holding precinct commanders personally responsible for crime reduction. A program called CompStat uses computer mapping to illuminate previously unseen crime trends, and the maps then serve as the basis for brainstorming sessions that hold commanders' feet to the fire. Bratton's successor, Howard Safir, has also enlisted federal agencies in offensives against drug gangs in neighborhoods like Washington Heights; Safir believes the drug trade is the root cause of much of the city's crime.

Despite the gains, some say the news is not quite as rosy as it appears. "Sure, crime is down," says UCLA professor emeritus James Q. Wilson, "but not compared to 35 years ago. We've made gains, but we're not back to the Garden of Eden yet." Others worry that the population of teens is now creeping up again, possibly ushering in another crime wave. These concerns are no doubt legitimate, but they can't obscure the bottom line: Thousands more people were alive to ring in another year.—*James Morrow*

the department to put more than 300 cops back on the street and raised hackles with his policy of rotating officers after four years in a post, such as the homicide unit. Some street cops don't seem to want to follow Frazier's program. "Baltimore is a little dysfunctional in a lot of ways," said one Maryland criminal-justice expert. "Frazier is a very innovative chief, but it's hard to get the department or city infrastructure to implement forward-thinking ideas, either because of a lack of cooperation or because you can't get your rank-and-file people to see the big picture."

That sort of friction may make it tougher to break the deadly cycle that begins with drugs. On a recent evening, officers Mike Kirschner and Antwuan Fletcher cruised in a white, unmarked car and stopped knots of men and women as light snow fell. The officers asked them to lift their shirts and coats as they searched for guns and drugs. Early in their rounds, they found a sad-eyed, 17-year-old youth who begged them to let him go; but he had 22 vials of crack and a wad of bills in his shirt. "How many times you been locked up?" Kirschner asked the teen. "Six times, sir," was the grim reply.

Whatever the strategy, it's that reality the cops face nightly. "You see so many more *boys* with guns," said Bill McCall, a 26-year cop who now normally rides a desk. The police are all searching for answers. One recent night, Col. Bert Shirey gave a pep talk at roll call before the troops headed out. The mood was somber. The officers knew the city had passed the 300 mark. "Don't let that disturb you," Shirey said. "There would have been a lot more if we hadn't been on the street. Everyone is doing a good job." He didn't need to say, "Better luck next year."

PERSPECTIVES

Drugs, Crime, Prison
and Treatment

**by Charles Blanchard, chief counsel, White House Office of National Drug Control Policy
(ONDCP); former Arizona state senator and CSG Toll Fellow, class of '91**

Talk to any police officer, judge or probation officer, or visit any prison. One fact becomes abundantly clear: there is a clear link between crime and drug use. While no one factor can explain criminal behavior, it is undeniable that drug addiction is an important factor in explaining crime and violence. Study after study confirms this link:

• Over half of the crime in this country is committed by individuals under the influence of drugs. The National Institute of Justice's ADAM drug-testing program found that more than 60 percent of adult male arrestees tested positive for drugs. In most cities, over half of young male arrestees are under the influence of marijuana. Importantly, the majority of these crimes result from the effects of the drug—and do not result from the fact that drugs are illegal.

• According to a study by the National Center on Addiction and Substance Abuse (CASA) at Columbia University, 80 percent of the men and women behind bars—about 1.4 million inmates—are seriously involved with alcohol and other drug abuse.

• A study published in the *Journal of American Medical Association* last year indicated that nondrug users who live in households where drugs (including marijuana) are used are 11 times as likely to be killed as those living in drug-free households. Drug abuse in a home increased a women's risk of being killed by a close relative by 28 times.

Despite this strong link between drugs and crime, few probationers and inmates receive drug or alcohol treatment. While states estimate that 70 to 85 percent of their inmates need some substance abuse treatment, only 13 percent of these inmates received any treatment in 1996. Sadly, even in those state prisons that do offer quality treatment, only a relatively small percentage of offenders take advantage of it.

It is time for state and federal leaders to take a closer look at funding substance abuse treatment in criminal justice systems. And, it is time to become more creative in using the coercive power of the criminal justice system (a system with many opportunities for rewards and punishments) to induce offenders to seek and remain in treatment.

Fortunately, in recent years many state and local governments and the federal government have experimented with drug treatment programs in the criminal justice system.

From *Spectrum*, Winter 1999, pp. 26-27. © 1999 by The Council of State Governments. Reprinted with permission from Spectrum.

Thanks to the evaluations of these innovative programs, we now have good evidence that using the coercive power of the criminal justice system to force probationers and inmates into treatment is a cost-effective means of reducing crime. Recent evaluations of a myriad of criminal justice treatment programs—ranging from diversion programs such as drug courts and the Brooklyn Drug Treatment Alternative-to-Prison program, and institutional drug treatment programs such as those in Delaware and the Federal Bureau of Prisons—have found that drug treatment reduces crime. These studies show that quality treatment programs of sufficient length that include transition services in the community reduce drug use and future criminal behavior.

Among inmates who completed residential drug treatment, only 3.3 percent were rearrested in the first six months, compared with 12.1 percent of inmates who did not receive treatment.

As a result of the Violent Crime Control and Law Enforcement Act of 1994, the Federal Bureau of Prisons now provides drug treatment to all eligible inmates prior to their release from custody. Last Spring, the Bureau of Prisons announced its first analysis of the success of this program. It shows that institution-based drug treatment can make a difference. Among inmates who completed residential drug treatment, only 3.3 percent were rearrested in the first six months, compared with 12.1 percent of inmates who did not receive treatment. Similarly, the Delaware Department of Corrections conducts outstanding drug treatment programs. A study of the Delaware program found that those inmates who received both institutional drug treatment and transitional support services had far fewer arrests and far less drug use after release than those inmates who had no such treatment. Eighteen months after arrest, 71 percent of the treated inmates were arrest-free, and 76 percent were drug-free. In contrast, only 30 percent of those inmates who had no treatment were arrest-free and only 19 percent were drug-free.

Perhaps the most innovative treatment programs, however, have not been in institutional settings. Instead, thanks in large measure to the ideas of scholars such as Mark Kleiman, several state and local leaders have begun to build treatment programs for offenders outside the prison system that are based on the concept of coerced abstinence. The idea is a simple one: use the coercive power of the criminal justice system to induce nonviolent offenders into treatment. Sadly, even when treatment is available, only a small number of offenders enter and remain in treatment. To remedy this problem, coerced abstinence programs use a "carrot and stick" approach—using drug testing, graduated sanctions and treatment—to induce offenders to take treatment seriously.

Surprisingly to some, these coerced abstinence programs work just as well as voluntary treatment programs in reducing the drug use and criminal activity of their graduates. Importantly, however, these coerced abstinence programs are more successful than voluntary programs both in inducing offenders to participate in treatment and in retaining offenders in treatment. For example, Charles J. Hynes, the Kings County (Brooklyn) District Attorney, has built a coerced treatment program known as the Drug Treatment Alternative-to-Prison (DTAP) program. Evaluations of the DTAP program found that the overall retention rate for offenders in the DTAP program was 64 percent—at least two times higher than the retention rate for most residential treatment programs. Moreover, after one year, DTAP offenders had less than half the arrest rate of drug offenders sent to prison.

Similarly, preliminary evaluations of drug courts have been encouraging. There are now about 300 drug courts in operation, with drug courts located in virtually every state. Using drug testing, treatment, and graduated sanctions, drug courts offer non-violent offenders the hope of a dismissal of charges if they successfully complete drug treatment. During the program, graduated sanctions (such as jail time) are used to punish offenders who test positive for drugs or who otherwise fail to participate in treatment. Offenders who fail the program altogether face time in prison. This combination of positive and negative incentives appears to work. Studies of the drug court programs in Brooklyn, Maricopa

County (Arizona), the District of Columbia, Portland (Oregon), and Dade County (Florida) all found high retention rates, low re-arrest rates and lower drug use. Participants in these programs had arrest and drug use rates far lower than similar offenders who did not participate in the program.

Substance abuse treatment of offenders will pay for itself. Indeed, the CASA study concluded that if just ten percent of inmates given one year of residential treatment stay sober and work during the first year after release, prison-based drug treatment would more than pay for itself in one year. This is because the costs of continued drug use by released offenders is tremendously expensive to society. By ensuring the availability of treatment in the entire continuum of criminal sanc-

tions—from diversion programs to probation to prison—states can reduce crime, reduce arrest and prosecution costs, reduce incarceration costs, reduce drug-related emergency room visits, and increase employment.

Of course, states must carefully construct quality treatment programs that are based on models—such as the Delaware prison treatment program and Brooklyn's DTAP program—that work. If they do so, however, there is every indication of a large payoff. By breaking the cycle of drugs and crime, we will have fewer victims, more productive citizens, and safer communities.

More infromation on criminal justice treatment programs can be found on the ONDCP web site: http://www.whitehousedrugpolicy.gov.

Doping Kids

Though shocked by bizarre shootings in schools, few Americans have noticed how many shooters were among the 6 million kids now on psychotropic drugs.

By Kelly Patricia O'Meara

Just three weeks after Eric Harris and Dylan Klebold went on their April 20 killing spree at Columbine High School in Littleton, Colo., President Clinton hosted a White House conference on youth violence. The president declared it a strategy session to seek "the best ideas from people who can really make a difference: parents and young people, teachers and religious leaders, law enforcement, gun manufacturers, representatives of the entertainment industry and those of us here in government."

There was, however, complete silence from the president when it came to including representatives from the mental-health community, whom many believe can provide important insight about the possible connection between the otherwise seemingly senseless acts of violence being committed by school-age children and prescription psychotropic drugs such as Ritalin, Luvox and Prozac.

There are nearly 6 million children in the United States between the ages of 6 and 18 taking mind-altering drugs prescribed for alleged mental illnesses that increasing numbers of mental-health professionals are questioning.

Although the list of school-age children who have gone on violent rampages is growing at a disturbing rate—and the shootings at Columbine became a national wake-up call—few in the mental-health community have been willing to talk about the possibility that the heavily prescribed drugs and violence may be linked. Those who try to investigate quickly learn that virtually all data concerning violence and psychotropic drugs are protected by the confidentiality provided minors. But in the highly publicized shootings

this spring, information has been made available to the public.

• **April 16:** Shawn Cooper, a 15-year-old sophomore at Notus Junior-Senior High School in Notus, Idaho, was taking Ritalin, the most commonly prescribed stimulant, for bipolar disorder when he fired two shotgun rounds, narrowly missing students and school staff.

• **April 20:** Harris, an 18-year-old senior at Columbine High School, killed a dozen students and a teacher before taking his own life. Prior to the shooting rampage, he had been under the influence of Luvox, one of the new selective serotonin reuptake inhibitor, or SSRI, antidepressants approved in 1997 by the Food and Drug Administration, or FDA, for children up to the age of 17 for treatment of obsessive-compulsive disorder, or OCD.

• **May 20:** T.J. Solomon, a 15-year-old at Heritage High School in Conyers, Ga., was being treated with Ritalin for depression when he opened fire on and wounded six classmates. Two other high-profile cases from last year show a similar pattern:

• **May 21, 1998:** Kip Kinkel, a 15-year-old at Thurston High School in Springfield, Ore., murdered his parents and then proceeded to school where he opened fire on students in the cafeteria, killing two and wounding 22. Kinkel had been prescribed both Ritalin and Prozac. Although widely used among adults, Prozac has not been approved by the FDA for pediatric use.

• **March 24, 1998:** Mitchell Johnson, 13, and Andrew Golden, 11, opened fire on their classmates at Westside Middle

School in Jonesboro, Ark. Johnson had been receiving psychiatric counseling and, although information about the psychotropic drugs that may have been prescribed for him has not been made public, his attorney, Val Price, responded when asked about it: "I think that is confidential information, and I don't want to reveal that."

A great deal has been written about all of these cases. There have, however, been no indications that all of these children watched the same TV programs or listened to the same music. Nor has it been established that they all used illegal drugs, suffered from alcohol abuse or had common difficulties with their families or peers. They did not share identical home lives, dress alike or participate in similar extracurricular activities. But all of the above were labeled as suffering from a mental illness and were being treated with psychotropic drugs that for years have been known to cause serious adverse effects when given to children.

At the top of the list of so-called "mental illnesses" among children is attention-deficit/hyperactivity disorder, or ADHD, which is diagnosed when a child meets six of the 18 criteria described in the *Diagnostic and Statistical Manual of Mental Disorders,* or *DSM-IV,* published by the American Psychiatric Association, or APA.

ADHD was determined by a vote of APA psychiatrists to be a "mental" illness and added to the *DSM-IIIR* in 1987. By definition, children with ADHD exhibit behaviors such as not paying attention in school, not listening when spoken to directly, failing to follow directions, losing things, being easily distracted and forgetful, fidgeting with hands or feet, talking excessively, blurting out answers or having

The boy had been prescribed Ritalin and Prozac. After killing his parents he went to school and opened fire in the cafeteria, killing two and wounding 22.

difficulty awaiting turn. The most common ADHD remedy among pediatricians and representatives of the mental-health community is, as noted, Ritalin.

First approved by the FDA in 1955, Ritalin (methylphenidate) had become widely used for behavioral control by the mid-1960s. It is produced by the Swiss pharmaceutical company Novartis. According to the Drug Enforcement Administration, or DEA, the United States buys and uses 90 percent of the world's Ritalin. A U.N. agency known as the International Narcotics Control Board, or INCB, reported in 1995 that "10 to 12 percent of all boys between the ages of 6 and 14 in the U.S. have been diagnosed as having ADD [attention-deficit disorder, now referred to as ADHD] and are being treated with methylphenidate."

But opponents are concerned about evidence they say confirms a close relationship between use of prescribed psychotropic drugs and subsequent use of illegal drugs, including cocaine and heroin. While the United States has spent more than $70 billion on the war on drugs, says Bruce Wiseman, president of the Citizens Commission on Human Rights, a California-based organization that investigates violations of human rights by mental-health practitioners, "if you think the Colombian drug cartel is the biggest drug dealer in the world, think again. It's your neighborhood psychiatrist . . . putting our kids on the highest level of addictive drugs."

This complaint is not new and there is a lengthy list of government agencies connecting the prescribed psychotropic drugs to use of illegal substances.

Twenty-eight years ago the World Health Organization, or WHO, concluded that Ritalin was pharmacologically similar to cocaine in its pattern of abuse and cited Ritalin as a Schedule II drug—the most addictive in medical usage. The Department of Justice followed the WHO by citing Ritalin in Schedule II of the Controlled Substances Act as having a very high potential for abuse. As a Schedule II drug, Ritalin joins morphine, opium, cocaine and the heroin substitute methadone.

According to a report in the 1995 *Archives of General Psychiatry*, "Cocaine is one of the most reinforcing and addicting of the abused drugs and has pharmacological actions that are very similar to those of Ritalin." In the same year the DEA also made the Ritalin/cocaine connection, saying, "It is clear that Ritalin substitutes for cocaine and d-amphetamine in a number of behavioral paradigms," expressing concern that "one in every 30 Americans between 5 and 19 years old has a prescription for the drug."

Despite decades of warnings about the potential for abuse of Ritalin, experts continue to argue that the benefits far outweigh the consequences. Yet the INCB has reported that "Methylphenidate's [Ritalin] pharmacological effects are essentially the same as those of amphetamine and methamphetamine. The abuse of methylphenidate [Ritalin] can lead to tolerance and severe psychological dependence. Psychotic episodes [and] violent and bizarre behavior have been reported."

These are, in fact, some of the same symptoms exhibited by Eric Harris.

David Fassler, a child and adolescent psychiatrist and chairman of the APA group on Children, Adolescents and Their Families, says he is unaware of any research to suggest a correlation between the recent cases of violent behavior in school-age children and the widespread prescription of psychotropic drugs. Fassler argues that the number of school-age children suffering from mental illnesses such as depression is "more than earlier believed and it is important that there be a comprehensive evaluation by a mental-health clinician trained in this area." He stresses that "treatment should be multimodal—not left to medications alone."

Mike Faenza, president and chief executive officer of the National Mental Health Association, the country's oldest and largest mental-health group, notes that "there is little known about how the drugs affect brain function." Faenza adds that "we do know that a hell of a lot of kids commit suicide because they aren't getting the help they need. It's irresponsible not to give them the help just because we don't know what causes the mental illness"

Opponents are quick to capitalize on this admission. "There is no such thing as ADHD" declares Wiseman. "It's not a deficiency of 'speed' that makes a kid act out. If you look at the criteria listed in the *DSM-IV* for ADHD, you'll see that they are taking normal childhood behavior and literally voting it a mental illness. This is a pseudoscience, entirely subjective. Unlike medical conditions that are proved scientifically, with these mental illnesses the only way you know you're better is if the psychiatrist says you're better. That's not science."

Pediatric neurologist Fred Baughman not only agrees that there is no such illness as ADHD, but says: "This is a contrived epidemic, where all 5 million to 6 million children on these drugs are normal. The country's been led to believe that all painful emotions are a mental illness and the leadership of the APA knows very well that they are representing it as a disease when there is no scientific data to confirm any mental illness."

Peter Breggin, a psychiatrist and director of the International Center for the Study of Psychiatry and Psychology and author of *Talking Back to Prozac, Toxic Psychiatry* and *Talking Back to Ritalin,* for years has waged a war with the APA about what he regards as its cavalier diagnoses of mental illnesses. "Psychiatry has never been driven by science. They have no biological or genetic basis for these illnesses and the National Institutes of Mental Health are totally committed to the pharmacological line." He is concerned that "there is a great deal of scientific evidence that stimulants cause brain damage with long-term

Despite decades of warnings about the potential for abuse of Ritalin, experts continue to argue that the benefits far outweigh the consequences.

Killer kids: Kipland Kinkel had been administered Ritalin and Prozac. Eric Harris was under the influence of Luvox, an antidepressant prescribed to treat obsessive-compulsive disorder, during murderous assault.

---

use, yet there is no evidence that these mental illnesses, such as ADHD, exist."

Breggin points out that the National Institutes of Health, or NIH, admitted as much at their 1998 Consensus Development Conference on the Diagnosis and Treatment of Attention Deficit Hyperactivity Disorder. Thirty-one individuals were selected by NIH to make scientific presentations to the panel on ADHD and its treatment. The panel made the following observations and conclusions: "We don't have an independent, valid test for ADHD; there are no data to indicate that ADHD is due to a brain malfunction; existing studies come to conflicting conclusions as to whether use of psychostimulants increases or decreases the risk of abuse, and finally after years of clinical research and experience with ADHD, our knowledge about the cause or causes of ADHD remains speculative."

If so, there is little evidence to support a scientific basis for classifying ADHD as a mental illness. On the other hand, there is an abundance of evidence that stimulants such as Ritalin can produce symptoms such as mania, insomnia, hallucinations, hyperactivity, impulsivity and inattention. And the DEA's list of potential adverse effects of Ritalin includes psychosis, depression, dizziness, insomnia,

nervousness, irritability and attacks of Tourette's or other tic syndromes.

While Ritalin is the drug of choice for treating ADHD, other mental illnesses such as depression and obsessive-compulsive disorder, or OCD, from which Columbine shooter Harris suffered, are being treated with new SSRI antidepressants. Harris' autopsy revealed that he had used Luvox (Fluvoxomine), an SSRI, prior to the shooting spree. And days earlier he had been rejected by the Marine Corps because he was taking the psychotropic drug.

Luvox, a cousin of Prozac, has been approved by the FDA for pediatric use, although research shows that a small percentage of patients experience adverse effects such as mania, bouts of irritability, aggression and hostility. But many physicians still prescribe it to children.

More disturbing to those who believe sufficient evidence exists that prescription psychotropic drugs may play a role in the violence being carried out by school-age children is the response of physicians to the issue. Rather than erring on the side of caution by reducing the number of kids on mind-altering drugs, physicians instead are prescribing psychotropic drugs even to infants and toddlers. The warning label states that "Ritalin should not be used in children under 6 years, since safety and efficacy for this age group has not been established" and "sufficient data on safety and efficacy of long-term use of Ritalin in children are not yet available."

A report in the July 1998 issue of the *Clinical Psychiatric News* revealed that in Michigan's Medicaid program, 223 children 3 years old or younger were diagnosed with ADHD as of December 1996. Amazingly, 57 percent of these children, many of whom are not

yet capable of putting together a complete sentence, were treated with one or more psychotropic drugs including Ritalin, Prozac, Dexedrine, Aventyl and Syban. Thirty-three percent were medicated with two or more of these drugs.

But it is Ritalin that is being prescribed to 6 million American children. Children's Hospital in Washington has been running television advertisements expressing concern. According to its spokeswoman, Lynn Cantwell, the ads were part of a series covering many medical issues. "We wanted to advocate that children get a comprehensive evaluation because we are finding that children were coming in who were taking Ritalin who actually did not have ADHD."

Wiseman has suggested that the only way to gain control of the situation is to expose widespread "fraudulent diagnoses" of psychiatrists. "Without the diagnoses, you can't get the drugs," he says. Baughman's answer isn't too far from Wiseman's. He says, "A big-time class-action lawsuit needs to be filed."

RITALIN and Novartis Stock-Market Value

Kids on Ritalin	*3,485,000
(×)	
$ spent for each kid	*$537
(=)	
Yearly gross sales	$1,873,117,800.
(×)	
% of gross sale price to Novartis	*50%
(=)	
Novartis' Ritalin sales	$936,558,900.
(×)	
Novartis' profit margin	*20%.
(=)	
Novartis' net profit	$187,311,780.
(×)	
Novartis's stock earnings multiple	*23X
(=)	
Novartis' Ritalin stock value	$4.3 billion
(÷)	
Kids on Ritalin	3,485,000
(=)	
Increase in Novartis stock for each kid on Ritalin	$1,236

*Estimate

Unit Selections

Key Points to Consider

❖ What do you believe to be the greatest drug-related threat facing our nation? Explain.

❖ How do drug-related threats and impacts differ from city to city and state to state? Why?

❖ It is often argued that Americans overreact and overemphasize the harm from illegal drugs while ignoring or underrepresenting the harm from legal drugs, namely alcohol and nicotine. Do you agree or disagree with this argument, and why?

❖ Has there been a significant shift in public concern over the abuse of legal drugs? Support your answer.

❖ Explain whether or not the harmful impacts from the abuse of drugs are greater today than they were a decade ago.

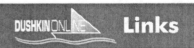 **Links** | **www.dushkin.com/online/**

These sites are annotated on pages 4 and 5.

The most devastating effect of drug use in America is the magnitude with which it affects the way we live. Much of its influence is not measurable. What is the cost of a son or daughter lost, a parent imprisoned, a life lived in a constant state of fear? The emotional costs alone are incomprehensible.

The social legacy of this country's drug crisis could easily be the subject of this entire book. The purpose here, however, can only be a cursory portrayal of drugs' tremendous costs. More than one American president has stated that drug use threatens our national security and personal well-being. The financial costs of maintaining the federal apparatus devoted to drug interdiction, enforcement, and treatment are staggering. Although yearly expenditures vary due to changes in political influence, strategy, and tactics, examples of the tremendous effects of drugs on government and the economy abound. The federal budget for drug control exceeds $10 billion. The Department of Justice devotes 50 percent of its budget to antidrug efforts, the Department of Health and Human Services almost $2 billion, and the Department of Defense $1 billion. Drugs are the business of the criminal justice system. The U.S. incarcerates more of its citizens than almost any other nation and the financial costs are staggering. In California, for example, it costs approximately $21,000 to house an inmate for one year. Including parolees, there are almost 300,000 felons under California Department of Corrections jurisdiction. Forty percent of those felons were incarcerated for violent crime, 23 percent for property crime, and 27 percent for drug-related crime. When one considers the relationship between violent crime and drug use and property crime and drug use, the resulting picture is numbing.

In addition to the highly visible criminal justice–related costs, numerous other institutions are affected. Housing, welfare, education, and health care provide excellent examples of critical institutions struggling to overcome the strain of drug-related impacts. In addition, annual loss of productivity in the workplace exceeds well over a $100 billion per year. Alcoholism, alone, causes 500 million lost work days each year. Add to this demographic shifts caused by people fleeing drug-impacted neighborhoods, schools, and businesses and one soon realizes that there is no victimless public or private institution. Housing and welfare departments struggle to distinguish between drug-related and nondrug-related assistance requests. Educational systems struggle to counter the availability of drugs and its associated victimization and fear. Teachers struggle to overcome the time sacrificed to drug-related disruptive behavior. Health-care systems struggle to treat drug-exposed newborns, at annual estimates of between 375,000 and 739,000 infants. Prenatal exposure to polydrug use exacts tremendous costs and no amount of debating, arguing, or denying the specific cause-and-effect scenarios really mean much in the face of reality.

Language acquisition delay, regardless of the degree to which it can be mitigated, is expensive. And it is just one of many problems that may arise when a child is exposed prenatally to drugs. Add injured, drug-related accident and crime victims, along with demands produced by a growing population of intravenous-drug users infected with AIDS, and a failing health care system frighteningly appears. A universally affordable health care plan capable of addressing drug-related impacts of such vast medical consequences may not be possible. Health care costs from drug-related ills are overwhelming. One of every $5 that Medicaid spends on hospital care is attributable to substance abuse.

It should be emphasized that the social costs exacted by drug use infiltrate every aspect of public and private life. The implications for thousands of families struggling with the adverse effects of drug-related woes may prove the greatest and most tragic of social costs. Children who lack emotional support, self-esteem, role models, a safe and secure environment, economic opportunity, and an education because of a parent on drugs suggest costs difficult to comprehend.

As you read the following articles, consider the costs associated with legal and illegal drugs. However, before joining the debate on which is the greater harbinger of pain and suffering, consider the diversity of impacts to which legal and illegal drugs contribute. Combining pharmacological, environmental, legal, and the multitude of other factors influencing drug-related impacts with cause and effect propositions soon produces a quagmire of major proportions. Although it is tempting to generalize while considering and lamenting the impacts of drug use on our society, it seldom produces the most salient observations. An incremental approach to assessing drug-related impacts and costs may produce a greater understanding of how to measure social costs than an attempt to make a case for a combination of impacts generated because of issues such as the legal status of a drug. For example, annual alcohol-related deaths far exceed those related to cocaine, but to say the reason for alcohol's disproportionate toll stems solely from alcohol's legal status is shortsighted. Certainly, the legality of a drug will enter the process of assessing drug-related impacts and their causes, but it is still just one component within an equation of many.

Lastly, as you read and think about the different articles in this unit, keep in mind the pervasiveness of drug-related impacts affecting American families. Subsequent reflection reveals that we don't just "change schools," "move to a different town," or flee drug-related issues, and that the most critical component of defense against drug ills, the family, is the most mercilessly pursued target. Most people recognize that the world's most powerful institutions merely buy time in hopes that family institutions will come together, endure, and prevail against drugs.

Measuring the Social Costs of Drugs

Editorial:

Substance Abuse and Addiction—the Need to Know

America has many social ills: crime and violence, poverty, teen pregnancy, domestic violence and child abuse, high health care costs, the spread of AIDS and other sexually transmitted diseases, and federal entitlement programs that defy reform. As a country, we have to take action to deal with all of these problems. However, unless we move to combat substance abuse and addiction, we are unlikely to succeed.

The statistical evidence gives substance abuse and addiction its status as public health enemy No. 1. Some 76 million Americans have experienced alcoholism in their families.[1] More than 61 million Americans smoke cigarettes.[2] Eleven million binge drink (five or more drinks on one occasion) at least once a week on average.[2] Almost 7 million use smokeless tobacco; more than 10 million smoke marijuana; more than 3 million abuse psychotherapeutic drugs such as tranquilizers, amphetamines, and sleeping pills; almost 2 million use cocaine; at least 1 million use hallucinogens such as PCP or LSD; and almost 1 million—many of them teenagers—report using inhalants.[2]

Of the 4 million women who give birth each year, some 820 000 smoke cigarettes, 760 000 drink alcohol, and 500 000 use illicit drugs during pregnancy.[3] These numbers cannot be added because many women use more than one substance. When a mother smokes, drinks, or uses drugs during pregnancy, the medical—and Medicaid—bill to deliver and care for her child can jump sharply.[4] For example, hospital charges for infants exposed to illicit drugs are up to four times greater than those for drug-free infants.[4]

More American children and adolescents are smoking cigarettes and using marijuana and inhalants, and at the youngest ages ever. Between 1992 and 1996, the proportion of eighth graders who reported smoking in the past month increased from 15.5% to 21% (L. Johnston et al., unpublished data, 1996). From 1992 to 1995, the proportion of eighth graders who said they had used marijuana during or before seventh grade rose from 7.7% to 12.7%, while the proportion of eighth graders who reported using inhalants during or before seventh grade grew from 14.5% to 17.7%.[5,6]

The gender gap in the use of alcohol, tobacco, and illicit drugs is disappearing as well. Among 12- to 17-year-olds, girls are now as likely as boys to experiment with alcohol and illicit drugs, although boys are still more likely than girls to become regular drinkers and users of illicit drugs.[3,7] In the past, girls who tried drugs did so at later ages than did boys. Today, however, girls and boys are wading into the sea of drug experimentation at the same early and vulnerable ages.[3]

Both the University of Michigan study Monitoring the Future and the tracking survey of The Partnership for a Drug-Free America have found a decline in the perception among adolescents that taking drugs is risky. The annual Center on Addiction and Substance Abuse National Survey of American Attitudes on Substance Abuse[8] revealed that the proportion of teens with friends and classmates who have used drugs such as cocaine and heroin jumped from 39% in 1996 to 56% in 1997. These disturbing trends come at a time when a generation of baby boomers, who grew up in an age when drug experimentation was widespread and fashionable,[2] is sending mixed messages to its children about the dangers of drugs.

The report by Johnson et al. in this issue of the Journal demonstrates how dramatic illicit drug use soared with the baby-boomer generation.[9] In 1996, the CASA Survey found that many baby-boomer parents appeared re-

---

Editor's Note. See related article by Chavkin et al. (p 117) in *American Journal of Public Health,* January 1998, Vol. 88, No. 1.

signed to drug use by their own children as well: 46% of them expect their teenagers to try drugs, and 65% of parents who regularly used marijuana in their youth believe their teens will try drugs.[10] Only 58% of boomer parents consider it a "crisis" when their child aged 15 years or younger smokes marijuana, compared with 83% of parents who never used marijuana. Yet, we know that adolescents who try drugs at such an early age use drugs more frequently, escalate to higher levels more quickly, are less likely to stop using them, and are more likely to move on from marijuana to drugs like cocaine and heroin.[9,11]

Recent neuroscientific studies have demonstrated in stunning detail the changes in brain chemistry that marijuana and cocaine cause, opening up exciting possibilities for new treatments.[12-14] They also challenge old beliefs about the supposed "safety" of marijuana use. The evidence indicates a biomedical link between use of alcohol, nicotine, marijuana, cocaine, and heroin, because all of these substances affect dopamine levels in the brain through common pathways.[12,13] Recent research also demonstrates that cessation of marijuana use brings on withdrawal symptoms,[12,13] which may encourage a user to resume marijuana use or to try other drugs such as cocaine or heroin.

We need to attack this problem on several fronts: research, prevention, treatment, and law enforcement. I believe that the greatest area of neglect has been research.

The National Center on Addiction and Substance Abuse at Columbia University has analyzed the United States Centers for Disease Control and Prevention 1995 Youth Risk Behavior Survey to determine whether smoking marijuana leads to more dangerous illegal drug use even in the absence of other problem behaviors such as criminal activity, truancy, eating disorders, poor school performance, and attempted suicides. We found that, among 12- to 17-year-old boys with no other problem behaviors, those who report drinking alcohol and/or smoking cigarettes at least once in the previous month are 28 times likelier to smoke marijuana than those who report neither smoking nor drinking alcohol. For girls 12 to 17 years old, the relationship is even stronger; those who report drinking alcohol and/or smoking cigarettes at least once in the previous month are 37 times likelier to smoke marijuana than those who report neither smoking nor drinking alcohol.

These statistical relationships are compelling. They are even more striking than findings in the first surgeon general's report on smoking and health that smokers were 9 to 10 times likelier to get lung cancer than nonsmokers.[15] The early returns from the Framingham Study showed that men with high cholesterol levels were 2 to 4 times likelier to have heart disease.[16] These findings on cancer and heart disease prompted massive investments in biomedical research programs.

In fiscal year 1997, the National Institutes of Health (NIH) spent more than $5 billion on research on cancer, cardiovascular disease, and AIDS (National Institutes of Health, written communication with Kimberly Garr-Ferguson, October 14, 1997). NIH spent about a seventh of that amount, just $787 million, on research on substance abuse and addiction, the largest single cause and exacerbator of those three crippling and killing conditions. Our nation should invest at least $1 billion a year on research on addiction, and there should be a significant increase in biomedical and social research on adolescence.

It is also important that research examine the nature and causes of substance abuse among men and women. A review of the research in this area by the National Center on Addiction and Substance Abuse suggests that the problem differs among men and women in important ways.[3] A better understanding of such differences could substantially improve prevention and treatment efforts.

The substance abuse and addiction problems of women are only beginning to receive the full attention they deserve. Although recent calls to include more women in study samples have met with some success, many researchers are not disaggregating their results by gender to search for differences that could inform prevention and treatment efforts. The studies on substance abuse in this issue of the Journal are encouraging exceptions.

For example, we need a better understanding of the nature of women's addiction to cigarettes. The finding by Husten et al.[17] that men are more likely than women to be intermittent smokers is provocative in light of increasing evidence that it is harder for women to quit than for men. In addition to being addicted to nicotine, women may also rely on cigarettes to manage depression or anxiety. Another factor that may make it harder for them to cut down or quit is that social rituals involving smoking may be particularly important to women.[18]

The report by Emmons et al.[19] also points to interesting differences in the correlates of smoking among women and men at college that could affect the success of prevention efforts. For example, the absence of religious beliefs is a stronger predicator of smoking for women, while not participating in athletics is a more powerful predictor for men.

We already know that weight concerns are a strong deterrent to women who want to quit.[3,20] The paper by Burnette et al.[21] demonstrates how the health risks associated with weight gain after smoking cessation are trivial relative to the health benefits of quitting. Yet, adolescent girls continue to take up the habit and women continue to struggle with quitting, and we do not fully understand why. Certainly, the entertainment industry, which is once again glamorizing smoking in movies as well as music videos,[22] and the fashion industry, whose love affair with a painfully thin image of women endures, send powerful messages to girls about how to be chic and popular in ways that may have deadly consequences.

As evidence mounts of the tragic consequences of smoking during pregnancy, the paper by Nafstad[23] demonstrates the damage done to the fetus when a pregnant woman is simply exposed to the smoke from other cigarette smokers. Despite such findings, however, state and local policy is largely focused on the consequences of prenatal use of illicit drugs such as cocaine. As reported by Chavkin et al.,[24] state interventions to combat drug use during pregnancy with punitive measures are increasing, while funding for substance abuse treatment is declining. To have an informed policy, we need greater investments in research on the nature and consequences of prenatal use of all substances—tobacco, alcohol, licit and illicit drugs—as well as the effectiveness of concerted prevention and treatment efforts.

Our nation's parsimonious investment in research on substance abuse and addiction is a critical mistake, because this public health epidemic destroys the lives and potential of millions of Americans. It is a chronic and costly disease without a cure in sight, making prevention all the more important. Perhaps most troubling, it is attracting our children in greater numbers to the potential ruin of their futures and ours. For this reason more than any other, we must devote resources to combating substance abuse and addiction that are commensurate with the devastating scope of the problem.

Joseph A. Califano, Jr
Chairman and President
National Center on Addiction
and Substance Abuse
at Columbia University

References

1. Schoenborn CA. Exposure to alcoholism in the family: United States, 1988. *Adv Data Vital Health Stat.* September 30, 1991; no. 205. US Government Printing Office; 1991–281821/-40008.

2. *Preliminary Results from the 1996 National Household Survey on Drug Abuse.* Rockville, Md: US Dept of Health and Human Services Administration; 1997:60.

3. *Substance Abuse and the American Woman.* New York, NY: National Center on Addiction and Substance Abuse; 1996.

4. *Drug-Exposed Infants: A Generation at Risk.* Washington, DC: US General Accounting Office; 1990.

5. Johnston LD, O'Malley PM, Bachman JG. *National Survey Results on Drug Use from The Monitoring the Future Study, 1975–1992. Volume I: Secondary School Students.* Rockville, Md: US Dept of Health and Human Services, National Institutes of Health; 1993:134.

6. Johnston LD, O'Malley PM, Bachman JG. *National Survey Results on Drug Use from The Monitoring the Future Study, 1975–1995. Volume I: Secondary School Students.* Rockville, Md: US Dept of Health and Human Services, National Institutes of Health; 1996:153.

7. *Substance Abuse among Women in the United States.* Rockville, Md: US Dept of Health and Human Services, Substance Abuse and Mental Health Services Administration: 1997.

8. *National Survey of American Attitudes on Substance Abuse III: Teens and Their Parents, Teachers and Principals.* New York, NY: National Center on Addiction and Substance Abuse; 1997.

9. Johnson RA, Gerstein DR. Initiation of use of alcohol, cigarettes, marijuana, cocaine, and other substances in US birth cohorts since 1919. *Am J Public Health.* 1998;88:27–33.

10. *National Survey of American Attitudes on Substance Abuse II: Teens and Their Parents.* New York, NY: National Center on Addiction and Substance Abuse; 1996.

11. *Cigarettes, Alcohol, Marijuana: Gateways to Illicit Drug Use.* New York, NY: National Center on Addiction and Substance Abuse; 1994.

12. Tanda G, Pontieri FE, Di Chiara G. Cannabinoid and heroin activation of mesolimbic dopamine transmission by a common opioid receptor mechanism. *Science.* 1997;276:2048–2050.

13. Rodriguez de Fonseca F, Carrera MRA, Navarro M, Koob GF, Weiss F. Activation of corticotropin-releasing factor in the limbic system during cannabinoid withdrawal. *Science.* 1997;276:2050–2054.

14. Volkow ND, Wang GJ, Fischman MW, et al. Relationship between subjective effects of cocaine and dopamine transporter occupancy. *Nature.* 1997;386:827–830.

15. *Smoking and Health: Report of the Advisory Committee to the Surgeon General of the Public Health Service.* Washington, DC: US Dept of Health, Education, and Welfare; 1964.

16. Dawber TR. The Framingham Study: the Epidemiology of Atherosclerotic Disease. Cambridge, Mass: Harvard University Press; 1980.

17. Husten CG, McCarty MC, Glovino GA, Christmon JH, Zhu B. Intermittent smokers: a descriptive analysis of persons who have never smoked daily. *Am J Public Health.* 1998;88:-86–89.

18. Perkins KA. Sex differences in nicotine versus nonnicotine reinforcement as determinants of tobacco smoking. *Exp Clin Psychopharmacol.* 1996;4:166–177.

19. Emmons KM, Wechsler H, Dowdall G. Abraham M. Predictors of smoking among college students. *Am J Public Health.* 1998;88:104–107.

20. Perkins KA, Levine MD, Marcus MD, Shiffman S. Addressing women's concerns about weight gain due to smoking cessation. *J Subst Abuse Treat.* 1997;14:173–182.

21. Burnette MM, Meilahn E, Wing RR, Kuller LH. Smoking cessation, weight gain and changes in cardiovascular risk factors during menopause: the Healthy Women Study. *Am J Public Health.* 1998;88:93–96.

22. Durant RH, Rome ES, Rich M, Allred E, Emans SJ, Woods ER. Tobacco and alcohol use behaviors portrayed in music videos: a content analysis. *Am J Public Health.* 1997;87:1131–1135.

23. Nafstad P. Nicotine concentration in the hair of nonsmoking mothers and the size of offspring. *Am J Public Health.* 1998;88:120–124.

24. Chavkin W, Breitbart V, Elman D, Wise P. National survey of the states: policies and practices regarding drug-using pregnant women. *Am J Public Health.* 1998;88:117–119.

Visualizing America's drug problems: an ethnographic content analysis of illegal drug stories on the nightly news

BY DAVID JERNIGAN AND LORI DORFMAN

David Jernigan, a sociologist on the staff of the Marin Institute for the Prevention of Alcohol and Other Drug Problems (24 Belvedere St., San Rafael, CA 94901), is currently studying the evolution of alcohol markets in developing countries. Lori Dorfman, of the Berkeley Media Studies Group, wrote her doctoral dissertation on how television reports health issues.

In 1986 President Ronald Reagan declared a national "War on Drugs." Three years later, President George Bush renewed the call to arms. The national media gave the War on Drugs their official blessing. On television, in news magazines and in newspapers, the media accepted and amplified the government's claim that illegal drug use was approaching epidemic proportions (Orcutt and Turner, 1993; Gitlin, 1989). Over the years from 1986 to 1992, U.S. citizens were treated to a barrage of news stories about illegal drugs. In 1992 drugs began to fade from the American agenda; by 1993 the federal government was moving to consolidate or eliminate the special agencies created or enhanced in 1986 to wage the drug war.

From 1986 to 1993 changes in actual drug use in America were fairly small. Between 1988 and 1990, the year under scrutiny in this paper, according to the National Household Survey on Drug Abuse, illegal drug use actually fell, as did use of cocaine. Crack use remained flat (U.S. Department of Health and Human Services, 1989, 1991). Others have argued that there never really was a drug crisis, at least in terms of an epidemic of illegal drug use (Reinarman and Levine, 1989;

Orcutt and Turner, 1993; Mosher and Yanagisako, 1991). And the War on Drugs actually had little impact on the use of illegal drugs. Meanwhile, use of the two most deadly drugs, alcohol and tobacco, either remained flat or dropped slightly.

There is a substantial body of literature offering explanations of why, although drug use in the U.S. was declining in the late 1980s and early 1990s, "drug war" rhetoric and punitive solutions to the "problem" ran rampant. A number of these works have attested to the importance of the news media in that process. Orcutt and Turner (1993) demonstrate how the news media distorted statistics to support the view that the problem was growing. Sharp (1992) shows how Presidential access to the media in this as in other historical periods enables political leaders to promote or demote drug issues in the media and hence in the public agenda. Jensen, Gerber and Babcock (1991) use surveys of newspaper and magazine coverage to demonstrate how initiatives by politicians preceded the formation of grassroots mobilization around illegal drugs, while Beckett (1994) employs OLS regression to show that television and print coverage, as well as public concern, were actually both functions of elite "state initiative," moves by political leaders to place illegal drugs on the public agenda. Iyengar (199) establishes a link between media coverage and public support for punitive solutions by combining content analysis with audience reaction studies.

Several of these authors use content analysis in their analyses. Yet all use written sources—news scripts or abstracts—as the source of the raw data that they analyze. Television is a visual medium. Although political leaders may drive the basic content of the news, news organizations themselves mediate that content, turning it into narratives with beginnings and endings, good characters and bad characters, and pictures that illustrate everything. The research described here attempts to go

AUTHORS' NOTE: *Preparation of this paper was funded in part by grants from the Beryl Buck Trust, the Western Consortium for Public Health, and the Center for Substance Abuse Prevention, Substance Abuse and Mental Health Services Administration, U.S. Department of Health and Human Services, Grant #U88SP03342. Views expressed in this paper are solely those of the authors and do not necessarily represent those of the funders.*

further than earlier studies in analyzing the visual as well as the textual content of television news stories about illegal drugs. Looking at a sample of stories aired in 1990, one of the high points of media coverage of illegal drugs, we aim to provide "thick description" of the mediated content, as well as the themes and patterns that lie within that coverage.

The importance of television news

Television news has become the chief source of information and analysis of major social problems for the overwhelming majority of Americans (Roper Organization, 1991). Cohen pointed out in the early 1960s, and later research has confirmed, that the news may not tell people what to think, but it definitely tells them what to think about (Cohen, 1963; Rogers and Dearing, 1988). This "agenda-setting" function of the mass media helps to explain why the War on Drugs became a national obsession in the late 1980s and early 1990s. But more than telling people what to think about, news "involves a selection, an analysis and, crucially, an evaluation of reality" (Glasgow Media Group, 1982:115). This selection process has a significant effect on people's political attitudes and behaviors. Issues highlighted by television news influence people's choice of political candidates (Iyengar and Kinder, 1985). Television news also influences public opinion: news shows that favor one side of an issue are associated with increases in popular support for that point of view (Page and Shapiro, 1987).

Iyengar's (1991) content analysis of television news divides news reports into two categories: episodic, stories that focus on a single episode or event; and thematic, stories that place events and issues in a broader context. Working from the abstracts provided by the Vanderbilt Television News Archive, Iyengar found that the vast majority of television news stories about crime (89%) and poverty (66%) fall into the episodic category. Stories about racial inequality and unemployment are more likely to be thematic: 60% and 67%, respectively.

Iyengar then went on to ask, What is the effect of this differential framing of issues on the viewing public? Testing episodic and thematic stories before audiences, he found that in all cases except unemployment, an episodic frame caused viewers to assign responsibility for both causing and treating the problem to the individual with the problem, whereas a thematic frame led to placement of responsibility at the feet of government or society. Furthermore, the dominance of episodic framing on issues such as crime and poverty leads Americans to think about these problems in isolation from other features of the social landscape. According to Iyengar:

> By simplifying complex issues to the level of anecdotal evidence, television news leads viewers to issue-specific attributions of responsibility, and these attributions tend to shield society and government from responsibility. Following exposure to episodic framing, Americans describe chronic problems such as poverty and crime not in terms of deep-seated social or economic conditions, but as mere idiosyncratic outcomes . . . viewers focus on individual and group characteristics rather than historical, social, political, or other such structural forces.

In this respect episodic framing encourages reasoning by resemblance—people settle upon causes and treatments that "fit" the observed problem. (1991:137)

Reasoning by resemblance is a particularly apt phrase with regard to television, since it is a visual medium. Because it is visual, the decisions made about pictures in the news are particularly important—sometimes more important than the verbal content of the story itself (Jamieson, 1988). Although in Iyengar's audience studies, participants watched actual news stories, his own analysis of the stories in his sample was based entirely on written abstracts, not on the visual stories themselves.

Graber (1990:152) suggests that people "trust what they see more than what they hear." In her study of audience interpretations of news stories, she found that visual themes were "remembered and learned more readily than verbal themes," particularly the "depiction of human beings" (1990:196). Her respondents believed "the visuals allowed them to form more complete and accurate impressions of people and events." Entman (1990, 1992) is one of the few authors to have used visual material as part of his analysis. From his study of local television news, he argued that typical news practices reinforce "modern racist" stereotypes of African-Americans as threatening, politically or socially demanding, and prone to complain about discrimination that in the "modern racist" view no longer exists.

Going beyond Iyengar's and others' text-based content analysis of television news, in our content analysis we sought to answer the following questions regarding the portrayal of drugs on television news: (1) how various drugs and drug problems are portrayed on television news; (2) whether these portrayals reflect public health data or a public health perspective; (3) what other themes emerge that relate to perspectives and policies on drugs in the United States. The content analysis was open-ended. We were looking for the news stories to show us their themes, rather than approaching them with preconceived ideas of what those themes would be. However, as Entman (1992) points out, analysis of visual elements of television news coverage continues to be largely uncharted territory in social science. Studies and measurement of audience reaction to visual images are rare, and there is no agreement and little investigation of standard coding methodologies. Our findings therefore are unavoidably speculative, but they are offered in the hopes of demonstrating the importance of this line of research.

Methods

This paper reports on a content analysis of network news reports on illegal drugs. The sample used for this study was part of a larger project examining how network news portrays health issues (Dorfman, 1994; Dorfman and Jernigan, 1992). To create the sample, 10% of the days of 1990 were randomly selected (with replacement) for a total of 36 sample days. All the network news stories relevant to health issues on the sample days, including all stories about illegal drugs, were then identified from the Vanderbilt Television News Archive Abstracts (Vanderbilt Television News Archive, 1990; Vanderbilt Television News Archive, 1991). The selected stories were compiled on videotapes by the Vanderbilt News Archive for a total of nearly three hours of news (02:52:35). This paper reports on the 43 minutes and 50 seconds taken up by the 24 illegal-drug stories from the randomly selected sample.

The Vanderbilt Television News Archive is the only place in the country to collect and index news broadcasts specifically for public access and research. Because at the time Vanderbilt collected only network news, we limited the content analysis to ABC World News Tonight, CBS Evening News, and NBC Nightly News. We examined 1990 because it was the latest complete year available from the Vanderbilt News Archives when we began the study. According to Beckett (1994), it also falls in the middle of the heaviest coverage of drug issues in the national media in the past decade.

The research done for this paper was extremely labor intensive, which is probably why this kind of content analysis is not done routinely. The text of the Vanderbilt tapes was transcribed verbatim. Each story was watched at least four times by the authors. With transcript in hand, each story was viewed first in real time to see the story; again to mark each new shot (cut); a third time in slow motion to record every image in every shot; and finally to review the story again in real time. One author viewed the total sample again twice to verify the number of shots in each story.

Stories were coded using ethnographic content analysis. Unlike a strictly quantitative content analysis, in which categories precede analysis of the data, in ethnographic content analysis quantifiable categories of analysis are supplemented by qualitative categories that are allowed to emerge from the data themselves (Altheide, 1987). This method is particularly well suited to textual and visual data such as those contained in news stories. Repeated viewings of the stories brought to light themes that would not have been obvious on a single viewing. Using the visual data as grist for the content analysis permitted a much more accurate analysis of the whole of what occurs in the experience of watching television than simply reviewing the abstracts or even transcripts of the stories would have allowed.

There are advantages and disadvantages both to how the sample was drawn and to how it was analyzed. The advantage of a random sample was that since the purpose was to look at the general shape of illegal drug coverage over the course of the year, we could draw from the year in an unbiased manner. We were not interested in following a single story, but rather in looking at what themes emerged in the breadth of coverage, regardless of the particular incident being reported.

However, random sampling has some drawbacks when applied to television news shows. The method takes the stories out of context, both as day-to-day unfolding stories and as part of a larger newscast. We did not look at what stories came before and after the stories of interest. These often set the stage and thus influence the frame of a story. The method also dictated that we view the news as a casual rather than a regular viewer. Some stories clearly had developed over time. Our method of sampling caught those stories midstream. Another possible research design would have been to follow two or three of the major illegal-drug stories over the course of the year. What would have been lost was the opportunity our sample provided to observe similar themes arising from stories on diverse aspects of the illegal drug issue.

The decision to sample national news rather than local news was tied to logistics: local coverage would have been much more difficult to sample; although the Vanderbilt Television News Archive is unique in its fastidious recording and archiving of news shows, it works only on a national basis. A similar study sampling local news coverage would be a useful avenue for further research.

The small size of our illegal-drug sample limits the validity of our findings. This small sample size is due largely to the amount of effort required in doing a qualitative content analysis of this kind. We also reviewed the text of all the abstracts categorized as illegal-drug stories for the first four months of 1990, the period of heaviest coverage, in an effort to lend greater validity to our analysis. Nonetheless, it should be emphasized that our small sample is capable only of suggesting certain themes and decisions that may have given a particular shape to television news coverage of illegal drugs in 1990.

Results

The sample yielded 43 stories about alcohol, tobacco, and illegal or pharmaceutical drugs. Seventeen of the stories aired on ABC, ten on CBS, and sixteen on NBC. Both in terms of time spent and in terms of number of stories, illegal-drug stories dominated the sample (see Figure 1). Twenty-four stories concerned illegal drugs, eight were about pharmaceuticals, seven covered tobacco, and seven discussed alcohol (three stories mentioned both alcohol and illegal drugs). In the breakdown of time spent on illegal-drug versus alcohol and tobacco stories, the sample was nearly representative of the entire year's stories.

Measuring by broadcast time (see Figure 2), alcohol stories in the sample took up 19% of the time, tobacco stories 8%, and illegal drug stories 73%. Tyndall (1991) tabulated the time spent on every major topic during 1990 on network news shows. He found that 77% of the broadcast minutes spent on alcohol, tobacco and illegal drugs went to stories about illegal drugs. (The three stories that mentioned both alcohol and illegal drugs focused primarily on illegal drugs. If time were broken down by amount within the stories spent discussing each drug rather than the total story time, then the sample would come even closer to Tyndall's. Since Tyndall did not measure coverage of prescription drugs, those stories were excluded from this comparison.)

Illegal drug story length averaged one minute 32 seconds (range = 10 seconds to four minutes 30 seconds). Using Iyengar's categories of episodic and thematic framing, the bulk of the illegal drug stories in the sample—71%—were framed episodically. Episodic stories focused on specific events such as drug busts or summits with foreign officials. The few thematic stories placed illegal drug use and problems in more of a context—e.g., teen health or the overall drug war effort.

Most stories fell into one of two overlapping categories. By far the smaller category was made up of stories on other issues that included an illegal drug component because of the dominance of the drug war frame at that time. This category included two stories on the U.N. World Summit on Children, both of which focused on "crack babies," and a very brief report on teen health issues that mentioned "drugs" in the lead-in but restricted subsequent discussion of drugs to statistics on teen deaths from alcohol use. The larger category was about the War on Drugs and how the government fights it here and abroad, and is sometimes undermined. Drug war stories covered the following topics: the War on Drugs in Colombia and Peru, a drug tunnel under the Mexican–U.S. border, a special television cartoon on the War on Drugs, drug smuggling in the Coast Guard, drug testing, suburban commuters buying drugs in the inner city, and Washington, DC, Mayor Marion Barry's trial on drug charges. A discrete set of visual and verbal messages and themes prevailed in these stories that depicted the fight against drugs as a heroic and ongoing battle of "us" against "them."

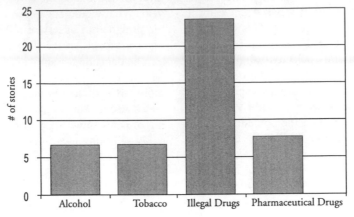

FIGURE 1

Drug stories on television news: distribution across drug categories

Fighting the drug war

One of the first illegal-drug stories of the year brings out the "war" in the War on Drugs. ABC on January 13 airs a four and a half minute "American Agenda" story on the drug war in Peru, produced as background for the drug summit planned for President Bush and the presidents of Colombia, Bolivia and Peru. The story begins with footage of the "war": helicopter gun ships patrolling over the jungles. Nine months later, this same footage shows up in ABC's "War on Drugs— One Year Later" story. The use of such file footage without identification reinforces the impression that the drug war is constant and ongoing.

The visuals in the two stories are reminiscent of Vietnam War-era coverage. Army units crash through jungles. Aerial shots show acres of unidentified crops, presumably coca. Peasants unload sacks of flour, to the accompaniment of mournful flute music. ABC correspondent Beth Nissen points out that the drug war's anti-coca cultivation campaign is pushing Peruvian peasants into the hands of the Shining Path guerrilla movement. Using a phrase made famous during the Vietnam War, she reports that the guerrillas are trying to "win the hearts

and minds of the peasants." And, according to Nissen, the Peruvian army, in the eyes of U.S. officials, is taking the road of appeasement: "To the dismay of U.S. officials, army units in the valley have decided not to interfere with coca until some substitute crops can be found."

All three networks covered the DEA's discovery and destruction of a drug tunnel running under the U.S.–Mexican border. ABC describes the tunnel as "something out of James Bond," and the NBC anchor says, "Nothing like it has ever been seen." The camera in two of the stories follows U.S. agents down the tunnel, peering over their shoulders down the length of it and then swooping dramatically up the shaft. A customs official warns drug smugglers everywhere: "We don't care whether you come over us, through us, or under us, we're going to be after you. . . ." This kind of statement obscures any domestic connection that the smugglers might have as well as the fact that the tunnel was effectively hidden for at least six months.

Near the end of the CBS story, over a sweeping shot of barren Arizona desert, the reporter says, "Officials are investigating the possibility of even more tunnels in the area, which is known as 'Cocaine Alley' because of the rampant drug trafficking." Two somewhat contradictory themes emerge: drugs are everywhere, and we are winning the drug war. Weaving these two together permitted television news to trumpet victories in the drug war, even as the figures on drug use showed little change. CBS reports that customs officials discovered the tunnel by following at truck from the warehouse at the U.S. terminus. The truck contained more than a ton of cocaine. Officials estimated the tunnel had been open at least six months. The story makes no effort to estimate how much cocaine got through before the tunnel was discovered. Such an investigation would have been a completely opposite frame: the futility of rather than victory in the drug war.

In a short "reader" immediately following the ABC Peruvian drug war story, anchor Peter Jennings reports that the annual survey of high school seniors in America has found that cocaine use has dropped to its lowest level since the mid-1970s, "even though, students say, there is more cocaine around." The juxtaposition of these two stories along with the content of the other War on Drugs stories suggests that the U.S. is doing its job in reducing demand and reinforces the view that the problem to be solved is at the supply end of the trade.

Us against them: foreigners

The "us against them" frame is evident in the stories about foreign involvement in the drug trade. These stories tended to be longer and to air nearer to the beginning of the newscast than other illegal-drug stories. Their prominence underscores this aspect of television's framing of the War on Drugs: it is a foreign problem, a matter of the U.S. fighting valiantly, with reluctant foreign cooperation or none, against a scourge that originates outside its borders and seeks to infiltrate it everywhere.

In its drug tunnel story, CBS reports that two Americans and two Mexicans have been apprehended, and that several houses, a ranch and two businesses have been confiscated. We never see these suspects or their U.S. holdings. Most of the focus is on dramatic visuals of the tunnel. Although a diagram shows that the bulk of the tunnel lies under U.S. soil, the focus of the story is on the Mexican involvement. CBS describes the Mexican terminus of the tunnel as being located in "an upper-class residence," "a luxury home in Mexico." The implication is that foreigners are making millions off the U.S. drug trade. At a press conference announcing the find, U.S. officials do the talking, while numerous Mexican officials are silent partners, shown seated quietly in the audience.

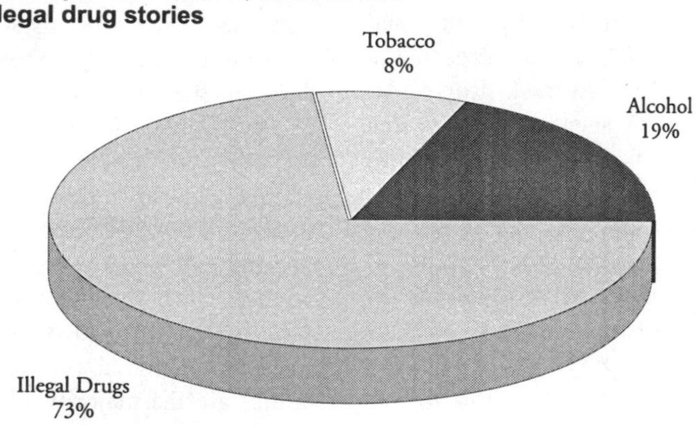

Similarly, the "us against foreigners" theme appears throughout the ABC story on the drug war in Peru. Nissen documents the plight of the Peruvian peasants, for whom coca cultivation is a rational economic choice. She reports that "in the presidential palace in Lima, the answer is clear: The U.S. must guarantee a market and better prices for legal Peruvian products." One of the longest stories in the sample, Nissen's report comes the closest of any of the drug war stories to a critical perspective, and to exploring deeper economic forces underlying the illegal drug trade. With the Vietnam-era references, both verbal and visual, it is difficult to predict how a U.S. audience would respond. Some might agree with Nissen's conclusion that "Peru is willing to be an ally in the drug war, but it wants development, not destruction. It wants a marked change in the battle plan." Others might see a repetition of another reading of the Vietnam experience: the U.S. pouring resources into a country that lacks the resolve to fight for its own freedom, in this case from drugs. In either interpretation, foreigners are the problem because they resist full cooperation with the U.S. tactics and so undermine the government's ability to fight the drug war.

A review of the Vanderbilt News Archive abstracts of all the illegal-drug stories aired on the three networks in the first four months of 1990 confirms the message coming through in the sample. Foreign stories attract the bulk of the coverage (51

of 94 stories in January alone). The stories emphasize a single theme: drugs are coming into the U.S. from outside, and foreign governments are not as committed to stopping this as the U.S. In the U.S.–Mexico drug tunnel story, U.S. Customs Commissioner Carol Hallett sums up the overall frame of the drug war stories: "When we work as a team, we're going to beat them. We're going to win. We're going to stop the druggers, and the good guys will win."

As for the role of U.S. citizens in the international drug trade, the stories in the sample reinforce the frame of drug smuggling being "un-American"—that is, an activity that comes from outside and is dominated by outsiders. Two stories on NBC report on that network's investigation of Coast Guard members' complicity in the drug trade. The first story, in May, has the tone of an exposé of government corruption. The "drugs are everywhere" theme is underlined by the revelation that one of the Guardsmen involved had been part of President Bush's protection detail on his summer vacation in Maine, with a visual of the President fishing accompanied by a Guardsman. The story ends on a comforting note, however, with quotes from Guardsmen. One says, "It relieves the rest of us at least that they were discovered and dealt with as the system allows." Another distances himself from the participants—"It's the lure of easy money. You just don't like to see it in your own back yard. I'm not familiar with the people." And the commandant at the base involved says it is "just a case of a few bad apples." The final shot is of a Coast Guard cutter going off into the sunset. The message is: All is well, the system is working.

By the time of the second story, in September, NBC tells us that the drug war "has been compromised by a scandal involving dozens of federal agents and Coast Guardsmen suspected of working for the drug smugglers." (The other two networks did not cover the story.) The wording of Brokaw's introduction is significant: The Guardsmen are not drug smugglers themselves, they work for "the drug smugglers." The "few bad apples" have become "an ongoing, well organized corruption ring at this Coast Guard base in Miami Beach and at other bases as far away as Boston." The story says at one point, "Whole boatloads of Coast Guardsmen supposedly on drug patrols became smugglers themselves." But the rest of the story makes a clear distinction between the (unidentified) drug smugglers and the (good) Coast Guardsmen. A government agent, his face checker-blocked out, says, "We are losing the drug war because of the fact that there are payoffs." In these news stories, the smugglers infiltrate "us" and undermine our efforts to enforce a moral order.

FIGURE 2

Time spent on alcohol, tobacco and illegal drug stories

Tobacco 8%

Alcohol 19%

Illegal Drugs 73%

Us against them: race

A "War on Drugs—One Year Later" story on ABC in September also employs the "us against them" frame, this time focused on race. The drug dealers, users and arrestees depicted are overwhelmingly African American. Below the words "Cocaine costs more and is less pure than a year ago," a black hand holds a large vial, cradling it as though offering it to someone. In the next shot, a much smaller vial lies in a white hand fingering it as if inspecting it. Below the words "Enforcement efforts," white hands inspect a plastic bag of white powder or rock. On the word "supply," a black man lights up a crack pipe. As the scene changes to a shot of a high school corridor, the camera focuses on a black student in the midst of a crowd of teenagers of a variety of ethnicities, following her and implying to the viewer that she is somehow central to the drug issue. White arrestees appear late in the story. They provide background footage as the reporter talks about "more arrests, maybe more deterrence, but not much more relief for the walking wounded."

A subtle pattern of images emerges driven by small and perhaps unconscious decisions that nonetheless are repeated in other stories. In a story about IRS efforts to track drug-trade-related money laundering, the arresting agents are white, the arrestees black. The reporter mentions that nine senior officials at two Texas banks have been indicted, but does not show them. Instead, the visual following these words is a pair of black hands, presumably a bank teller, counting out money at a teller's booth. In a story about the purchase of a new police dog in Berkeley, California, four out of five Berkeley residents interviewed are black. The frame of the story assumes that the reason the new dog is controversial is because its job will be sniffing out and attacking black people, in scenes reminiscent of Sheriff Bull Connor and the battles for civil rights.

A story about an anti-drug cartoon special broadcast by all three networks reinforces the frame through the coloring of the cartoon itself. The main character in the cartoon, a child, is colored Caucasian. The figures offering the child drugs are colored in dark gray tones. Drugs are shown as vapors arising from the sewers; the dark-colored drug dealers slip in and out of the vapors, camouflaged, seemingly an integral part of the big city environment.

The stories about Washington, DC, Mayor Marion Barry's trial for buying cocaine in an FBI sting illustrate how drug users are depicted as an "other." The fact that Barry happens to be African American may have served to underscore the "us against them" racial frame. The sample picked up six stories about his trial, including all three networks' coverage of Barry accuser Rashida Moore's first day in court. The stories refer to Barry with phrases like "crack addict and womanizer." Other language used establishes that Barry lives outside of acceptable moral bounds. Two of the stories report Moore's claim that Barry even used cocaine at "her mother's house, on Mother's Day." One of them adds, "While her mother played the organ at church . . . the mayor met [Moore] for drugs and

sex." The stories allude briefly to the warm support Barry seemed to be receiving from the African American community at this time, and show him wearing a kinte cloth stole, but do not follow these up—a possible indication not only that the community supporting him is not the primary audience for the stories, but that Barry is telling another story to that community, a story about victimization of and the need for solidarity among African Americans in the drug war.

The "us against them" racial frame is evident even when the drug users depicted are white. This story reports that inner city drug sales are not just an inner city problem—suburbanites are buying drugs here as well. NBC profiles a New Jersey woman killed buying drugs in Harlem as a cautionary tale, warning suburban viewers to steer clear of the inner city drug trade. The story is news because it involves people in the drug trade who are outside of the news media's standard frame for illegal drugs: white suburbanites. The inner city residents (shown in shots of drug dealers on street corners) are black; the suburbanites in the story are white. The reporter blames the commuters for interfering with efforts to gain control of the "rampant narcotics trade in the nation's inner cities." In terms of the frame being presented, white suburbanites are out of place in the drug trade, and this is what makes this story news.

A more accurate view of actual drug use in the U.S. appears twice in the story. The reporter states that 60%–90% of the arrests in police sting operations in poor black neighborhoods are white suburbanites. Then a Drug Enforcement Agency (DEA) spokesman says, " . . . the majority of drug money that goes to the cartels comes not from the crack user but from the cocaine user. And a significant percentage of those users are in the suburbs, not necessarily in the inner city or poor." In fact, as Figure 3 shows, according to the National Household Survey on Drug Abuse and the FBI's Uniform Crime Reports, whites are the majority of both drug users and arrestees. But the implication of the story is both that white, suburban drug users are extraordinary, and therefore news, and that the corollary is also true: black characters in the story are not an anomaly—they are expected to be involved in the drug trade.

Through their images and words, the 24 stories on illegal drugs in the sample present a consistent story line. Illegal drugs are everywhere, an omnipresent threat to America. "Addicts" are generally portrayed as innocent victims, while "dealers" are evil and are most often shown as African American or foreign. The U.S. government and its agents are presented as heroes, while foreign governments are at best silent partners and at worst are reluctant and undependable partners in the U.S.'s heroic efforts to stop the world drug trade. In the entire sample of health and alcohol, tobacco and other drug stories, the U.S. government for the most part shows up as a negative force, something to be reined in, inefficient or inept (Dorfman and Jernigan, 1992). But in the illegal-drug stories, government officials are rarely questioned or doubted.

The War on Drugs, then, was an "us against them" story for television, a story primarily about others. "Us" is the audience that identifies with white suburbanites, with young, corruptible and contrite (white) Coast Guardsmen, with white children being offered drugs by dark and evil cartoon figures from the sewers of the city. "Them" domestically was African Americans or corrupted whites, who, according to television news, are the main actors in the domestic drug trade. In the foreign stories, "them" is foreigners, whether faceless drug smugglers or Latin American governments, who do not share "our" commitment to eradicating drugs and who are depicted as invaders and threats to the American moral order. Importantly, it is the unusual white—the bad apple—who is implicated negatively regarding drugs. No such distinction is made when African Americans or foreigners are implicated.

Discussion

This analysis of news stories about illegal drugs on television network news suggests that the news coverage "otherized" the U.S. drug problem in 1990. The drugs used by and killing most Americans—alcohol and tobacco (McGinnis and Foege, 1993)—received little coverage from television news. The drugs used by a very small group in society, a group that by definition is an "other" to most Americans, since statistically fewer Americans are likely to know an illegal drug user than a drinker, a smoker or a pharmaceutical user, appeared shrouded in evil.

Why did the news depict the drug war in this way? Two classic studies of the production and content of news argued that the news does not reflect reality; it "reconstitutes the everyday world" (Tuchman, 1978:107) and reflects the values it assumes its audience holds (Gans, 1979). It imposes order on the raw material of daily life, and reduces idiosyncrasy into formula. It creates and the reinforces standard stories. It "reports on those at or near the top of the hierarchies [we call nation and society] and on those, particularly at the bottom, who threaten them, to an audience, most of whom are located in the vast middle range between top and bottom" (Gans, 1979:284). According to Gans, the news "supports the social order of public, business and professional, upper-middle class, middle-aged, and white male sectors of society" (1979:60).

The dominance of illegal-drug stories, in terms of both numbers and placement in the newscast, may be attributed to television's much greater concern with social disorder and violation of the norms of the dominant group than with epidemiological evidence (Gans, 1979). The reliance of the news on official sources also explains the emphasis on illegal drugs as opposed to other drug problems. The drug story on television news provides yet another example of how easily the news is led by official framings of social problems (Sharp, 1992; Beckett, 1994). Events staged by and for major public officials, such as the "drug summit" held in Colombia in February 1990, hold powerful sway over the news media and predictably influence the content of news coverage (Gans, 1979). The Bush administration's decision to define the War on Drugs

FIGURE 3
Illegal-drug-related data by ethnicity

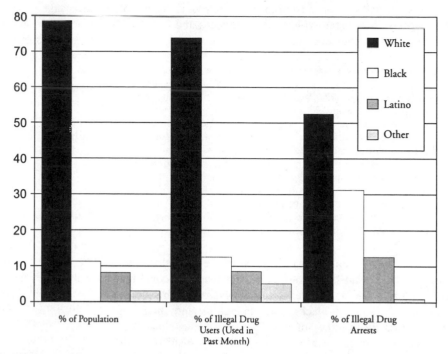

as the province of the Drug Enforcement Agency more than the Department of Health and Human Services drove reporters' decisions to look to the DEA rather than to DHHS for War on Drugs stories.

Gans points to ethnocentrism as one of the eight core values reflected in news in the U.S. This goes some way toward explaining the nature of the coverage of foreign nations attitudes toward or efforts to join the U.S. War on Drugs. But the impact of ethnocentrism in this case is simply to reinforce the dominant frame on the illegal-drug story: illegal drugs are problems of an "other," outside the American mainstream, foreign to American shores and values.

The burial of the story of white drug use and consequences—that is, the fact that by far the highest percentage of drug users and drug arrestees are white—reflects the upper-middle-class values and bias of the news media. If illegal drug use is outside the current experience of those reporting the news—and for all populations, illegal drug use is centered in a very small minority—then news professionals might easily fall prey to locating this use in an "other," in persons or communities with which they are unfamiliar. The paucity of African American or other racial/ethnic minority staff in network news operations reinforces this bias (Smith, 1991). The presence of African American reporters or editors might also have made some difference in the apparently routine practice of using (often unidentified) file footage of black suspects, dealers and users in drug stories to provide a visual backdrop for "America's drug problem." However, the visual needs of television also perpetuate this practice. The fact that shooting footage of African Americans doing or dealing illegal drugs openly in the streets is easier than filming European Americans with drugs in their homes means that television will rely on the former to illustrate illegal drug use.

In his analysis of stories from local newscasts, Entman took the relationship between typical news practices and depictions of African Americans even farther:

> TV favors middle- or upper-class persons when they appear in the news, because those persons have the skills and resources to manipulate television's production practices. To counter this slant, journalists would have to understand the class bias and take steps to counteract it—suggesting that black lawbreakers put on business suits, for example, or asking police to allow them to walk freely for the news camera [rather than shackled]. But such overt intervention in the construction of the subject's image would be impractical and would be viewed by editors as staging the news or editorializing. In the absence of such steps, crime coverage may compound whites' fear of blacks by showing black criminals more than white criminals surrounded with symbols of menace (1990:337).

These findings can easily be applied to the drug stories we studied. The central theme of "us against them" is consistent with Entman's finding that depictions of blacks in crime stories reinforce the idea of blacks as a dangerous and menacing "other." And the routines of television news mean that drug offenders without the protection of upper-class insulation will remain easy targets for news cameras. The ongoing problem is not only that typical depictions of drug users distance them from the majority white audience, but that similar depictions of whites are rare.

Because of the paucity of studies of audience reactions to news stories, only limited conjecture is possible regarding the political and social effects of such coverage. Graber (1990) found that close-ups of unfamiliar people in exotic circumstances were among the most likely visuals to be remembered by her respondents. This suggests that these "otherizing" visuals of the drug war had an effect. Her respondents believed that "the visuals allowed them to form more complete and accurate representations of people and events" (1990:49). The visuals add credibility to television news, according to Graber, because people feel that they can see for themselves what is happening and so draw their own conclusions. In an analysis that parallels Iyengar's (1991) findings, Graber suggests that the implications of people's tendency to remember visuals of people means that personal roles are emphasized over other factors in news stories. The emphasis on roles "enshrine[s] the politics of personality at the expense of considering the influence of the broader political system and at the expense of dispassionate factual analysis" (1990:153).

Iyengar's work focused on the attribution of responsibility for social problems as a result of viewing news stories. Episodic framing, combined with the tendency of television news to fragment social problems from their contexts, leads to news stories that place the blame primarily on individuals rather than on social or structural causes such as poverty, unemployment, or the economic development needs of poor agrarian nations (Iyengar, 1991). Iyengar also discovered that regardless of whether stories were framed episodically or thematically, for black crime and illegal drugs the subject matter of the news had a greater impact than the frame. Across all framings, his audiences were twice as likely to hold society responsible for the cause of crime in the case of white violent crime versus black violent crime. Similarly, illegal-drug stories in his sample (regardless of frame) evoked individualistic attributions of responsibility. In terms of responsibility for treating the problem, illegal-drug stories were only half as likely to evoke attributions of societal responsibility as stories of black crime. Thus a preponderance of illegal-drug stories featuring black violent crime, such as appeared in our sample, would be expected to influence public attitudes about both issues in the direction of attributions of individual responsibility, and in favor of punitive treatment.

Conclusion

Regardless of questions of television journalists' intent, analysis of this sample of stories suggests that through application of such "business as usual" practices as use of uncredited file footage and heavy reliance on official sources, and reflecting both the ethnocentric and the moral values of upper-middle-class America, the supposed illegal drug epidemic appeared on the evening news as primarily the fault and the scourge of African Americans and Latin Americans.

This finding shows race to be a category of continued significance in American life, with meanings separate from statistical evidence and powerful enough to distort it regarding the significance of race, at least in terms of actual use of and problems associated with illegal drugs. If this finding is accurate, it suggests that the drug war of the 1990s replicates in U.S. history the pattern of drug wars as a means of social control over racial and ethnic minorities: Chinese, in the case of the opium scare of the late 19th century (Morgan et al., 1988; Musto, 1973); Native Americans, in much of the anti-alcohol legislation of the American frontier (Mosher, 1975); African Americans in the backlash against cocaine use following Reconstruction (Morgan et al., 1988); and Mexicans, in the campaign against marijuana in the 1930s (Morgan et al., 1988; Mosher, 1990; Bonnie and Whitbread, 1974).

Close observation of the stories in our sample, combined with the research findings of other social scientists regarding the power and impact of television news, suggests that television coverage of the War on Drugs not only helped it to be a "war on some drugs" and a "war on some populations" but also supported the nation's single-minded reliance on punitive approaches to the illegal drug problem. This may have fueled public support for a largely ineffectual response to illegal drug use. It may also have supported social control of a very specific kind: to the extent that blacks are overrepresented among the population of drug users—and they are, although in sheer numbers white users far outnumber them—the building of support for and subsequent creation of extraordinarily punitive responses to illegal drug problems (stiff mandatory sentences) increased the already disproportionate number of African Americans incarcerated in the United States (Beck and Gilliard, 1995).

Visual analysis of even a small sample of network television news stories about illegal drugs illustrates that there is more going on in television news than meets the ear. This kind of analysis is expensive and time-consuming, and the size of the sample analyzed here limits the generalizability of our findings. Given the predominance of television news as a source of information for the public, and the emerging body of evidence about the power of the news to shape people's perceptions of and prescriptions for social problems, a key part of the agenda and method for future social science research on illegal drug problems may be summed up in a single short sentence: Television bears watching.

References

Altheide, David, L. "Ethnographic content analysis." *Qualitative Sociology* 10:65–77, 1987.

Beck, Allen J. and Darrell K. Gilliard, "Prisoners in 1994." *Bureau of Justice Statistics Bulletin* NCJ-151654, August 1995.

Beckett, Katherine, "Setting the public agenda: 'Street crime' and drug use in American politics." *Social Problems* 41 (3):425–447, 1994.

Bonnie, Richard J. and Charles Whitbread II, *The Marijuana Conviction: Marijuana Prohibition in the United States.* Charlottesville: University Press of Virginia, 1974.

Cohen, Bernard, *The Press and Foreign Policy.* Princeton, NJ: Princeton University Press, 1963.

Dorfman, Lori, "News operations: How television reports health issues." Doctoral dissertation, University of California at Berkeley, 1994.

Dorfman, Lori and David Jernigan, "How television news frames health." Presentation given at the 120th annual meeting of the American Public Health Association, Washington, DC, 1992.

Entman, Robert, "Modern racism and the images of blacks in local television news." *Critical Studies in Mass Communication* 7(4):332–345, 1990.

____, "Blacks in the news: Television, modern racism and cultural change." *Journalism Quarterly* 69(2):341–361, 1992.

Gans, Herbert, *Deciding What's News.* New York: Vintage Books, 1979.

Gitlin, Todd, "The war on drugs and the enlisted press." *Columbia Journalism Review* November–December:17–18, 1989.

Glasgow Media Group (G. Philo, J. Hewitt, P. Beharrell, and H. Davis), *Really Bad News.* London: Writers and Readers, 1982.

Graber, Doris A., "Seeing is remembering: How visuals contribute to learning from television news." *Journal of Communication* 40(3):134–155, Summer 1990.

Iyengar, Shanto and Donald R. Kinder, "Psychological accounts of agenda-setting." Pp. 117–140 in Richard Perloff and Sidney Kraus, eds., *Mass Media and Political Thought.* Beverly Hills: Sage Publications, 1985.

Iyengar, Shanto, *Is Anyone Responsible? How Television Frames Political Issues.* Chicago: University of Chicago Press, 1991.

Jamieson, K., *Eloquence in an Electronic Age: The Transformation of Political Speechmaking.* New York: Oxford University Press, 1988.

Jensen, Eric L., Jurg Gerber and Ginna M. Babcock, "The new war on drugs: Grass-roots movement or political construction?" *Journal of Drug Issues* 3.651–667, 1991.

McGinnis, J. Michael and William H. Foege, "Actual causes of death in the United States." *Journal of the American Medical Association* 270:2207–2212, 1993.

Morgan, Patricia, Lawrence Wallack and David Buchanan, "Waging drug wars: Prevention strategy or politics as usual." *Drugs and Society* 3(1/2):99–124, 1988.

Mosher, James F., "Drug availability in a public health perspective." Pp. 129–168 in Hank Resnick, ed. *Youth and Drugs: Society's Mixed Messages.* Washington, DC: Office for Substance Abuse Prevention, 1990.

____, "Liquor Legislation and Native Americans: History and Perspective." Unpublished manuscript. Berkeley, CA: Alcohol Research Group, 1975.

Mosher, James F. and Karen Yanagisako, "Public health, not social warfare: A public health approach to illegal drug policy." *Journal of Public Health Policy* 12:278–323, 1991.

Musto, David, *The American Disease: Origins of Narcotic Control.* New York: Oxford Press, 1973.

Orcutt, James D. and J. Blake Turner, "Shocking numbers and graphic accounts: Quantified images of drug problems in the print media." *Social Problems* 40:190–206, 1993.

Page, Benjamin I. and Robert Y. Shapiro, "What moves public opinion?" *American Political Science Review* 81:23–43, 1987.

Reinarman, Craig and Harry G. Levine, "The crack attack: Politics and media in America's latest drug scare." Pp. 115–134 in Joel Best, ed., *Images of Issues: Typifying Contemporary Social Problems.* New York: Aldine de Gruyter, 1989.

Rogers, Everett M. and James W. Dearing, "Agenda-setting research: Where has it been, and where is it going?" Pp. 555–594 in James A. Anderson, ed., *Communication Yearbook,* Vol 11. Beverly Hills: Sage Publications, 1988.

Roper Organization, *Roper's The Public Pulse* 6, Research Supplement:1, 1991.

Sharp, Elaine, "Agenda-setting and policy results: Lessons from three drug policy episodes." *Policy Studies Journal* 20:538–551, 1992.

Smith, Erna, *What Color Is the News? An Ethnic Content Analysis of Bay Area News Media.* San Francisco: New California Alliance, Public Research Institute, San Francisco State University, 1991.

Tuchman, Gaye, *Making News: A Study in the Construction of Reality.* New York: The Free Press, 1978.

Tyndall, Andrew, "The review of the year." *Tyndall Report,* January 1991.

U.S. Department of Health and Human Services, *National Household Survey on Drug Abuse: Populations Estimates 1988.* Rockville, MD: National Institute on Drug Abuse, Division of Epidemiology and Prevention Research, 1989.

____, *National Household Survey on Drug Abuse: Populations Estimates 1990.* Rockville, MD: National Institute on Drug Abuse, Division of Epidemiology and Prevention Research, 1991.

Vanderbilt Television News Archive, *Television News Index and Abstracts.* Nashville, TN: Vanderbilt Television News Archive, 1990.

____, *Television News Index and Abstracts.* Nashville, TN: Vanderbilt Television News Archive, 1991.

The Casualties of War

Using prisons to solve the drug problem hurts not just the black and Latino communities that have suffered the most, but all of America

By Ellis Cose

IN SEARCH OF STORIES, WE SNIFF THE Sewer Of Scandal; and aroused by the scent, we fearless journalists strike. So tell us, George W., did you snort it? Did you smoke it? And assuming that you did, tell us when. Somehow we make of this a test of character. And in some minor sense it is. But in the end it doesn't tell us much about whether a man deserves to be president. Irrespective of what George W. Bush might have done in his wilder, daring days, he and other presidential candidates have a responsibility to reflect on this so-called war on drugs. Largely because of that so-called war, more Americans than ever are behind bars. The federal prison population quintupled in less than two decades, as the number of people sentenced for federal drug offenses multiplied more than 11 times. A huge proportion of those convicted have come from places such as Watts in Los Angeles that are predominantly black and Latino. Part of the reason is that drug dealing in poor inner-city communities is more likely to be out in the open than it is in the suburbs, where it generally takes place behind closed doors. Another reason is that residents of such neighborhoods are less likely to have sophisticated legal help—or to get the benefit of the doubt from prosecutors. They are also more likely to be caught with crack cocaine, an offense that carries much stiffer penalties than possessing the powdered kind.

Connie Rice, cofounder of a Los Angeles-based advocacy group called The Advancement Project, estimates the number of prisoners and ex-prisoners among men from certain parts of Watts at nearly 50 percent. "I don't understand the lack of alarm about it," she says. Dina Rose, a sociologist at John Jay College of Criminal Justice in New York, notes that in such communities prison time is so prevalent it has become a natural and expected part of life. And she questions whether arresting such large numbers of people really drives down crime. Rose's preliminary research in Tallahassee, Fla., has found that arrest levels soon reach a "tipping point" beyond which a community becomes so destabilized that the crime rate goes up instead of down as more people are imprisoned.

It would be one thing if we could be confident that this focus on imprisonment was solving the drug problem. But the evidence is, at best, mixed. Overall drug use is down from its peak in 1979 (cocaine use peaked six years later, in 1985). But there is little evidence that incarceration policies had much to do with it. In the get-tough state of Texas, for example, cocaine use is rising. Among students, it is at its highest level since the annual survey of the Texas Commission on Alcohol and Drug Abuse began in 1988. Meanwhile, heroin overdoses in Texas have risen, as has the percentage of adolescents testing positive for marijuana upon arrest—and all this despite the fact that Texas has the second highest incarceration rate (724 per 100,000 residents) of any state in the nation (just after Louisiana).

Texas's prison-focused policy has been a failure. And so, in large measure, has the nation's "war." It has left us with overcrowded prisons, and with hundreds of thousands of people who have lost the right to vote, and have little chance at a job and a slim prayer of being reconnected to the larger society. It has also left many Americans, particularly black Americans, with the sense the judicial system is "the new Jim Crow," in the words of Eric Sterling, president of the Criminal Justice Policy Foundation. For all that, taxpayers foot a huge bill for prisons as the convict population swells.

Obviously, some people are so violent and incorrigible that prison is the only fit place for them. The problem is that we are spending less and less time figuring out who those people are; and we are devoting precious little energy to reclaiming those lives that can be reclaimed. We have also given up on the very idea of rehabilitation, of providing prisoners with skills and hope. Instead, we warehouse the fallen in dismal places that produce nothing more useful, for the most part, than license plates and ruined souls. One reason is that the war rhetoric and the war mentality allow us to create "collateral casualties," in the words of William Mofitt, president of the National Association of Criminal Defense Lawyers. The tragedy is that many of those collateral casualties are potentially productive human beings.

America needs desperately to break its addiction to this witch's brew of angry language, absurd (often dishonest) assumptions and ineffective policy that is poisoning the nation from within. Since presidential-campaign rhetoric—going back at least to Richard Nixon's celebrated war on crime—is a large part of what got us into this fix, it's only fair to expect that anyone seriously aspiring to the presidency be committed to getting us out.

Ultimately, however, the problem is not just one for politicians—whether they are suspected of using drugs or not—but for those who elect them; for all, in other words, who have responded too readily to the whoops of bloodthirsty generals waging war with a strategy that will never win.

Pregnant, Hooked & Booked

Pregnant substance abusers face challenges and charges that others don't

By Eileen Moon

Anna Smith (not her real name), a 32-year-old California resident, received some bad news on the day she was to leave the hospital where she had just given birth to a daughter. Traces of marijuana had been found in her placenta during routine hospital testing. The state immediately took custody of the child.

Had Anna Smith been a South Carolina resident, things could have been much worse. She might well be serving a jail sentence right now.

That's what happened to Cornelia Whitner, 34. Six years ago, Whitner, a resident of Seneca, South Carolina, lost custody of her newborn son after hospital tests detected cocaine in his bloodstream. Four days after the birth, she was arrested—one of more than 40 new mothers in South Carolina who were taken from their hospital beds by police to face charges of child neglect and abuse. She is now serving an eight-year prison sentence.

South Carolina is the only state in the union whose highest court has sanctioned the criminal prosecution of pregnant substance abusers under child abuse statutes. Although as many as 30 states have had similar cases brought to their highest court, only South Carolina has held the legality of using child abuse statutes to prosecute women for their behavior while pregnant.

As state Attorney General Charlie Condon has said, "Every viable fetus is a fellow South Carolinian." In his prior role as a prosecutor in Charleston, Condon was the first to launch a legal attack on pregnant addicts.

"The attorney general has made his career prosecuting these women," said Lynn Paltrow, a reproductive rights attorney now affiliated with the Women's Law Project in New York City, noting that the only women targeted in Condon's initiative were economically disadvantaged and minority women. "He started arresting only black women, taking them out in chains and shackles, and not offering any treatment."

Conciliation Courts—have expressed similar concerns.

The practice of using punishment to attack the problem of addiction is not new. For decades, judges and lawmakers have favored punitive measures over efforts at rehabilitation, and in doing so have held pregnant women to a higher standard.

"Can you believe they've come up with another thing to punish women for?" said Jackie Hudak, a psychotherapist practicing in Red Bank, New Jersey. "This is a sickness, not a crime."

As Paltrow points out, the South Carolina policies that require the reporting of pregnant women suspected of substance abuse

that women at all economic levels, whether they seek medical care in public facilities or with personal physicians, are subject to the same criteria for maternal and newborn drug screening.

According to state protocol, "newborn drug screens for cocaine, LSD, heroin, amphetamines, and marijuana may be ordered at the discretion of the physician based on the totality of the circumstances surrounding an individual patient's history and medical condition on presentation. The chart should appropriately document the reasons why the testing was ordered."

"You have to be really careful about even having the appearance of discrimination," Christohillis says.

The state has adopted a system of "layers and intervention" that utilize a team approach in determining what options are appropriate in dealing with a substance-abusing mother.

Christohillis says the protocol is treatment-oriented, and adds that the state's involvement may begin with a referral to the Department of Social Services, as well as with attempts to persuade the woman to seek voluntary treatment. Pregnant women who don't cooperate may face a hearing in family court. "It's a perfect vehicle to use to get a court order for treatment," she said. "We're using that criminal approach as a very last resort."

South Carolina has increased its treatment facilities for addicted mothers, but Christohillis admitted that the state is still in desperate need of more. "We've gone forward a big step in that we have created more residential options," she said. "The bottom line is that treatment is cheaper than jail, but you have to have some form of the arm of the law involved with it."

> *"For decades, judges and lawmakers have favored punitive measures over efforts at rehabilitation, and in doing so have held pregnant women to a higher standard."*

If South Carolina's aim is to end substance abuse through criminal prosecution, Paltrow says, they should be expanding their arrests to include all levels of society. They don't, she says, because the policy is inherently racist and elitist. "There is no question that there is an incredible targeting of race and class."

An attorney with the New York City-based Center for Constitutional Rights, a national, nonprofit, public-interest law firm, Paltrow fought Whitner's conviction all the way to the state Supreme Court. Whitner's attorneys have now petitioned the U.S. Supreme Court to review her case and others like it.

Aftershock

Criticized by medical and mental health professionals nationwide, the precedent-setting decision in South Carolina has had repercussions throughout the addiction treatment field.

The American Society of Addiction Medicine has called the criminal prosecution of pregnant women "counterproductive," noting that the policy inevitably will deter women from seeking prenatal care and treatment for chemical dependency. Dozens of other public health organizations and advocacy groups—including the American Medical Association, the American Nurse's Association, the American Public Health Association and the Association of Family and

are in direct conflict with federal confidentiality statutes that protect the privacy of anyone seeking addiction treatment. "It absolutely puts treatment providers in conflict over their state obligation to report, and their federal obligation not to," she said.

"These are patients that a lot of people don't want to work with because of the potential lawsuits," said New York City psychotherapist Esther Miller. "They go from treatment center to treatment center without getting the help they need."

Catharine Christohillis, the head of South Carolina's Drug Prosecution Unit, does not argue with those who say that treatment is obviously the best remedy for the problem of substance abuse in pregnancy. But she is convinced that the law can be a very persuasive tool in persuading women who are pregnant and addicted to enter treatment.

"It's treatment with a stick," she said. "You have to do both. I would love to have these women just come in voluntarily, but that isn't going to happen."

South Carolina's initiatives in handling the problem of pregnant addicts have been revised substantially since the first headline-making incidents in which poor women in a Charleston hospital were charged under child abuse statutes before going home with their newborns. Those incidents were exaggerated and, in some cases, mischaracterized by the media, Christohillis says, noting that few women actually went to jail.

The state's approach has been modified and screening policies have been revised so

Prescription for disaster

Those who propose imprisoning pregnant women, as a means of forcing them into treatment or keeping them from continuing their substance abuse, are dangerously naive about the realities of life behind bars, say many experts.

According to San Francisco attorney Ellen Barry, founder and director of Legal Services for Women with Children, and an advocate for women prisoners for more than 20 years, few prisons offer effective drug and alcohol treatment. Women are often forced to withdraw from drugs "cold turkey," endangering their own health and that of their unborn children as they go through withdrawal.

"It's a prescription for disaster," said Barry. "We've had cases where women in jail have lost their babies very late term."

Nor do women prisoners receive adequate maternity care, Barry says. In fact, a statewide study in California concluded that prenatal care for inmates in the state's two

> *"Who will watch their children while they are in treatment? What will they use for transportation? How will they pay their bills?"*

largest prisons and one large urban county jail was "drastically inadequate." Other studies came to the same conclusion, Barry said.

Those who believe that putting women in prison cuts off their access to drugs are also mistaken, Barry says.

"It is extremely naive for policymakers to maintain that prisoners with substance abuse problems are cut off from the sources of their addiction by incarceration," Barry wrote in an article entitled, "Pregnant, Addicted and Sentenced (ABA Criminal Justice, Winter, 1991). "In some instances, illegal substances are even more readily available in correctional facilities than on the streets."

While many policymakers cling to the idea that imprisoning pregnant drug abusers is the only option, Barry strongly supports the expansion of model programs that open the doors of recovery for these women, instead of close them. Two programs she cited are Mandela House in Oakland, California, and Jeleni House in San Francisco, both of which offer intensive, long-term, residential treatment.

"It is, in fact, possible to create a setting where women can safely detox and stay clean away from drugs, [so they can] rebuild their lives and give birth to healthy infants," Barry said. "They've actually taken women who were crack dependent, who have gone into recovery and turned their lives around. Without those types of programs, there are really not a lot of options."

Anna Smith is currently rebuilding her life and working on her recovery at a similar intensive residential treatment program, the Prototypes facility in Pomona, California. The facility's director, Dr. Vivian A. Brown, PhD, called the practice of imprisoning pregnant women "archaic and brutal." "I think the ruling should be that women should be given treatment on demand," Brown said, noting that the demand for such all-encompassing treatment centers far exceeds the supply. "We have not even come close to providing the slots necessary."

Substance-abusing women who are economically disadvantaged typically have a myriad of problems associated with their addiction. "The majority of these women have had histories of physical and sexual abuse

from early childhood. They also have emotional problems. They may live with a current batterer."

In order for their addiction treatment to be effective, Brown says, they also need help with a constellation of practical problems. Who will watch their children while they are in treatment? What will they use for transportation? How will they pay their bills?

"The answer to those problems is to provide all the treatment services these women need in one location, where the women can address their problems in a supportive environment while living with their children," Brown said. "They need parenting training; they need vocational training. What we've done is bring everything onto the campus."

Prototypes have 85 women and 50 children in residence, with another 50 families receiving outpatient services. The families may remain in residence at Prototypes for up to 18 months as they take the steps necessary to become sober and self-sufficient. "We are always filled," Brown said. "We always have a waiting list."

At every level

Although the pregnant substance abuser is commonly stereotyped as urban, crack-addicted, and poor, the fact is that pregnant women at all levels of society frequently use drugs (both legal and illicit), alcohol and tobacco.

"Lots of people are drinking while they are pregnant," says U.S. Public Health Nurse Dr. Genevieve Monahan, PhD, a research associate with the UCLA Drug Abuse Research Center in Los Angeles. "I think tobacco and alcohol are far worse problems... than crack cocaine. That's not the thing that's affecting 90 percent of America."

The difference between the middle-class addict using prescription drugs, alcohol, or marijuana, and the "street-level" addict taking heroin or smoking crack, often comes in her ability to conceal her disease, and escape the attention of those who believe that arrest is the answer.

What they have in common is that they are all endangering the developing fetus. As a result of their continued substance abuse,

they may suffer a psychic crisis, says Helen McGivney Glassman, coordinator of the Addiction Recovery Program at the Postgraduate Center for Mental Health in New York City, and a therapist in private practice.

"Most women cherish this life inside them. They want their children to be happy and healthy, and they bond with them. They don't want to hurt them. There is a very, very deep conflict about wanting to love this child and not wanting to hurt it. I think what is going on inside them is terrible."

Early intervention is the only answer that makes sense when it comes to treating pregnant substance abusers, Glassman says. That means access not only to addiction services but also to free and nonjudgmental prenatal and obstetrical care.

Santa Monica counselor Laurie Tanner, author of *The Mother's Survival Guide to Recovery,* says that the first thing she does for a pregnant addict who seeks help is offer her understanding, "The number one thing that works for women is to have a one-on-one relationship with a nurse, a counselor, or a therapist. All they need is one person, who says, 'You can do this. I am here for you.'"

"The main thing I say to her is, 'I know you don't mean to hurt your baby, and I know you are using and drinking. There is not a woman on earth who would have chosen this path.'"

A former prenatal counselor working with poor women in the Santa Monica area, Tanner said women who take that first step toward recovery will confront a number of obstacles as they journey toward sobriety. Husbands and boyfriends may endanger their recovery. They may have to leave those relationships and stand on their own two feet for the first time in their lives. They need an opportunity to learn how to live in a new way.

Tanner advocates for more treatment centers for pregnant/addicted women that can provide the intensive care these women need for recovery.

"Once-a-week outpatient treatment for an hour doesn't work when you have screaming kids," she says. "These women need help. These suffering families can't wait."

After all, she said, the disease that gets women arrested in South Carolina is exactly the same as "alcohol and pills in Beverly Hills. Their disease is the same as Betty Ford's. It's the same as any movie star's. The disease isn't worse because it's a Native American alcoholic or a cocaine user."

Eileen Moon is a freelance writer from Atlantic Highlands, New Jersey.

Alcoholism in Women

by Sheila B. Blume

The average American, when asked to picture an alcoholic, will conjure up a male image, whether it is a businessman lingering over a three-martini lunch, a skid row derelict begging for the price of a bottle, or the romanticized drunken writer played by Ray Milland in *The Lost Weekend*. But alcoholism is also a major problem among American women.

This is not a new phenomenon, a product of the jazz age or the atomic age. The biblical book of Samuel relates the story of Hannah, who moved her lips when she asked God for a child while praying silently at a temple. A passing priest, assuming that she was intoxicated, advised her to give up drinking. Aristotle mentioned the tendency of drunken women to produce defective offspring. In early Rome, the law forbade the use of alcohol by women on penalty of death, but heavy drinking among women became widespread in the late Roman Empire. Alcohol consumption by both sexes was high in colonial and early 19th century America.

Nevertheless, men have always consumed more alcohol than women. The average drinking man's intake (one and a half drinks a day) is about twice that of the average drinking woman. Furthermore, women are more likely to be abstainers at all ages. Some 13% of men qualify for a diagnosis of current alcohol abuse or dependence, as compared to 4% of women. The rate of alcoholism is highest among women in their 20s and declines steadily with age. Women in their 20s and early 30s are most at risk if they are childless, never married, and not employed full time; possibly they have not fully assumed adult social roles. In their late 30s and 40s, women are at highest risk when they are divorced and unemployed, with no children living at home. Some may have sustained these losses in part because of drinking. In the 50s and 60s, the risk is highest for married women who are not working outside the home and have no children at home—suggesting an "empty nest" syndrome.

A family history of alcoholism is common among female as well as male alcoholics, and recent research has established that heredity accounts for nearly 50% of the risk of contracting the disease. But alcoholism may be less genetically influenced in women than in men. Researchers have described a highly heritable type of alcoholism, associated with antisocial behavior, that passes mainly from father to son. The less heritable, more environmentally influenced type occurs in both sexes and predominates among women.

Women are physiologically more sensitive to alcohol than men. At a given dose, their blood level of alcohol is higher and they are more intoxicated, even after adjustment for body weight. Thus a woman will be incapacitated for driving by fewer drinks than a man of the same height and weight. There are two reasons for this difference. One is that women's bodies have a higher proportion of fat and a lower proportion of water, so alcohol is less diluted when they drink. The other is that men's stomachs secrete more of an enzyme that breaks alcohol down before it reaches the bloodstream. Unfortunately, these differences are generally not recognized. We serve the same dose of alcohol to all adults, regardless of sex or body size. Furthermore, the alcoholic beverage industry is trying to make female drinking more socially acceptable with glamorous images linking it to liberation and independence. If women are ever induced to drink as much as men, they will surely have a higher rate of alcohol problems.

The female metabolism of alcohol also affects the progression of alcoholism. Women develop all the symptoms faster, but especially physical complications such as liver disease, high blood pressure, peptic ulcers, and weakening of the heart and skeletal muscles. In a Swedish study of 5,000 people treated for alcoholism, the death rate was three times the average among men and five times the average among women. In an 11-year follow-up study of 103 women treated for alcoholism at a St. Louis hospital, their death rate was 4.5 times higher than average and their lives were shortened by an average of 15 years. The good news is that women who recovered from alcoholism had a normal life expectancy.

Women who drink heavily during pregnancy risk premature labor and other obstetric complications, and their infants often have birth defects. The most severe is fetal

From *The Harvard Mental Health Letter*, March 1998, pp. 5-7. © 1998 by the President and Fellows of Harvard College. Reprinted by permission.

alcohol syndrome, which includes mental retardation and other symptoms such as growth deficiencies, poor motor coordination, behavior problems, abnormalities of the heart, skin, and skeleton, and a characteristic facial deformity. Less severe effects are a reduced birth weight and a lower IQ.

Research has shown the utter falsity of the ancient and still common belief that alcohol heightens sexual responsiveness in women. In fact, it interferes with their sexual functioning in a variety of ways. A single dose has little effect on female sex hormone levels, but sustained heavy drinking is associated with irregular menstrual periods, infertility, early menopause, lack of sexual interest, and painful intercourse. In one experiment, women underwent physiological tests after drinking either an alcoholic or a nonalcoholic beverage; the results showed that depression of sexual arousal and orgasm were directly correlated with blood alcohol level.

The mistaken belief that alcohol induces female sexual arousal has created a special stigma: women who drink are seen as lustful "fallen women." A woman pictured with a bottle of beer is judged more sexually available than the same woman with a nonalcoholic drink. This belief promotes sexual assault, including date rape, since drunkenness is unreasonably and unfairly thought to make the rapist less responsible and the victim more responsible. Alcoholic women sometimes think they need alcohol for sex and are afraid to resume their sex lives when they stop drinking. They should be reassured that recovery will enhance rather than reduce their enjoyment of sex.

Alcoholic women are more likely than alcoholic men to suffer from other psychiatric disorders—especially depression, anxiety, and eating disorders. In women these disorders are also more likely to appear before the alcohol abuse rather than afterward. That means depression or anxiety in a woman will less often go away when the drinking stops and more often requires independent treatment. Relieving the primary depression or anxiety disorder will not cure the alcoholism either; both must be treated.

But early treatment of depression and other psychiatric disorders may help to prevent alcoholism from developing in the first place. Childhood sexual abuse triples the risk of alcohol abuse or dependence in women, perhaps because of the resulting low self-esteem, depression, sexual problems, and post-traumatic stress symptoms. A 27-year follow-up study found that college women were more likely to develop an alcohol problem later in life if they drank during their undergraduate years to combat shyness or to become intoxicated. Drinking as a solution to personal problems can lead to alcohol dependence. Divorced, separated, and widowed women, women caring for the elderly or chronically ill, and others who are under stress need to develop coping skills rather than rely on alcohol for relief.

Because most alcoholic women do not resemble the stereotype in most people's minds, their own denial and the denial of their families may be reinforced while they seek other explanations for their problems. Social stigma may also prevent accurate diagnosis by health professionals, especially in the early stages. As a result, alcoholic women may be given sedatives, tranquilizers, or opiate painkillers and become dependent on prescription drugs as well as alcohol. Fortunately, nonaddictive medications are also available to treat their symptoms.

Although alcoholism treatment programs were originally designed to meet the needs of men, many women now participate as well, and the outcome is about the same for both sexes. Women make up a third of the membership of the best-known self-help group, Alcoholics Anonymous, and 40% of the membership under 30 years of age. Some alcoholism programs have added all-female therapy groups, female staff members who serve as role models, and other features to serve women. A self-help group, Women for Sobriety, is available in some parts of the country, and all-female halfway houses and outpatient facilities may be especially useful: a report on one such program in Sweden showed better outcomes than standard treatment. Women are still somewhat underrepresented in treatment programs, and few programs provide child care or accommodate both mothers and children. Women with alcohol problems still need better screening and access to treatment.

Sheila B. Blume, M.D., C.A.C., is Clinical Professor of Psychiatry at the State University of New York at Stony Brook and Medical Director of the Alcoholism, Chemical Dependency, and Compulsive Gambling Programs at the South Oaks Hospital in Amityville, Long Island.

The facts about women, alcohol

Pioneering research explodes myths about female drinkers

By Marilyn Elias
USA TODAY

When Sharon Wilsnack searched the Harvard library in 1968 for scientific studies on women and alcohol, she found six. "There were thousands on men," recalls the University of North Dakota psychologist. Experts assumed drinking was a male problem.

Thirty years later, although awareness and research have expanded, far more still is known about men's drinking habits than women's. And some of the widely believed "folk wisdom" about how and why women use alcohol is dead wrong, suggests a pioneering 15-year study co-led by Wilsnack. The surveys, on nationally representative samples of U.S. women, have involved about 1,100, including 354 followed since 1981. The newest findings also reflect interviews with 369 male spouses or partners.

"It's a landmark study—the best and only one of its kind. We just don't have anything on women and alcohol this large or long-term," says Mary Dufour, deputy director of the National Institute on Alcohol Abuse and Alcoholism (NIAAA). The agency funded Wilsnack and her husband and co-author, sociologist Richard Wilsnack, hoping to fill some of the huge gaps in understanding about women and alcohol.

The anonymous, in-person interviews, conducted by the University of Chicago's National Opinion Research Center, produced some key surprises, Sharon Wilsnack says. Among popular assumptions challenged by the new report:

➤ **Men influence women to become heavy drinkers.** No, it's mutual. Following women over time shows "kindred marries kindred," Wilsnack says. Women who already drink a lot marry men like themselves, and vice versa.

➤ **The stress of juggling several roles makes women heavier drinkers; a more low-key life leads to less drinking.** The more roles women play—wife, mother, worker—the less likely they are to have drinking problems. "They may be getting more emotional support, more surveillance or perhaps they just have less time and higher self-esteem," Wilsnack speculates.

➤ **Getting a divorce prompts more alcohol use for women.** It can be just the opposite. Leaving an unhappy marriage marred by problem drinking—alcohol creates trouble at home, on the job, driving, etc.—apparently improves women's chances of ending an alcohol habit. After five years, 44% of women with drinking problems who stay married still have alcohol dependency symptoms; 31% who get divorced are still alcohol dependent.

Other findings from the survey aren't as surprising. Women of all ages who live with partners rather than marrying tend to drink more and have more alcohol-related hassles than women who choose to marry. Other studies on alcohol and drug use by both sexes have found this, too. Live-in partners are just less traditional in general than spouses are. "They may come into the relationship already drinking more than average," Wilsnack says.

The survey also confirms findings that both sexes tend to "mature out" of serious alcohol problems. The 20s look wild for a sizable minority of women, but by their 50s most aren't having serious drinking problems. For example, in the new report:

• 29% of women age 21 to 34 say they've had six or more drinks in a single day at least four times during the past year;

only 14% who are 50 to 64 years old have binged.

• 26% who are 21 to 34 report symptoms of alcohol dependency—blackouts, inability to control themselves or remember events while drinking—compared with 6% of women age 50 to 64.

Some details on the survey are reported in the Wilsnacks' new book, *Gender and Alcohol* (Rutgers Center of Alcohol Studies, $29.95).

While women's drinking habits aren't shaped by male partners on the home front, they do use more alcohol if employed in male-dominated careers. Female lawyers, doctors, construction workers and airline pilots drink more than teachers, nurses or librarians. "This may be a matter of, 'If you're going to work with the boys, you'll have to drink with the boys,' " Wilsnack says. Women far outnumbered by men on the job also may feel stressed and drink to cope.

As is true for men, women's alcohol habits are linked to parents' approach to drinking, but for women the mother is somewhat more influential. "It may be part of their female modeling," Wilsnack suggests.

The study also reveals a tie between alcohol use and sexual function. About 60% of women say alcohol makes them feel less sexually inhibited; 80% of frequent bingers (six or more drinks a day) say alcohol helps them shed hesitance about sex.

More isn't necessarily better for their sex lives, though. Women with the lowest rates of sexual dysfunction are moderate drinkers—13 or fewer drinks a week. Abstainers and heavier drinkers have the most sexual problems, such as trouble reaching orgasm and lack of desire.

Also, for women whose drinking generates problems, the worse their sexual dysfunction is, the less likely they are to end their problem drinking over time. "Sexual function is one of the strongest predictors we have of whether women will get better or continue to have alcohol problems," Wilsnack says.

"It doesn't look like a poor sex life gets them started drinking, but it keeps them going at it," she says. These women might be using alcohol in an attempt to loosen up sexually or to "self-medicate" by deadening their awareness of unsatisfying sex, Wilsnack says. If sexual function improves, they may be more able to let go of the alcohol.

Perhaps the most explosive finding from the survey so far is that childhood sexual abuse raises the risk for alcohol dependency in adulthood. Some 24% of women who have alcohol problems reported experiences of abuse in their childhood, a rate about the same as found in national incidence studies done by the federal government.

The finding has clear ramifications for prevention and treatment programs, says

Where you can find out more

Information on women and alcohol is offered by the National Clearinghouse for Alcohol and Drug Information (NCADI).

For free brochures phone NCADI at 800-729-6686, 8 a.m. to 7 p.m. ET. Among brochures available: *Drinking and Pregnancy; Making the Link: Alcohol, Tobacco and Other Drugs & Women's Health; Making the Link: Domestic Violence & Alcohol and Other Drugs; and The Genetics of Alcoholism.*

Additional reports, studies and publications are at the NCADI Web site: www.health.org.

Ulonda Shamwell of the federal Substance Abuse and Mental Health Services Administration. "When we do prevention programs with young girls," she says, "we have to understand sex abuse is a much wider problem than we've appreciated before. It must be addressed. And if we can prevent the sex abuse, it could lower their risk for other problems down the line, the alcohol and mental health problems."

Indeed, sexual abuse might make it particularly hard to overcome an alcohol problem, says psychiatrist Frank Putnam of the National Institutes of Mental Health, who researches how abuse affects girls biologically. Although there are no formal studies, "a lot of people who run treatment programs say abused women are resistant to treatment, they just have a poorer prognosis than others. . . . When they're detoxed, they'll often tell their counselors, 'I need alcohol, it's the only way I feel normal.'"

Some frontier studies suggest childhood sex abuse might cause brain or hormonal changes that lead to post traumatic stress disorder and the need for alcohol to lower stress. But research is just beginning in this area.

MEDICAL CARE OF HEROIN USERS

Jeannette Y. Wick, RPh, MBA

Scientists learned to separate drugs chemically from plants in the 1800s, and life has never been the same. Certainly life has improved for almost everyone, especially when it comes to treatment of pain and disease. But for the small number who become addicted to opiates, life has been considerably more difficult. The first epidemics of addiction occurred in the late 1800s, when there were no laws guiding the use of drugs with addictive potential. Drug refinement advanced, and drugs became more available and potent. As society became aware that many over-the-counter medications contained addictive drugs, including morphine and laudanum, legislators moved toward restricting use. Over the decades, U.S. laws became stricter and more specific. Beginning with the Food and Drug Act of 1906 and the Harrison Act of 1914, laws were enacted to tighten control and limit access to the newly designated *controlled substances.*

The tenacious hold of diacetylmorphine, or heroin, presents a huge challenge to health care providers. This article addresses the problems heroin addicts encounter when they must seek medical care, and the trials, tribulations, and apprehensions health care providers must overcome to provide good, or even adequate, care.

Trial 1: The Patient

Many health care providers know little about heroin users. The stereotype of the user, while sometimes accurate, obscures the individual and often clouds consideration of the patient's unique circumstances. In general, health care providers who practice in emergency rooms, correction facilities, and addiction programs have the most current and applicable skills when dealing with addicts. As the patient becomes more removed from these practice locations, resistance, misunderstanding and reluctance to treat become greater. Adequate care becomes a goal that can't be achieved without collaborative efforts on the part of all health care providers, the patient, and the patient's family or closest contacts.

The heroin user presents special problems. Preoccupation with the need for the next dose contributes to dishonesty and manipulation. Health care providers will need to sort *purposive symptoms* from *nonpurposive symptoms.* Purposive symptoms are those reported by the patients for the purpose of obtaining opiates, other drugs, or sympathy, or of meeting other self-serving needs. Nonpurposive symptoms are observable manifestations of withdrawal. Treatment of any health crisis should be based on assessment of actual problems—nonpurposive symptoms. The user may have poor insight into his own problems, or ulterior motives that lead to deception. Often (and only if the patient consents), inclusion of family members or other health care providers in the decision-making process can lend clarity and direction to the treatment plan.

Trial 2: The Drug

Heroin users often enter the health care system via emergency rooms or jails. Once their addiction has been identified, the health care provider is faced with a problem: No prescription vial, pharmacist or prescriber can be found

Box 1: Quinine

Indications:

- An antiprotozoal used to treat malaria
- An antimyotonic used to decrease muscle cramps

Contraindicated in these people:

- Patients whose electrocardiogram shows a defect called QT prolongation (can cause sudden death)
- Patients diagnosed as deficient in the enzyme glucose-6-phosphate dehydrogenase (causes blood disorder)
- Diabetes (causes low blood sugar)

Quinine overdose can cause these problems:

- Cardiovascular toxicity, including low blood pressure, slowed heart, irregular heartbeat, and cardiac arrest.
- Central nervous system toxicity. Delirium, seizures, coma, respiratory arrest, restlessness, somnolence, and confusion have been reported.
- Ocular toxicity (a hallmark of quinine toxicity), including visual defects, blindness, and cinchonism (blurred vision or changes in color vision).
- Gastrointestinal disturbances. Stomach cramps, pain, diarrhea, nausea, and vomiting are most common.

Reprinted with permission from *The Counselor,* May/June 1998, pp. 15-19. © 1998 by the National Association of Alcoholism and Drug Abuse Counselors, www.naadac.org.

or contacted to determine the purity and characteristics of the drug.

In addition, the chances are good that the patient has been exposed to several substances other than heroin. Street grade heroin is usually 5% to 10% pure. The remainder of its weight comes from a variety of diluents chosen mainly for whiteness, solubility, low cost, and availability. Diluents may be added to increase volume, enhance effect, or even to kill or torture the user. Common diluents include lactose, quinine, and cornstarch—others are strychnine or dirt—and other contaminants, drugs, and toxins are also found with alarming frequency. Quinine is one of the most frequent, and most troublesome, of diluents. (See "Quinine.")

Though heroin has the reputation of being the ultimate high, new substances rumored to be stronger or better appear from time to time. They often contain fentanyl or derivatives of meperidine (Demerol ®). Epidemics of drug-induced morbidity or mortality are reported occasionally, when molecular manipulation leads to unintentional but severe destruction of brain cells, symptoms of Parkinson's disease, accelerated aging, paralysis, or death. (See "History of Heroin-Related Problems.")

One recent epidemic deserves note. In 1995–96, at least 325 cases of drug overdose in heroin users were identified in several major cities on the east coast. The patients had consumed heroin mixed with scopolamine, a strong drug from the family called anticholinergics. In high doses scopolamine causes rapid heartbeat, elevated blood pressure, dry skin and mucous membranes, and hallucinations. Treatment of anticholinergic poisoning is entirely different from treatment of heroin overdose. Such epidemics are frightening, and difficult to track and treat.

Trial 3: The Route

Heroin is used in several ways, and each presents its own problems. Injection of heroin is probably the most common route, and also the most dangerous. Injection is quick and irreversible, increasing the chance of overdose. The drug enters the bloodstream directly, and its full effect is felt within minutes. Any impurities also enter the drug stream directly, increasing the potential for sepsis (infection).

It is not unusual to find venous damage at the injection site. Addicts often use dirty or blunt needles, increasing trauma to the skin and veins. Health care providers in large cities attest that the recent popularity of cocaine-heroin mixtures have caused complicated wounds

and sores at the injection site that are far more difficult to treat than those caused by either drug alone.

Heroin can also be sniffed or snorted, and there is some evidence that this method is gaining popularity. This method is somewhat slower than injection; overdose is less likely because the user has some opportunity to gauge effect and slow administration. However, sniffing creates other problems, notably pneumonia, when impurities become lodged in the lungs.

Smoking heroin presents a long list of problems, usually compounded by the high rate of cigarette smoking among addicts. Many of the complications of smoking heroin are discussed below.

Trial 4: Increased Risk of Death

The health problems of heroin users are both chronic and acute. The acute problems, usually associated with either overdose or withdrawal, put them at increased risk for emergency services or death. Chronic problems decrease overall quality of life, increase morbidity of coexisting problems, and contribute to social problems.

In 1988, heroin users accounted for 38,000 emergency room visits; in 1993, for 63,000. Risk of death in heroin users is considerably higher than in similar age groups in the general population. Approximately 1% of heroin users die each year. Since heroin is an illegal drug, estimates of its use are based on the number of overdose fatalities, the number of

arrests associated with is use, the admission rate in detoxification programs, and the number of cases of hepatitis reported.

Trial 5: Communicable Diseases

The lifestyle of the heroin user contains many high-risk behaviors. Communicable diseases of concern in this population include HIV/AIDS, hepatitis, tetanus, botulism, syphilis, gonorrhea, chlamydia, and tuberculosis. High rates of these diseases make heroin users a treatment challenge and increase the complexity and cost of care.

In many criminal justice and emergency care facilities, heroin users are considered immunocompromised until determined otherwise. Certain tests can be conducted to assess immune status, but HIV testing can be conducted only with the patient's consent. This can be a problem, as many users refuse the test. Poor insight, impaired judgment, and a drug-seeking agenda can make heroin users a public health risk, and each state has laws governing how these patients are to be treated. Counselors who treat heroin addicts should familiarize themselves with relevant laws.

Trial 6: Overall Health Status

The heroin user's overall health status is usually poor. Beginning with malnutrition, these patients often have chronic conditions that have been neglected for too long. Hypertension, if it

Box 2: History of Heroin-Related Problems

1930–1945	Intravenous heroin use becomes widespread.
1950–Mid '60s	Many cities experience low levels of heroin use.
1960	U.S. reports about 60,000 heroin users.
1960–70	Heroin claimed 4,254 lives in New York state. The Vietnam War took 3,191 lives from heroin.
1967	U.S. reports about 108,000 heroin users.
1973–74	Epidemic of heroin use nationwide.
February 1975	A suspected heroin epidemic turns out to be etorphine, a very potent morphine derivative.
1977–78	Epidemic of heroin use nationwide.
Fall 1980	An epidemic of "China white" use is discovered to be fentanyl instead.
1981	AIDS is first described in the literature.
Mid-1980s	U.S. reports about 500,000 heroin users.
1988	About 38,000 emergency room visits are related to heroin use.
1993	About 62,000 emergency room visits are related to heroin use.
1995–96	A scopolamine poisoning epidemic is identified in major east coast cities.
1997	U.S. reports about 600,000 heroin users. A total of 115,000 methadone maintenance slots are DEA-approved.

> ### Box 3: Signs and Symptoms of
> ### Pulmonary Disorder Secondary
> ### to Heroin Use
>
> - Usually occurs after IV heroin use but is not limited to this route.
> - Not dose-related or restricted to overdose situations.
> - Patient usually presents in coma, with depressed respiration or respiratory distress. May include shallow or rapid breathing, low blood pressure, cyanosis, rapid heartbeat, and low blood oxygen.
> - Onset is one to two hours after drug use, and major problems clear within two days.
> - Complete recovery may be prolonged. Treatment includes naloxone (Narcan®), respiratory support, and oxygen. Secondary pneumonias (bacterial or aspiration) may follow.

exists, is usually uncontrolled and complicated. The user's skin, already compromised by serious vitamin deficiencies, lacks resiliency and provides little protection from the elements and bacteria. Rash, injection site necrosis and infection, and burns are common and require complicated, long-term treatment. Dental problems result from neglect and malnutrition, and can seriously threaten overall health. Compliance with treatment for any of these conditions is often compromised by the user's need to seek heroin.

Cardiomyopathy is a common problem induced by repeated exposure to heroin and a variety of diluents. Both quinine and scopolamine can affect cardiac health, and exposure to other drugs of abuse predispose this group to hypertension, cardiac arrhythmias, and poor circulation.

Lung care presents a range of challenges. Foreign bodies, infiltrates and damage appear after heroin is inhaled or smoked. Pneumonia develops frequently. Acute pulmonary disorders have a mortality rate of about 10% in this group; they usually occur after IV administration of heroin, but can occur after inhalation or smoking. Pulmonary complications usually present as coma, decreased respiration or respiratory distress, and if the patient survives the acute problem, there is a high likelihood that bacterial or aspiration pneumonia will follow. "Signs and Symptoms of Pulmonary Disorder Secondary to Heroin Use" describes some of the signs and symptoms of pulmonary disorder secondary to heroin use.

Most mental health clinicians and addiction counselors recognize that mental illness and addiction are common co-morbidities. Both problems must be addressed for optimal treatment success.

Cotton fever exemplifies the complications of heroin use. It occurs when heroin is unavailable to the addict, who then tries to extract a remnant of drug from used cotton filters with water or other solvents. The reaction that may follow, called cotton fever, is an allergic reaction. Most experts believe it is a reaction to tiny cotton fibers. It begins with fever, chills, shallow breathing, low blood pressure and irregular heartbeat. Untreated, it usually improves noticeably within four hours, and disappears within a day. However, sepsis (generalized infection of the blood) can follow.

Other infectious diseases are also possible. Bacterial endocarditis, pneumonia, cellulitis, septic arthritis, abscess, thrombophlebitis, and embolism have been reported. These diagnoses refer to the heart, lungs, skin, joints, and veins; abscesses and emboli can settle almost anywhere, increasing the possibility of death.

Trial 7: The Law

While heroin use is forbidden throughout the United States, detoxification and the legality and protocols of treatment programs vary, particularly concerning replacement therapy with methadone or similar drugs. Methadone maintenance programs offer respite to some heroin users, but present problems of their own.

Methadone programs must be approved and licensed by the Drug Enforcement Administration and the local jurisdiction. Not all states allow methadone maintenance; see "States That Bar Methadone Maintenance." Slots are lim-

ited, and in most states, enrollees must report daily for doses, making access difficult.

Laws vary greatly, and health care providers who do not practice in addiction, prevention or psychiatry are often unfamiliar with the law, and hesitant to use methadone. In situations other than approved maintenance programs, federal law allows methadone use for detoxification only; there is no provision for maintaining the patient who is enrolled in a methadone maintenance program but needs hospitalization. Consequently, methadone program enrollees may be deprived of needed doses, and travel is almost impossible, since few states offer "guest doses."

Some states, New York in particular, are taking steps to make methadone maintenance and other types of treatment programs more accessible. Some boroughs of New York City are implementing a system of managed care for Medicaid recipients who are known drug users. This program will restrict serious drug users to one health care facility, limiting their ability to shop for services or manipulate care. In the past, programs, like this have been prohibited because Medicaid regulations prevent choice restriction. Federal Medicaid administrators have waived this regulation in an attempt to reduce emergency visits and hospitalizations, decrease multiple visits for the same problem, and add structure to the user's health care program. As with all new programs, only time will show if this plan works better for users, but all indications are that it will.

> ### Box 4: States That Bar
> ### Methadone Maintenance
>
> | | |
> |---|---|
> | Idaho | North Dakota |
> | Mississippi | South Dakota |
> | Montana | West Virginia |
> | New Hampshire | Vermont |

Trial 8: The Questions

Lack of experience, a society that considers addiction criminal, and cultural experiences that are diverse but not necessarily understanding, raise questions for health care providers who must treat heroin users.

Those who are afflicted with addictive illnesses are not exempt from concurrent illnesses or accidental injury. Addiction can cause the user to neglect or aggravate pre-existing conditions. In addition, the user may try to manipulate the system to obtain desirable drugs, with clonidine, benzodiazepines and pain medication high on the list.

When heroin or methadone users are injured or experience pain, there are always questions about treatment. Many clinicians believe that addicts should abstain from any substance with addictive potential. This is not always possible especially when the pain is acute and menacing. If the patient is a heroin user, it is usually best to consult with an addiction expert, if time permits. If the patient is maintained on methadone, the methadone maintenance program should be involved in treatment.

In cases where nonopiate analgesics cannot be used or do not relieve the pain, opiates can be prescribed. Larger than normal doses may be needed because the user will have developed cross-tolerance. Adequate doses should be scheduled (as opposed to given as needed) if possible, dosing intervals should be established and adhered to, and the medication should be tapered off and discontinued after the period of acute pain is over. The methadone user may enter a period of controlled relapse, losing the ability to make rational decisions about medication even after the pain has subdued. Pain mismanagement by well-intentioned clinicians can cause relapse; whenever possible, nonopiate drugs and other methods of pain relief should be employed.

The Solutions

Society is moving, albeit slowly, toward a better understanding of addiction and its simultaneous health problems. The following steps can help heroin or methadone users receive better health care:

- Education at all levels is essential. Many users are knowledgeable about their problem and their needs, but reluctant to reveal themselves to health care professionals. Users must be encouraged to present their situations in a forthright and honest manner. If the user has serious health problems, encouraging him to wear a Med-alert bracelet or carry a summary of health problems in his wallet can save time when treatment is needed.

- Clinicians often lack knowledge about specific addictions, but will listen to other professionals and to patients. Counselors should make sure their clients know they should involve their treatment program whenever they are seen for emergency treatment or a serious health crisis.

- If your client is a current user, make sure he knows he should bring the illicit substance and any apparatus he's used with him to the emergency room in the event of overdose or crisis. This may help the health care professional determine the exact nature of the problem much more quickly, and help identify epidemics and new drugs earlier.

- There is a misperception that inhaling or smoking heroin is less onerous and safer than injecting. Remind clients that all routes of heroin administration have extremely serious risks.

- Establish screening programs for communicable disease in your program. Annual or biannual screening for the most serious—tuberculosis, hepatitis and HIV/AIDS—can protect the client and the public. Periodic screening for sexually transmitted diseases and other communicable diseases can prevent disease progression or transmission.

- Help clients deal with concurrent illnesses by making medical care available. Many states include a medical component in their addiction, prevention and recovery programs. A combined, multidisciplinary medical, psychological, vocational and social approach is the most successful.

- Know the law in your area, and prepare a handout that is available for health professionals or concerned lay people quickly. Make sure you address not only the law, but other frequently-asked questions or points of confusion.

Conclusion

Opiate abuse has been around for more than 6,000 years. With a history like this, we should be able to draw some conclusions. First, there appear to be epidemics of abuse periodically, and they tend to abate when confronted and publicized. Second, heroin use never disappears completely, and has been growing in the past decade. Third, rate of relapse is almost 100% in heroin users, and those interventions that work are not widely available. Fourth, new routes of administration, combinations of drugs and molecular manipulations change the milieu constantly and complicate treatment.

Open communication, documentation and publication of new or different issues, and education of the public are essential if we are to help current heroin users and prevent the spread of this epidemic. As a counselor, you can help. Watch for changes in patterns of use. Observe clients who succeed for subtle interventions that work. And encourage good medical care.

Jeannette Y. Wick, RPh, MBA, is chief pharmacist at the District of Columbia Commission on Mental Health Services in Washington, DC.

Unit Selections

Key Points to Consider

❖ As you read the following articles, attempt to identify additional questions and issues that mold public opinion and shape public policy on drugs. Some examples worthy of discussion are: How serious is the drug problem perceived to be? Is it getting worse?

❖ What are the impacts of drugs on children and schools? How do drugs drive crime? What are the impacts of drugs on policing, the courts, and corrections?

❖ How are public opinion and public policy affected by public events, drug education campaigns, announced government policies, and media coverage?

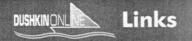 **Links** **www.dushkin.com/online/**

These sites are annotated on pages 4 and 5.

The drug problem consistently competes with all major public policy issues, including the economy, education, and foreign policy. Formulating and implementing effective drug control policy is a troublesome task. Some would argue that the consequences of policy failures have been worse than the problems they were attempting to address. Others would argue that although the world of shaping drug policy is an imperfect one, the process has worked generally as well as could be expected. Although the majority of Americans believe that failures and breakdowns in the fight against drug abuse have occurred in spite of various drug policies, not because of them, there is public pressure to rethink the get-tough, stay-tough enforcement-oriented ideas of the last two decades.

Policy formulation is not a process of aimless wandering. Various levels of government have responsibility for responding to problems of drug abuse. At the center of most policy debate is the premise that the manufacture, possession, use, and distribution of psychoactive drugs without government authorization is illegal. This premise is targeted frequently as misguided due to the consequences it is felt to perpetuate, such as syndicated crime and violent competition among criminal organizations and individuals alike. Media hype and the fervor it generates are powerful influences in the public's perception of any drug problem. The fact remains, however, that present-day drug control policy revolves around the majority consensus of prohibition.

One exception to prevailing public views that generally support drug prohibition may be the perceived softening of attitudes regarding the medical use of marijuana. Proponents of medical use propositions approved in California and Arizona argue that these decriminalizing laws reflect the common sense lacking in other drug policies. Opponents argue that these loosely written laws were misleading, albeit successful, attempts to simply legalize marijuana. Opponents further argue that public support of pro-marijuana attitudes encourages ambivalent youth attitudes toward the risks associated with marijuana use.

Still, surveys typically report that 80 percent of Americans think that legalizing dangerous drugs is a bad idea. The fear of increased crime, increased drug use, and the potential threat to children are the most often stated reasons. Citing the devastating consequences of alcohol and tobacco use, most Americans question society's ability to use any addictive, mind-altering drug responsibly. Currently, the public favors both supply reduction and demand reduction as effective strategies in combating the drug problem. Concomitantly, policy analysts struggle with objectives. Shaping public policy is a critical function that greatly relies upon public input. Policy-making apparatus is influenced by public opinion, and public opinion is in turn influenced by public policy. When Presidents Bush and Clinton referred to crack and methamphetamine, respectively, as threats to national security, the impact on public opinion was tremendous.

The prevailing characteristic of today's drug policy still reflects a punitive, "get tough" approach to control. The leveling off of both adult as well as youth drug use over the past 2 years serves to sustain this policy and there are, in fact, about 10 million fewer drug users now than existed in 1985 during the height of the crack epidemic. The prison experience is primarily one of retribution, not rehabilitation. There is typically little opportunity for treatment afforded to the vast majority of prisoners suffering from drug problems. A drug-abusing prisoner, initially committed to the prison system for drug offenses, who receives no drug treatment while in custody, is a virtual guarantee to re-offend. Correctional settings that are offering drug treatment to qualified offenders are reducing recidivism significantly. Court-directed coercion of drug offenders, as a mechanism to force offenders into treatment, is generally meeting with positive results. And in some cases, successful treatment and rehabilitation accompanies the incentive to have arrests ultimately expunged and be rewarded with re-entering society as a citizen, not a felon. A state of California study found that every dollar spent on treatment saved $7 in hospital admissions and law-enforcement costs. Nevertheless, the degree to which Americans are willing to support and sustain a less enforcement-oriented response to drug policy questions remains to be seen. There is concern that even with a shift in policy toward education, prevention, and treatment, an intense, enforcement-oriented perspective will remain on the nation's poor, inner-urban, largely minority subpopulations.

Another complicated aspect of creating national as well as local drug policy is consideration of the growing body of research on the subject. The past 20 years have produced numerous public and private investigations, surveys, and conclusions relative to the dynamic of drug use in American society. Most literature reflects, however, an indirect influence of research on large-scale policy decisions. There is a saying that "policy makers use research like a drunk uses a lamppost—for support, rather than illumination."

Further complicating the research/policy-making relationship is that the policy-making community is largely composed of persons of diverse backgrounds, professional capacities, and political interests. Some are elected officials, others are civil servants, and many are private citizens from the medical and educational communities. In some cases, such as with alcohol and tobacco, powerful industry players assert a tremendous influence on policy. As you read on, consider the new research-related implications for drug policy, such as those addressing the incarceration of drug offenders.

167

"For too long, United States drug policy has been driven by the need to appear 'tough' on drugs, regardless of results. The United States should leave behind the distinction between 'tough' and 'soft' approaches to drug abuse and concentrate its attention, research, and resources on determining what actually works."

America's Drug Problem and Its Policy of Denial

MATHEA FALCO

For almost 100 years, Americans have considered other countries the primary source of their drug problems. When the first drug laws were adopted in the early decades of this century, the public associated drugs with immigrant groups and minorities: opium with Chinese laborers in the west, cocaine with blacks, and marijuana with Mexican immigrants in the southwest. These drugs were seen as foreign threats to the social fabric, undermining traditional moral values and political stability. Today this link between foreigners and illicit drugs continues to influence United States international drug policy, prompting the government to use diplomacy, economic assistance, coercion, and military force to try to stop drugs from entering the country.

Americans strongly support government efforts to cut off foreign drug supplies. More than two-thirds of the respondents in a 1997 poll by the Pew Research Center for the People and the Press considered drug control to be a "top priority" goal of United States foreign policy; only protecting American jobs and preventing the spread of nuclear weapons received higher scores. Similar views have prevailed in other surveys. A 1995 Chicago Council on Foreign Relations nationwide poll found that 86 percent of Americans consider "stopping the flow of drugs" one of the country's most important foreign policy goals. The close connection in the public mind between international initiatives and drug abuse, which is often experienced as an intensely local problem involving families, schools, and communities, gives this issue particular resonance in public views of foreign policy.

SUPPLYING AMERICA'S DEMAND

America's drug habit has historically been supplied from foreign sources: cocaine and marijuana from Latin America and the Caribbean; heroin from Southeast Asia's Golden Triangle (Burma, Laos, and Thailand) and South Asia's Golden Crescent (Afghanistan, Pakistan, and Iran). However, in recent years a substantial percentage of illicit drug consumption in the United States has been met by illegal domestic production. In particular, many of the drugs gaining popularity among teenagers—marijuana, methamphetamines, and LSD—are produced at home as well as imported.

While much of the marijuana the country uses continues to be imported through Mexico and the Caribbean, domestic production now supplies an estimated one-third to one-half of America's consumption. Although a complete nationwide survey of illegal marijuana cultivation has never been made, government officials report major cultivation areas in states as diverse as New York, Kentucky, California, and Hawaii. Increased indoor cultivation, which allows for more selective hybridization, has accelerated the trend toward higher-potency marijuana. In 1996, the THC (tetrahydrocannabinol) content of high-grade "sinsemilla" (seedless) marijuana ranged from 12 to 24 percent, according to the Drug Enforcement Administration (DEA), compared to less than 2 percent THC in marijuana cultivated in the early 1970s. Even as potency has increased, marijuana prices, after rising during the 1980s, have in the

MATHEA FALCO *is president of Drug Strategies, a nonprofit research institute in Washington, D.C. The author of* The Making of a Drug-Free America: Programs that Work *(New York: Times Books, 1994), she served as assistant secretary of state for international narcotics matters from 1977 to 1981.*

1990s fallen back to levels of the early 1980s. Depending on its quality, marijuana now sells for roughly the same as in 1982—as little as $40 per ounce, although prices for high-quality "boutique" marijuana strains can reach $900 per ounce.

The historic view that America's drug problems are pre-dominantly foreign in origin is thus harder to sustain, given increasing domestic illegal drug production, not only of marijuana, LSD, and amphetamines but also of newer "designer" psychoactive drugs such as MDMA (known as Ecstasy). None-theless, United States drug policy continues to concentrate on trying to reduce the foreign supply of drugs, both through efforts to reduce drug cultivation in other countries and to interdict drug traffic before it crosses America's borders. Unfortunately, the strategy of trying to reduce United States drug use by attacking drug supplies overseas is fundamentally flawed.

CERTIFICATION: THE "TOUGH" APPROACH

Emblematic of this focus on foreign sources is the United States government's annual "certification" process. Imposed by Congress on the executive branch in 1986, the concept of cer-tification reflects a worldview that still classifies countries into producer, consumer, and transit categories. The intent of Con-gress was to put teeth into United States efforts to compel cooperation as well as to make the president accountable for enforcing a more vigorous international drug policy.

The certification legislation requires the president to identify annually those countries that are "significant direct or indirect sources" of illicit drugs "significantly affecting the United States." Inclusion on this list, which currently comprises 30 countries, automat-ically triggers certain sanctions unless the president decides to "certify" the country. Those deemed to have fully cooperated in drug control efforts are certified. Those deemed less cooperative are decertified, which results in the termination of United States as-sistance (except for humanitarian and drug control funds), United States opposition to multilateral development loans for that coun-try, and the stigma of being branded a drug-trafficking nation. This may carry negative economic repercussions beyond the aid-re-lated sanctions included in the law; *The Wall Street Journal* reported in August 1997 that Colombia's decertification had contributed to an atmosphere of uncertainty, causing investors to put off new projects.

A "national interest" waiver is used to justify suspending the penalties for a country that would otherwise have been decertified—a way to improve performance without actually cutting off assistance. Congress has the authority to overturn presidential decisions by passing a joint resolution within 30 days, but has never done so.

The idea of being formally judged by the United States remains objectionable to many countries.

Under Presidents Ronald Reagan and George Bush, the cer-tification process was predictable and went largely unnoticed. Decertification was reserved for countries like Iran and Syria, with which the United States had limited or no relations, as well as Burma and Afghanistan, which together produce 90 percent of the world's illicit opium. Lebanon was consistently granted a national interest waiver. In 1988 and 1989, Panama was added to the decertification list, just before the United States intervened militarily to remove President Manuel Nori-ega for his involvement in drug trafficking.

Under President Bill Clinton, certification has become more rigorous. In 1994, Nigeria, a key trafficking country and a significant source of oil for the United States, was decertified for the first time. Also, Bolivia and Peru, the world's largest coca producers, joined a growing list of countries given a na-tional interest waiver. In 1995, Colombia, a major source of cocaine and heroin; Paraguay, a cocaine transit country; and Pakistan, a prime producer of heroin, were added to the waiver list.

By 1996, certification had emerged as a major source of tension between the United States and its Latin American neighbors. The administration decertified Colombia for the first time because of alleged links between President Ernesto Samper and the drug cartels, which were believed to have con-tributed to his presidential campaign. Colombia was again decer-tified in 1997; Mexico, however, was certified, despite revelations of extensive drug-related government corruption that, as some observers noted, paralleled the situation in Colombia.

Critics both in the United States and Latin America argued that the certification process harmed relations with Mexico and Colombia without producing any measurable benefits. Moreover, a double standard appeared to in-fluence the ultimate decisions. In 1996, trade between the United States and Colombia to-taled $9 billion, while United States–Mexico trade reached $130 billion. Additionally, Mex-ico shares a border with the United States, making Mexican cooperation on a range of issues such as crime, immigration, and envi-ronmental protection essential to Washington.

Media coverage of the certification deci-sions was intense, especially in Latin Amer-ica, where the decisions were widely viewed as demonstrations of United States imperial-ism. The idea of being formally judged by the United States remains objectionable to many countries. During the 1997 certification de-bate, the Mexican government rejected the concept of certifi-cation, pointing out that the United States is responsible for its own drug problem and has no right to pass unilateral judg-ment on other countries when it does not also judge its own performance. Although Congress did not overturn the admini-stration's 1997 decision to certify Mexico, some members of the House of Representatives have indicated that a similar de-cision in 1998 will be met with stiff congressional opposition.

In practice, the consequences of decertification vary widely, depending on a country's reliance on United States and international aid. For major producer countries such as Burma, which is already isolated from the international community (and subject to United States sanctions on investment), the material consequences of decertification are virtually zero. However, for some countries, such as Bolivia, Haiti, Laos, and Cambodia, annual United States and multilateral bank aid amounts to a significant proportion of their GDP, making them especially vulnerable to the threat of decertification.

Relative vulnerability is only one part of the equation as to whether United States pressure will affect cooperation; even more important is the government's capacity to address illicit drug production and trafficking, as well as the sheer scale of the problem. The degree of United States leverage does not determine whether pressure will compel action. For example, the United States has considerable influence over a country like Haiti, but the Haitian government is so weak, particularly in the area of law enforcement, that it is largely incapable of producing drug control results, regardless of United States pressure.

A CERTIFIED FAILURE?

What impact has certification had in its 11-year history? From the United States perspective, the primary measure of the success of drug control efforts overseas would be reduction in foreign opium, coca, and marijuana cultivation as well as declining availability of foreign drug supplies coming into the United States. Reductions would presumably lead to higher domestic drug prices. However, worldwide opium production has doubled in the past decade, while coca production has nearly doubled.

The price and purity of drugs in the United States market are also traditional measures of drug control success. Reduction in supplies should make drugs more expensive and less pure (as dealers dilute purity to maintain profit margins). This in turn should prevent new drug use and drive addicts to go "cold turkey" or find treatment. However, since 1981, heroin's average retail price has fallen by more than half while its purity now approaches 50 percent, compared to only 16 percent in 1986. During the same period, the price of cocaine has dropped by almost half.

Administration officials point to some successes from the certification process: increased numbers of arrests of major traffickers in Colombia following decertification; reorganization of the antinarcotics police in Mexico after indications of widespread corruption made decertification a strong possibility in 1997; more vigorous efforts to reduce coca cultivation by the Bolivian government following national interest waivers in 1994 and 1995. However, these examples of government action that may have been influenced by the certification process have not produced measurable results in terms of reduced drug availability in the United States, the ultimate goal of United States international drug control efforts.

The certification process also has negative consequences for other United States interests. Focusing on one aspect of often complex bilateral relations can distort the management of foreign policy. In Latin America, where the process has been es-

pecially acrimonious, relations with half a dozen countries are dominated by United States narcotics control concerns. The unilateral nature of certification—where the United States passes judgment on other countries—undermines the administration's position that the nations of the Western Hemisphere should look to the United States as a partner in a broader effort to establish a community of democracies.

In the past year, momentum has been building for finding alternatives to the current certification process. Both the administration and the Organization of American States (OAS) are exploring new multilateral approaches to determining whether countries are fully cooperating in international drug control efforts. Discussion of these new approaches is on the agenda for the April 1998 Summit of the Americas meeting in Santiago, Chile. A more comprehensive system that would include an assessment of United States efforts along with those of other drug producing, consuming, and transiting countries, could be administered through an independent organization, perhaps linked to the OAS or the United Nations. This would broaden the approach beyond its current unilateral context as well as encourage political recognition of the global nature of the drug problem.

A KEY TO LASTING PROGRESS

The United States is the world's largest drug market in terms of revenue. According to the National Household Survey on Drug Abuse, 22 million Americans reported using illicit drugs at least once in 1996, while 12 million used drugs regularly (once a month or more). During the past five years, drug use among teens, especially of marijuana, has climbed dramatically.

What progress has been made in the past decade has come from reduced demand, which has declined in the face of increasing supplies of ever cheaper drugs. Between 1986 and 1992, marijuana and cocaine use dropped by half, reflecting the power of health concerns and negative social attitudes toward drugs (accelerated by the sudden cocaine overdose death of sports star Len Bias in 1986). However, public perceptions of the dangers of drugs have changed, and both adults and teens are more tolerant of drug use than they were five years ago. Reversing this trend will require intensive prevention and education efforts that build on the research of the past decade.

Extensive studies have found that school prevention programs can reduce use by half and new alcohol use by a third among young teens. These programs, built on social-learning theory, teach children to recognize the internal and external pressures that influence them to smoke, drink, and use drugs. Children also learn how to resist these pressures through role-playing in the classroom. The cost of these programs ranges from $15 to $25 per pupil, including classroom materials and teacher training. Program results are stronger when prevention includes families, media, and the community in a comprehensive attack on alcohol, tobacco, and drug use. Anti-drug ads by the Partnership for a Drug Free America have intensified negative attitudes toward illegal drugs, particularly in markets where the ads appear frequently.

Treatment has also proved effective in reducing drug abuse and drug crime. National studies that have followed tens of thousands of addicts through different kinds of programs report that the single most important factor in measuring a program's success is length of time in treatment. One-third of those who stay in treatment longer than three months are drug-free a year after leaving treatment. The success rate jumps to two-thirds when treatment lasts a year or longer. Programs that provide intensive, highly structured treatment with supportive follow-up services, such as job training and housing referral, report even better results.

Treatment is less expensive than the alternatives. An untreated addict can cost society an estimated $44,000 annually, compared with an average of $19,000 for a year of residential treatment or $2,500 for an outpatient program. A 1994 state-wide study in California found that $1 invested in alcohol and drug treatment saved taxpayers $7.14 in future costs. Drug courts, which divert nonviolent drug offenders from prison to court-supervised treatment, are also cost-effective. Studies report that drug courts cut recidivism by half among treated offenders at a small fraction of the cost of incarceration, which runs about $30,000 a year.

Treatment is also more cost-effective than supply reduction efforts. According to a 1994 RAND Corporation study, $34 million invested in treatment reduces cocaine use in the United States as much as $783 million spent for foreign source country supply control programs or $366 million spent for interdiction. Domestic enforcement produces equivalent results for about seven times the amount invested in treatment; $246 million in domestic enforcement reduces cocaine use as much as $34 million in treatment.

MORE MONEY, FEWER RESULTS?

In the past decade, the government's drug control spending has more than tripled, climbing from $4.7 billion in 1987 to $16 billion in 1997. Most of this growth has supported domestic drug enforcement and international interdiction, which account for more than half the total $105 billion spent on federal drug control since 1989.

The single largest enforcement expenditure is for prisons. Increasing prison costs stem not only from climbing drug arrests but also from mandatory federal minimum sentences that have resulted in longer prison stays for drug offenders. More than 1.7 million people are behind bars in America. More than two-thirds have serious drug problems, yet intensive, rigorous treatment is available for less than 10 percent of these offenders. In 1997, the federal drug budget spent more for prisons than for prevention.

Although President Clinton has clearly articulated the importance of reducing the demand for drugs in the 1997 and 1998 National Drug Control Strategy reports, federal spending priorities have remained essentially unchanged. Efforts to cut off supplies of drugs through interdiction and enforcement continue to dominate the government's drug budget, accounting for two-thirds of total spending.

Despite impressive seizures at the border, on the high seas, and in other countries, foreign drugs are cheaper and more readily available today than two decades ago. Domestic production of illegal drugs such as marijuana and methamphetamines is increasing, further reducing the potential impact of interdiction on United States drug use. United States foreign supply reduction efforts have also caused problems of their own, especially in Latin America, where narcotics control dominates the diplomatic agenda with the United States. The unintended consequences of these programs have sometimes been severe, including political unrest among peasant farmers who rely on drug crops for their livelihood; human rights abuses as governments try to suppress drug cultivation; increased corruption among police and military forces; and expanding roles for the military in drug enforcement and internal security in countries where democracy is still fragile.

Ultimately, the costs incurred—both in the United States and overseas—in pursuing the supply-side drug strategy will not produce the promised benefits of reduced drug availability and higher drug prices. The largest drug profits are made within the United States at street-level sales, not in foreign poppy or coca fields or on the high seas. The total cost of cultivating, refining, and smuggling cocaine to the United States accounts for less than 15 percent of domestic retail prices. Recent anecdotal evidence from the southwestern United States suggests that smuggling costs may have increased as a result of intensified border interdiction: Mexican traffickers are said to be offering as much as half their cocaine shipments in exchange for safe passage. Still, the value of drugs at that point is only a fraction of their retail price on American streets. As one DEA official explained, "The average drug organization can afford to lose as much as 80 percent of its product and still be profitable."

MAKING DEMAND THE FOCUS

The nation's drug control strategy should shift from a primary focus on reducing drug supplies to reducing the demand for drugs through prevention, education, treatment, and community anti-drug coalitions. Law enforcement has a critically important role to play; studies indicate that street-level enforcement is more effective in driving up drug prices and has the added benefit of making neighborhoods safer. In the international arena, greater emphasis should be placed on attacking the growing power of the drug cartels that challenge the integrity of political, financial, and judicial institutions in this country and abroad. The United States should concentrate on efforts both to strengthen democratic governments and to combat money laundering, drug-related corruption, and violence through bilateral and multilateral initiatives. For too long, United States drug policy has been driven by the need to appear "tough" on drugs, regardless of results. The United States should leave behind the distinction between "tough" and "soft" approaches to drug abuse and concentrate its attention, research, and resources on determining what actually works.

Strange Bedfellows: Ideology, Politics, and Drug Legalization

Erich Goode

The political landscape is a maze of contradictions; politics, we are told, make for "strange bedfellows." Perhaps nowhere is this more apparent than in the issue of drug legalization. In a recent letter to the editor to *The New York Times,* anti-drug crusader William Bennett charged the pro-legalization forces with being "strange bedfellows." What Bennett does not say is that advocates of *all* positions on the drug legalization question crawl under the sheets with ideologies they would reject in other areas. Positions that are very close to one another *in general* may actually have drastically differing views on drug policy; likewise, positions that seem poles apart on most *other* issues may snuggle up on the question of what to do about drugs. Here, the distinction between advocates of legalization and prohibitionists are frequently fractured by cross-cutting political views. Seen politically, positions on legalization may be regarded as the secondary manifestation of deeper and more compelling ideological commitments.

To be specific about it, most conservatives *oppose* a relaxation of the drug laws, but many *extreme* conservatives favor a program of complete decriminalization; at the other end of the spectrum, many radicals oppose certain forms of legalization as state control—and in that view, agree with many extreme conservatives, who propose something of a laissez-faire policy. Black politicians, usually well at the liberal end of the political spectrum, are (with a tiny number of exceptions) *staunchly* opposed to drug legalization. Moving toward the center, advocates of legalization (taken as a whole) and prohibitionists (again, lumped together) stand on opposite sides of the great divide on the issue of legalization, but a more nuanced view of their positions suggests that "progressive" advocates of legalization and "progressive" prohibitionists share much more in common than the first does with the more extreme or "hard core" advocates of legalization and the latter does with the more extreme

or "hard core" prohibitionists. Consequently, the usual political spectrum is not a very useful road map for finding out where someone stands on drug policy.

How do we divide up the drug legalization debate pie? What are the most prominent positions on this issue? Who stands where on the question of legalization? Peter Reuter made use of a warfare analogy in locating "doves," "hawks," and "owls." In limning the ideological landscape of the debate over what to do about the drug problem, Franklin Zimring and Gordon Hawkins find *generalists* (those who apply the same standards to all psychoactive substances, regardless of their legal status), *legalists* (who say a drug is what the law says is a drug), and *cost-benefit specifists* (pragmatists who set aside issues of morality and consider only harm reduction). Ethan Nadelmann, an outspoken, prolific, and high-profile advocate of legalization, delineates "legalizers, prohibitionists, and the common ground," suggesting that some adherents of positions on either side of this divide may share more with one another than with their presumed allies. What sort of "strange bedfellows" perplexities do we find spread across the drug legalization canvas?

The more high-profile views on the drug legalization issue may be crystallized out as follows: *cultural conservatives; free-[market] libertarians; radical constructionists; progressive legalizers;* and *progressive prohibitionists.*

Cultural conservatives. Cultural conservatives believe in "old fashioned" values; they feel that what is wrong with the country, drug abuse included, is that too many people have strayed too far from age-old custom and tradition. We should return to mainstream religion; the traditional family; conventional sexual practices; the "basics" in education; strong communities where neighbors care about one another; conformity to traditional values; moderation in our consumption of alcohol, complete abstention from illegal psychoactive substances; and so on.

Reprinted by permission from *Society,* May/June 1998, pp. 18-27. © 1998 by Transaction Publishers. All rights reserved.

What is bad about the country is that there is too much freedom, rampant individuality, hedonism, selfishness, a lack of concern for our fellow human beings, godlessness, lack of a communitarian spirit, a too-heavy reliance on the federal government to do things for us, not enough self-control—all of which lead to divorce, abortion, pornography, illegitimacy, crime, violence, and drug abuse.

Cultural conservatives believe that everyone is responsible for his or her own actions, that all behavior is an individual moral choice. No one has the right to hide behind social "factors" or "conditions" which, others will claim, cause or influence people to do things. For instance, the cultural conservative would see the conflict sociologist's argument that drug abuse is related to a lack of power, residence in certain neighborhoods, and low socioeconomic status as little more than an *excuse* for illegal and immoral behavior. To the cultural conservative, strengthening morality means *defeating* illegal and immoral behavior, drug use included; when morality fails to take hold, law enforcement must step in and take over. In fact, law enforcement is an *agent* of morality, since it *teaches* violators that they cannot get away with breaking the law. Just as important, it is the job of law enforcement to ensure that *justice* is meted out, because justice is trampled on whenever the law is violated.

Cultural conservatives adopt what Zimring and Hawkins refer to as a *legalistic* definition of drugs and drug abuse: A drug is an *illegal* psychoactive substance, and drug abuse is use of a drug *outside a medical context.* Advocates of legalization draw a sharp distinction between alcohol, on the one hand, and all currently illegal drugs, on the other; alcohol is not a drug, nor is alcoholism a type of drug abuse. For the cultural conservative, drug abuse is immoral, a repugnant vice. (So is the immoderate abuse of alcohol—although, again, it does not qualify as *drug* abuse.) By its very nature, indulgence in drugs degrades human life. Drugs should be outlawed because using them represents a repudiation of the status quo—that is, tradition, conservative values, all that is good and true. Intoxication represents an unhealthy decadance, an expression of degeneracy, a quest for a spurious, insidious, ill-gotten, *illegitimate* pleasure. It is *incompatible* with a decent life; drug intoxication and the decent life are a contradiction in terms.

Interestingly, cultural conservatives believe that there is *too much* government spending and intervention in nearly all areas of life, but with some major exceptions—where there is *too little.* One exception is that far more money should be spent, in Bennett's words, for a "more effective and tough-minded criminal justice system, including more prisons, judges, and prosecutors." Juveniles who commit violent crimes should be tried as adults; convicts should serve out at least half their sentences, and less parole should be granted; fewer cases should be dismissed on technicalities; less probation and fewer suspended sentences should be handed out; and

so on. Cultural conservatives are *adamantly* opposed to the legalization of the currently illegal drugs. Bennett refers to arguments for legalization as "morally scandalous," "irresponsible nonsense." Again, note that the ravages of the *legal* drugs do not enter into the cultural conservative's equation at all; James Q. Wilson argues that while tobacco *shortens* human life, cocaine *debases* it. A clear-cut example of the cultural conservative point of view on the drug question was expressed by Senator Jesse Helms in 1995; in attempting to derail a bill designed to allocate more federal dollars to AIDS sufferers, Helms argued that, instead, we should *reduce* funding for AIDS, because those who contracted the disease did so as a result of their own "deliberate, disgusting, revolting conduct." He was, of course, referring mainly to homosexuals and drug addicts (and not hemophiliacs, contaminated blood transfusion victims, or children of infected mothers). The fact that Senator Helms is the tobacco industry's staunchest and most powerful ally—and that tobacco kills as a result of the "deliberate" actions of smokers—underscores the selective vision of the cultural conservative.

The answer to the drug problem for the cultural conservative, then, is a return to traditional values. Law enforcement is seen as an ally in this struggle. Victory cannot be achieved without government intervention, and that means, mainly, long sentences for violations and increased allocations for the police and for building jails and prisons. There should be "zero tolerance" for drug use—zero tolerance in the schools, the workplace, the government sector, on the highway, in the street, in public, even in the home—anywhere and everywhere intervention is feasible. If private parties can bring this about, so much the better, but the government must be enlisted in this fight because it has the resources, the power, and the influence to exert a major impact.

Cultural conservatives have a great deal of faith in the "War on Drugs"; Richard Nixon, Ronald Reagan, and George Bush, all used the expression often and were zealous generals in this "war." Carrying on this tradition in his campaign speeches, presidential candidate Bob Dole vowed to re-ignite the drug war, which had lapsed, he claimed, under Bill Clinton—whom he designated politically and culturally far to his left. More specifically, cultural conservatives have a great deal of faith in a principle we might refer to as *absolute deterrence.* That is, they do not believe simply that law enforcement is more likely to "contain" or keep a given activity in check or at a lower level than no enforcement at all; instead, they argue, that war can—absolutely—defeat the enemy. Further, they believe (or, at least, in their speeches and writings, they state) that law enforcement, if not restrained by loopholes, technicalities, and restrictions, will actually reduce that activity, ideally, nearly to zero. We *can* win the war on drugs, the cultural conservative asserts, if we have sufficient will, determination, and unity.

Cultural conservatives are not particularly interested in calculating costs and benefits to minimize the harms that the current drug policy might inflict, nor do they consider the impact of alternate drug policies, since that would open the door to thinking about some forms of legalization. What counts is crushing the monster of drug abuse. Pragmatism enters into this picture only through the back door. What we have here is a kind of holy war, a struggle of good against evil—and winning it represents an end, a goal, and a good in itself. There can be no compromise with evil. It is simply *assumed* that harsher penalties translates into less use, but it is not especially important if it does not. What counts is being on the right side and being tough and uncompromising against the enemy.

Not all supporters of the present system of drug criminalization are cultural conservatives. Somewhere in between cultural conservatives and progressive prohibitionists (a denizen we will encounter shortly) lies a position which may encompass a majority of Americans. Their position may be dubbed "meat and potatoes" or "garden variety" criminalization. Its endorsers do not bring the heavy ideological and moral baggage to the drug legalization debate that the cultural conservatives bring, but they are not as pragmatic or as dedicated to "cost benefit analysis" or "harm reduction" as the progressive criminalizers or the progressive legalizers, either. They are opposed to legalization because it does not sound like a good idea. They are wary of change and do not want to seem to encourage the use of the illegal drugs by legalizing them. They think this would send the wrong message to potential users, and they do not think the government has any business dispensing heroin or cocaine. They think that drug violators should be arrested—especially dealers. They do not think that sending addicts to jail is a great idea, but they do not have a clear idea of what should be done with them. They favor treatment, but are skeptical about its efficacy. In short, they borrow elements of positions that stretch on either side of their own. They do not have a strong or clear-cut view on the question. Still, ultimately, it is their voice that will be listened to most in the debate, since their numbers are so great. On many issues, politicians have a way of listening to the majority, and the drug legalization debate is no exception to this rule.

Free-market libertarians. Both cultural conservatives and free-market libertarians are at the conservative end of the political spectrum, but they disagree on almost everything else pertaining to drug legalization. For one thing, while cultural conservatives believe that there are real differences between legal and illegal drugs, free-market libertarians believe that the legal-illegal distinction is artificial and should be dismantled. Technically, free-market libertarians are opposed to legalization, but for exactly the *opposite* reason as the cultural conservatives. While the cultural conservatives feel that legalization would represent a dangerous step toward *too little* government inter-

vention and control, for the free-market libertarian, legalization would result in *too much* government intervention and control. The libertarian wants a laissez-faire or "hands off" government policy—no government-administered methadone maintenance programs, no government "drug stores" or "supermarkets," no Alcohol Beverage Control package stores, no laws telling citizens what they can and can't do, no medical prescriptions for imaginary neuroses or mental illnesses, no restrictions, controls, legislation, or regulations whatsoever.

No one should be *forced* to take drugs, they say, and no one should be forced *not* to take drugs. One major exception for many in this camp—a condition for which a law is necessary—is the *age* of the purchaser: An adult should not be allowed to sell drugs to a minor. Otherwise, more or less "anything goes." What free-market libertarians want is *complete decriminalization*, not state-controlled, state-supervised legalization. Psychiatrist Thomas Szasz and economist Milton Friedman stand foursquare in this tradition; their coauthored volume, *On Liberty and Drugs*, contains a chapter, penned by Friedman, entitled "The Drug War as a Socialist Enterprise." Interestingly, they also believe that *legalization* would represent a "socialist enterprise."

An important concept here is *caveat emptor*—"let the buyer beware." No seller should be held responsible for selling anything that might be potentially dangerous to any legally competent adult; free-market libertarians take the principle that we are all responsible for our own actions to a far more extreme position than the cultural conservative does. Just as we do not blame the seller of food for the obesity of a customer, we should not blame the "drug habits" of the addict on the drug dealer. While falsely listing the contents of what one sells should not be permitted, *not disclosing* its contents is acceptable and should be legal—even if it is dangerous and harmful—again, because the buyer should "beware" of what he or she purchases. And if the contents do harm people, well, after awhile, sellers of such products will lose their customers. After all, forcing sellers to disclose the contents of what they sell represents too much government intervention.

Free-market libertarians argue that freedom from government constraint *inevitably* produces the greatest good for the greatest number of people. This sounds like a pragmatic, consequentialist, or empirical argument—that is, that government nonintervention is good *because* it produces positive, measurable results. But more closely examined, it becomes clear that this is a *moral* and *ideological* argument, that libertarians are in favor of nonintervention as a good *in and of itself*. If, in a specific instance, a particular case of government intervention results in producing a result all would agree is good, the libertarian would nonetheless oppose it because, *by its very nature*, and *as a general principle*, government intervention is undesirable. In fact, in the introduction to *Our Right to Drugs*, Szasz states explicitly that his criticism of the war on drugs is not based on pharmacological or therapeutic arguments, but on "political-philosophical considerations." To draw a parallel, William Bennett's strong endorsement of 1960s civil rights legislation as laws that have had a positive consequence, would be *anathema* to free-market libertarians, who believe *any* effort to legislate people's behavior is wrong—*the less government, the better* is their motto.

In *Our Right to Drugs*, Thomas Szasz argues that government taxation is "legalized robbery"; politicians and other officials are "government parasites with a comfortable living"; a system of government-controlled medical licensing, he says, results in a "loss of personal freedom," whose results have been "undesirable"; the system whereby drugs are reviewed by the Food and Drug Administration to determine whether they are safe and effective is "therapeutic slavery"; support for government funding for medical research is a product of "crowd madness," "dogma," and a "pharmacological phobia and pharmacological hubris"; any effort to control drugs is "chemical socialism (or communism)"; advocates of drug legalization, he says, are in fact "medicalizers and thus, de facto, paternalistic prohibitionists." Once again, government intervention not only *does* harm—it *is* harm *by its very nature*. The government has no right to intervene in the lives of its citizens, nor should the government set up controls or regulations that attempt to protect citizens from their own behavior, nor should the government institute programs that are designed to do good of any kind. Left to their own devices, the people will get together and do what is best for themselves. If we make mistakes as a result of exercising our freedom, we will inevitably learn from them. All citizens have the right to do and to purchase anything they wish, so long as this does not harm someone else; it is the government's job to stay out of the people's business, which is exercising our freedoms and maximizing our individual potential.

For the free-market libertarians, the fundamental point is that drugs represent a form of property; they feel that the ownership of property is sacred, not to be tampered with by the government in any way. Only under extremely limited circumstances does the government have the right to step in and take away such a basic and fundamental right. Under most circumstances, they believe, where such restrictions are practically non-existent, the public good will be maximized; where [nonintervention] results in harm to some people, nonetheless, the *general principle,* in and of itself, of nonintervention must be preserved. There are very few instances, many free-market libertarians feel, where this principle is so blatantly violated as with the drug laws. And legalization is not much better, they believe; it simply results in ever more state intervention.

To the free-market libertarian the ideal solution is complete decriminalization of currently illegal drugs. Free-market libertarians do not delude themselves into thinking that decriminalization will eliminate either drug use or the medical harm that drug use causes; to them, this is beside the point. But they do believe that instilling a sense of personal responsibility in a citizenry for their own actions is more likely to result in them choosing the most reasonable path than if the government forces them to do something against their will, or prevents them from doing what they might otherwise choose to do. Such paternalism breeds the very dependency that we (mistakenly) attribute to drugs. Our aim should not be, in Szasz's words, a "drug-free America" but an "America free of drug laws." In the 19th century, there were no legal controls on drugs; in our century, we must "return to a free market in drugs. We need not reinvent the wheel to solve our drug problem. All we need to do is to stop acting like timid children, grow up, and stand on our own two feet."

Radical constructionists. To some degree, all social scientists are constructionists; all of us are interested in how interpretations of reality are constructed, what functions they serve, how they grow out of broader political and ideological views, and what consequences they have. However, these days, some of us seem to be arguing that the brute facts of the material world count for very little in these social and cultural constructs, that almost any interpretation of reality can be dished up and accepted as true, no matter how much it may run counter to the facts, if it serves the interests of certain privileged segments of the society. Observers with these views could be called *radical constructionists.* Radical constructionists are not so much in favor of legalization as opposed to the "war on drugs." They argue that, objectively speaking, there *is* no real drug crisis. The government has targeted drugs and drug users because they serve as a convenient scapegoat: Most are poor and powerless, many are members of racial and ethnic minorities, they do not have the resources with which to fight back, or they are members of a despised, stigmatized deviant category, and hence, they are inconvenient for the affluent, hegemonic segments of the society. Attention to the phony drug "crisis" serves the function of diverting attention away from the real problems of the day—problems which either cannot be solved within the existing institutional framework or which, if they were solved, would snatch privileges away from the affluent, the powerful, and the privileged.

Consider the drug "crisis" that gripped American society between 1986 and 1992. In a series of speeches between June and September 1986, Ronald Reagan called for a "nationwide crusade against drugs." Federal bills were passed in 1986, 1988, and 1992, increasing allocations for fighting the drug war several-fold. Media attention to the drug problem increased by 20 times between the early to the late 1980s. Public opinion polls revealed that the proportion of Americans who regarded drug abuse as the "number one problem facing the country today" increased from the 2 to 3 percent range in the early to mid-1980s to *64 percent* in September 1989. (After

1989, the percentage declined; it declined again after 1992.) In a *constructed* or *subjective* sense, there was, indeed, a drug crisis between the late 1980s into the early 1990s. Perhaps never before in the country's history had so many Americans felt such an intense concern about drug abuse. Even more important, never before was law enforcement so vigorously involved in incarcerating drug violators. Between 1980 and 1992, the number of new commitments to state prisons on drug charges increased by *ten times,* at a time when the number of violent offenders increased by only 50 percent. In the last presidential election, Bob Dole promised to reinvigorate a holy crusade against drugs—which has, supposedly, lapsed a bit under President Clinton.

But radical constructionists argue that this public concern, and the repression that accompanied it, were based on an exaggerated fear; they were not based on any corresponding increase in objective harm caused by drug abuse. In fact, they argue, the use of illegal drugs actually *declined* in the 1980–1990 period, and by a good amount. Why was there an *increase* in concern over drugs at the very moment when *rates of drug use* and, presumably, the magnitude of the drug problem, were decreasing? In fact, fear and concern over drugs in the late 1980s turned out to be a "panic," a "scare"—not a true crisis at all. Why? Why this exaggerated concern over illegal drug abuse—a declining problem objectively speaking? Why the sudden rush to imprison drug users, addicts, and dealers, at a time when drug abuse posed little threat to American society? Why the intense, biased, hysterical, sensationalistic depiction of illegal drug use in the media?

The scare was generated, radical constructionists contend, for political, bureaucratic, and financial purposes. The rise of the New Right, and the need to protect the interests of the rich and the powerful, was behind the drug scare. In the words of sociologists Craig Reinarman and Harry Gene Levine, instead of focusing on the real problems—poverty, urban decay, unemployment, an unjust distribution of society's resources—these social problems were blamed on "chemical bogyman," a "scapegoat," an "ideological fig leaf." Poverty is blamed on character flaws in the poor; drug abuse is also a product of these self-same character flaws, while, in turn, further contributing to poverty. If the actual structural conditions and disastrous conservative policies were pinpointed as the true causes of poverty, the affluent would have to relinquish some of their privileges. The drug scare of the late 1980s, in the words of Reinarman and Levine, was "concocted by the press, politicians, and moral entrepreneurs to serve other agendas." It appealed to "racism, bureaucratic self-interest, economics, and mongering by the media." In addition, "the issue of illicit drug use . . . focuses attention away from structural ills like economic inequality, injustice, and lack of meaningful roles for young people. A crusade against drug use allows conservative politicians to be law-and-order minded; it also permits them to give the appearance of caring about social ills without commit-

ting them to do or spend very much to help people." The social construction of drug abuse as a major social problem in the late 1980s and early 1990s, radical constructionists argue, served a political agenda for the powers that be (including the media). Maintain the status quo and profit from doing it. If and when that crusade becomes top priority once again, the same political motives may be detected lurking in the shadows. Notice that the radical constructionists do *not* deny that drug abuse is a problem for the society. But they do argue that it is a less serious problem than a number of *far* more damaging conditions, about which very little fuss is made—such as alcoholism and tobacco addiction, not to mention poverty, racism, and gross inequalities in the distribution of society's resources. Moreover, they say, the recent "war on drugs" emerged specifically at a time when the severity of the drug problem was declining and hence, it must have served symbolic functions; it was, in fact, a war against the poor.

The radical constructionist sees law enforcement and the media as working hand-in-hand with one another; in the "war on drugs," they are *allies.* Both reinforce existing power and economic arrangements. In fact, in a drug "panic" such as that which erupted in the United States during the 1986 to 1990 (or so) period, lawmakers and law enforcement on the one hand and media attention on the other can be seen as two separate indicators or measures of the same thing: concern about a given problem or condition. In effect, they are both devoted to the same cause: persecuting a scapegoat. Just as police priorities are misplaced in targeting drug violators, media coverage is "cracked" or biased against drug abusers. They are two ingredients in the same recipe. Media critics Jimmie Reeves and Richard Campbell charge that the "drug control establishment" and "mainstream journalism" are partners in advancing a hysterical witch-hunt that, during the late 1980s, "helped mask the economic devastation of deindustrialization, aggravated black-white tensions . . . , and, ultimately, helped solidify middle-class support for policies that favored the rich over the poor." Although the heat of the drug "panic" of the late 1980s died down by the early 1990s, fundamentally the same processes are continuing today on a more institutionalized and less frenzied basis. And one ingredient in that institutionalization is more and longer prison sentences for drug violators.

Radical constructionists do not see drugs as the enemy. Most argue that drug abuse is the *symptom* of a problem, not the cause of it. The problem is, of course, the gross inequity in society's resources: poverty, unemployment, urban decay, the powerlessness of the poor and racial minorities, racism, a lack of economic opportunities in the inner cities, combined with the grotesque affluence of the very rich. Drug selling, at least at the street level, is caused not by a character flaw but by a lack of economic opportunity; drug abuse is not an expression of being weak-willed but of hopelessness brought on by urban decay.

The solution to the drug problem is not legalization by itself, which will do nothing to solve the ills and injustices of poverty or the grossly unfair distribution of society's resources. Clarence Lusane, in *Pipe Dream Blues* writes: "As long as economic and racial inequities exist, abuse will continue whether drugs are legal or illegal." Hence, a "radical redistribution of wealth" and "fundamental economic reform" must be at the heart of any meaningful response to the drug crisis. After this, more crucial but less grandiose measures must be taken. High on any reform agenda: "establishing new approaches to policing and law enforcement." Communities must take back their streets; the police must listen to and be responsive to the needs of the people, and discontinue stereotyping, stigmatizing, and harassing poor, inner city minorities. Alternatives to prison must be instituted, such as community service; prisons are already overcrowded, and African-Americans are hugely over-represented—and growing—in the prison population. The "war on drugs" should cease. Law enforcement should stop criminalizing the junkie; drug addiction should be seen as a medical not a criminal matter. Treatment facilities, especially those that involve the community and are drug-free, should be hugely expanded. At the same time, high-level dealers who conspire to poison poor and minority communities should be handed long prison sentences. In conjunction with these changes, alcohol and tobacco could be restricted in a variety of ways; their sale is profitable to their manufacturers and harmful disproportionately to the poor. Above all, what is needed is *empowerment*—a vastly greater and more effective participation in the political process by the poor, the under-represented, and members of racial and ethnic minorities. With empowerment will come economic redistribution which, in turn, will bring about a defeat of drug abuse as a major problem in American society.

Progressive Advocates of Legalization. Unlike the cultural conservatives, progressive advocates of legalization are generalists; they hold a definition of drugs that is based on their psychoactive quality, not their legality. In fact, such advocates wish to dismantle or at least radically restructure the legal-illegal distinction. Unlike the free-market libertarian, the progressive advocate of legalization does believe in state control of the dispensation of psychoactive substances. Unlike the radical constructionist, the progressive advocate of legalization argues that the drug laws *are* the problem. Matters of reforming the economy, the political system, and redistributing society's resources are important in themselves, but the reform of drug policy, too, is a crucial issue in its own right. Progressive advocates of legalization are more concerned with what to do about drugs than about reformulating the political and economic system generally. They think that there are many things that are seriously wrong with the present system, but that the laws prohibiting drugs represent one of them; they wish to reform them, so that there will be less pain and suffering in the world.

How does the progressive formulate or *frame* the drug legalization issue? What is the nature of the drug problem, and what is the solution? For the most part, progressive advocates of legalization see the drug problem as a *human rights* issue. What they are talking about when they discuss drug reforms is treating drug addiction as a health problem, much like schizophrenia or alcoholism—not as a crime or law enforcement problem. Above all, society should, in Ethan Nadelmann's words, "stop demonizing illicit drug users"; "they are citizens and human beings." Criminalizing the possession and use of the currently illegal drugs is *unjust, oppressive,* and *inhumane*; it has no moral justification. It represents a kind of witch-hunt, and it penalizes the unfortunate. Innumerable young lives are being ruined by imprisonment for what are essentially victimless crimes. It is the suffering *of the drug user* that is foremost on the progressive's mind in demanding a reform of drug policy. Nadelmann, the progressives' foremost and most well-known spokesperson concludes: "Harm reduction means leaving casual drug users alone and treating addicts like they're still human beings." "My strongest argument for legalization," he adds, "is a moral one. Enforcement of drug laws makes a mockery of an essential principle of a free society—that those who do no harm to others should not be harmed by others, particularly by the state . . . To me, [this] is the greatest societal cost of our current drug prohibition system."

A key to the thinking of progressive advocates of legalization is their belief that drug use is a sphere of behavior that is influenced by much the same rules of human nature as any other activity. They feel that drug users are no more irrational or self-destructive than are participants in such routine—and far less legally controlled—activities as skiing, boating, eating, drinking, walking, talking, and so on. There is, in other words, no special or *unique* power in psychoactive drugs that makes it necessary for the society to erect laws to control and penalize their use. Why do we penalize people who use drugs, and harm no one (perhaps not even themselves), but leave the stamp-collecting, chess-playing, and television-watching addict untouched? It is a philosophical tenet of these progressives that it is *unjust* to penalize one activity in which the participant harms no one while, at the same time, other, not significantly safer, activities are left legally uncontrolled. The assumption that drugs possess *uniquely enslaving* and *uniquely damaging* qualities is not only widely held in American society, it is also sharply challenged by the progressive advocates of legalization. No special or uniquely negative qualities means that there are no extraordinarily compelling reasons why drugs should be singled out to be criminalized or prohibited. Most drug users are every bit as rational as, for example, chess players; society has no more cause to penalize the former for their pursuits than the latter.

Progressive advocates of legalization claim to be serious in considering a cost-benefit analysis, but insist that others who also make that claim leave out at least one crucial element in this equation: *pleasure*. Few other perspectives that weigh losses and gains are willing to count the psychoactive effects that users seek—and attain—when they get high as a benefit. But why don't they? Sheer bias, the progressive advocate of legalization would respond. Most people take drugs because they enjoy their effects; this must be counted as a benefit to the society. If we are serious about counting positives and negatives, why ignore the most central positive of all—the enjoyment of drug taking? It is what motivates users, and it must be counted as a benefit. Clearly, such a consideration would be challenged by cultural conservatives, who see hedonism and the pursuit of ecstasy as signs of decay and degeneracy—part of what is wrong with the country.

The position of progressive advocates of legalization can best be appreciated by a contrast with that of the *progressive prohibitionists*. Advocates of both positions urge reforms in the drug laws, both are, or claim to be, concerned with harm reduction, both attempt to weigh costs and benefits carefully and empirically in any evaluation of drug policy, and both believe that users of the illegal drugs are treated too harshly, and that the legal drugs are too readily available. But the differences between these two positions are as important as their similarities.

There are three major and profound dissimilarities between the progressive advocates of legalization and the progressive prohibitionists: First, in their evaluation of costs and benefits, progressive advocates of legalization weigh the *moral* values of individual liberty, privacy, and tolerance of the addict very heavily, while the progressive prohibitionist to some degree sets these values aside and emphasizes concrete, material values—specifically public health—much more heavily. Second, in considering the impact of legalization—more specifically, whether it will increase use or not—progressive advocates of legalization are *optimists* (they believe that use will not increase significantly), while progressive prohibitionists are *pessimists* (they believe that use will increase, possibly even dramatically). Even if use does increase, the progressive advocates of legalization say, legalization is likely to result in increased use of *less* harmful drugs and decreased use of *more* harmful substances.

And third, progressive advocates of legalization believe that most of the harms from the use of the currently illegal drugs stems from criminalization, while the progressive prohibitionists believe that such harms are more a product of use per se than of the criminalization of those drugs. Harm from contaminated drugs, the grip of organized crime, the crime and violence that infects the drug scene, AIDS, medical maladies from addiction—all

secondary, not primary effects of drugs. And all will decline or disappear under legalization. Progressive prohibitionists are skeptical.

With very few exceptions, progressive advocates of legalization have not spent a great deal of time or space spelling out what their particular form of legalization would look like. Still, they do *not* mean by legalization what free-market libertarians mean by decriminalization, nor, indeed, what their critics mean by legalization. "When we talk about legalization, we don't mean selling crack in candy stores," says Nadelmann. Unlike free-market libertarians, most progressive advocates of legalization realize that selling drugs in a kind of "supermarket," where any and all psychoactive substances would be as readily available as heads of lettuce and cans of soup, is not feasible for the foreseeable future. Many point to harm reduction strategies that seem (to some observers) to have worked in the Netherlands, Switzerland, and England. All support steps in that direction: legalize or decriminalize marijuana, increase methadone maintenance programs, reschedule many Schedule I drugs (such as LSD, ecstasy, and heroin) that may have therapeutic utility, stop arresting addicts, get them into treatment programs, and so on. However, they see these as only stopgap or transitional steps. If not the supermarket model, then what would full legalization look like? Nadelmann suggests that the *mail order model* might work: sell drugs in limited quantities through the mail. While not the ideal solution, it is the best compromise "between individual rights and communitarian interests." It must be noted that, while all progressive advocates of legalization emphasize the unanticipated consequences of prohibition, they do not spend much time or space considering the possible unanticipated consequences that *legalization* itself might have.

Progressive prohibitionists. Progressive prohibitionists (such as Mark Kleiman, Mark Moore, Franklin Zimring and Gordon Hawkins), urge many of the same reforms that progressive advocates of legalization argue for; most of them, for instance, would support most of the following: needle exchange, condom distribution, an expansion of methadone maintenance, no incarceration of the addict, rescheduling of many Schedule I drugs, a consideration of legalization or decriminalization of marijuana, higher taxes and more controls on alcohol and tobacco. (Interestingly, as I said, there are far more similarities between progressive prohibitionists and progressive advocates of legalization than there are between the former and "hard-line" criminalizers on the one hand, and between the latter and "radical" or "extreme" free-market libertarians, on the other.) The progressive prohibitionists draw the line, however, at the legal, over-the-counter or even mail-order sale of drugs such as heroin, cocaine, and amphetamine.

Progressive prohibitionists are not as distressed by the moral incongruity of criminalizing the possession and sale of powerful psychoactive agents and legally tolerating substances or activities that also cause harm. Once again, to demarcate their position from that of the progressive advocates of legalization, they say, to *some* degree, there *is* a special and unique quality in certain drugs that compels *some* users of them to become abusers. Not a majority of the society, they say, but a sufficient minority to warrant concern for the public health of the entire society. In fact, to step back and look at their political, ideological, and moral position more generally, progressive prohibitionists are far more *communitarian* than *individualistic*. While the touchstone of the progressive advocate of legalization is the *rights of the individual,* for the progressive prohibitionist, the guiding principle is *the health of the community.* The individual, they would say, does not have the right to harm the society; certain rights have to be curbed for the good of the society as a whole. If injured, the individual has to be cared for by the community; foolish acts engaged in by the individual are purchased at the price of a very substantial cost to the rest of us. The individual *does not have the legal or moral right* to ignore the seat belt laws, the helmet laws, or rules and regulations against permitting him or her to be placed in extreme danger—or any other laws, rules, or regulations that attempt to protect individuals from harming themselves. Any humane society must balance freedom over and against harm, and in this equation, quite often, certain freedoms must be curtailed. In short, compared with progressive advocates of legalization, progressive prohibitionists are much more concerned with a potential gain in public health than with the moral issue of which human rights are, allegedly abridged. For instance, coercing addicts and drug abusers into drug rehabilitation programs by arresting them and giving them a choice between imprisonment and treatment is not a moral problem for the progressive prohibitionist as it would be for the progressive advocate of legalization.

It is almost in the very nature of the progressive prohibitionist's argument that there is an assumption of greater use under any possible legalization plan. (Marijuana may very well represent an exception.) This position views the American population—or a segment of it, at any rate—as being *vulnerable* to the temptation of harmful psychoactive drugs. Progressive prohibitionists are *pessimists* when it comes to contemplating the extent of use under legalization. They do not necessarily see the dire and catastrophic "worst case" scenario predicted by the cultural conservatives—for instance, the tens of millions of new cocaine and heroin addicts and abusers predicted by William Bennett under legalization. But many progressive advocates of legalization do see a doubling, tripling, or a quadrupling of hard drug abuse in the United States as an entirely possible outcome of many of the currently-proposed legalization schemes. And they find that unacceptable. *Most* Americans will resist the temptations and blandishments of these seductive, dependency-producing substances. But focusing on the potential behavior of "most" Americans is a distrac-

tion and irrelevant in any case. What counts is whether the *small minority* who use drugs destructively is likely to grow. Most distressing: The volume of drug abuse *of current addicts and abusers* is likely to increase, and along with it, the harm that flows from it.

And finally, the progressive prohibitionist sees more *direct* harm from use of the hard drugs, such as cocaine, amphetamine, and heroin, than the progressive advocate of legalization does. There are, it is true, they say, some secondary harms and complications caused mainly by the legal status of these drugs; certainly HIV/AIDS ranks high among them. But most of these secondary or indirect harms can be attacked through modifications of the current system that fall far short of outright legalization. Certainly needle exchange and condom distribution programs would go a long way in combating the problem of HIV contamination. The fact is, cocaine and heroin are a great deal more harmful than the progressive advocates of legalization claim, say the prohibitionists. Harm has been kept low by the very fact of the drug laws, because far fewer people use [drugs] currently than would be the case under legalization. Alcohol and tobacco kill many Americans in part because their use is *intrinsically* harmful (at least, given the way they are used) and in part because they are widely used. Cocaine and heroin—considering the many possible ways that drugs can be harmful—are *also* intrinsically harmful drugs, though, they are harmful in very different respects. *And* they are taken, recklessly, by segments of the population who are far more likely to take extreme risks with their health than others. If they were to be used as widely and as commonly as alcohol and tobacco are used today—not a real possibility—many, many users would die as a result of their use. As many as those who die as a result of using these legal drugs? Possibly. It is foolish and unrealistic, the progressive prohibitionist says, to imagine that these illegal drugs are harmful today *entirely* or even *mainly* simply because they are illegal. While the progressive advocate of legalization stresses the *secondary* harms and dangers of the illegal drugs, the progressive prohibitionist stresses their *primary* harms and dangers.

Again, while the more progressive prohibitionists and the more moderate or progressive advocates of legalization share many items in their drug policy agenda, they differ on these three major issues: how much they stress individual liberty versus public health; their prediction of whether drug abuse, and its attendant harms, will increase significantly under legalization; and their notion of whether the currently illegal drugs are more intrinsically or directly harmful or harmful indirectly, that is, mainly because they are illegal. Ironically, although the progressive advocates of legalization and the progressive prohibitionists stand on opposite sides of the great legalization divide, they share more particulars of their drug policy proposals than any two major positions in this debate. If major changes in drug policy do take place in the next century, they are likely to be drawn from the substantial overlap in these two positions.

The various approaches to drug legalization fit more or less comfortably into, and have relevance and resonance for, quite distinct political views or orientations. Drug legalization may be said to be a specific *instance* of, or a specific *issue* for, a more general political, ideological, and moral position. The issue is thought about in terms of a broader image or world-view expressing how things ought to be. In this sense, then, it is misleading to think about the debate strictly in pragmatic or empirical terms. In many ways, it is an ideological debate about which political perspective will dominate policy on drugs in the years to come.

Moreover, it is illogical to picture the drug legalization debate as an either-or proposition. What counts is the particulars of a given proposal; the position taken by some observers—Arnold Trebach is an outstanding example—that nothing could be worse than what we have now, therefore, let us legalize at once and take care of the specifics as we go along, is irresponsible in the extreme. *All policy changes represent a minefield of potential unanticipated—and undesired—consequences. Both God and the devil are "in the details."*

Erich Goode is professor of sociology at the State University of New York at Stony Brook. He is the author of Between Politics and Reason: The Drug Legalization Debate, *by St. Martin's Press, from which this article has been adapted.*

Governments and Drugs

Germany: A Strict Approach

Any legalization trends must be firmly opposed.

EDUARD LINTNER

Germany will continue its life-without-drugs stance and resist all demands for illicit drugs to be legalized. The International Narcotics Control Board shares the view that the European states must more firmly oppose legalization trends and must promote cooperation in the area of illicit-drug control, specifically precursor control.

Our government has always been, within the European Union, a guarantor for a consistent drug policy and, more importantly, for a policy that is consistent with public health policy objectives.

The greatest cause for concern in Germany is the growing willingness of adolescents and young adults to pop what they falsely believe are "happiness pills." The trend drug of the nineties, Ecstasy, is taken because it appears to provide "more fun and pleasure," thanks to the physical and emotional high it produces. For the past two years, it was consumed mostly by middle class, socially integrated young persons from 16 to 25 years of age. The "techno scene" setting plays an important role, although being a techno fan does not automat-ically imply consumption of synthetic drugs.

Although Ecstasy is harmful and involves a high risk of dependence, while at the same time the pleasant effects markedly weaken and the negative physical impact worsens, regular users (those who take more than one pill a week) seem relatively unwilling to quit. This is despite survey results suggesting that the majority of users know that the drug is illicit.

Studies show that in most cases cannabis and alcohol consumption precedes Ecstasy use. Young people tend to try cannabis and alcohol for the first time between the ages of 13 and 15, and Ecstasy between 16 and 18 years of age. According to recent studies, those who use Ecstasy usually take other drugs as well. Staples of the widely prevalent polydrug use are cannabis, LSD, and cocaine, with heroin being rather rare. These practices exponentially increase the health risks.

Periodically debates on drug liberalization, which in one case culminated in the western state of Schleswig-Holstein demanding that hashish be dispensed via pharmacies, are rekindled.

Although these aspirations have not been pursued any further since then, the aftereffect has been a persistent and continuously growing carelessness in dealing with drugs, especially the so-called soft drugs. This attitude is attended by a dangerous misjudgment of the risk inherent in using narcotics of any type.

A look at the annual statistics of the nonresidential addict support institutions in Germany reveals that cannabis abuse is on the rise, accounting for 3.2 percent of all diagnoses recorded in 1996, a growth of 24 percent over the previous year. This ranks cannabis third after alcohol and opioid peptide abuse.

In 1997 the overall number of hard-drug users who came to the police's attention for the first time was up by almost 20 percent from 1996 figures: from 17,197 to 20,594. The highest rate of increase was among amphetamine users, at 37 percent, followed by cocaine users, which rose 31 percent.

The number of recorded first-time heroin users grew by approximately

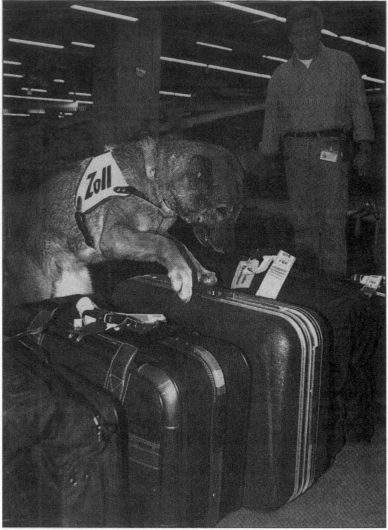

WIDE WORLD

■ *On the job:* Customs officials at Frankfurt Airport uncovered three tons of drugs in 1997.

phetamine labs, were raided (18 narcotics labs were raided the previous year).

Thus, the relative quantities seized suggest that users tend to prefer substances with activity-boosting and euphoric effects such as cocaine, amphetamine, LSD, and Ecstasy. It shows there is an enormous demand for cannabis products. And today as in the past, upward of 90 percent of the LSD, amphetamine, and Ecstasy seized in Germany originates (production and/or transit) in the Netherlands.

The demand for narcotics, of whatever type, can be successfully and effectively curbed only by forging a prevention alliance endorsed by and coordinated with the whole population—involving parents, teachers, associations, and others with a particular concern about the health and well-being of society.

Our primary goal must be to prevent addictions from developing in the first place by educating young people step by step as early in life as possible. In this regard, all of us—whether as parents, educators, friends, or relatives are called upon to be positive role models by critically reexamining our own habits, be they in the area of drugs or any other aspect of life.

The key is to approach young people in their own environment and help them understand how to enjoy a drug-free life. Fine examples are projects in which their own peers are able to make them see the positive aspects of having fun without drugs and, where necessary, point to counseling and assistance services. Hot lines are also useful in rounding off youth-related prevention efforts.

The effectiveness and consistency of any prevention endeavor is certain to be undermined, however, if we continue to publicly debate an endless stream of new projects for liberalizing narcotics. This goes also for the current debate over the so-called drug checking before techno events and at discos, where illicit drugs are analyzed for their composition.

18 percent, while the number of LSD users increased by about 14 percent over the previous year. The total first-time Ecstasy users rose some 5 percent: from 3,609 to 3,799. For the first half of 1998, trends are going in the same direction.

Owing to modifications in the police's recording practice, recent figures for first-time hard-drug users cannot be compared with those of the year before.

However, it can be reasonably assumed that the increased use of individual substances is in fact due to stepped-up demand and not merely because of a change in recording criteria. This is especially true for synthetic drugs, where the striking uptrend in consumption persists. That is also borne out by the sheer quantities seized in Germany, which has obviously shown a high demand market for such substances.

In 1997, police and customs seized 46 percent more amphetamines, 25 percent more cocaine, 17 percent more LSD trips, as well as approximately 126 percent more cannabis resin. At the same time, seizures of heroin dropped by about 20 percent and marijuana by about 31 percent. The amount of Ecstasy seized in 1997 (694,281 consumption units) remained just as high as the year before (692,397 units). In 1997, some 16 narcotics labs, 9 of them am-

Such tests, by their very existence, suggest that a drug, if checked, can be more safely consumed. Yet such a safety would ultimately be only an illusion. After all, recent studies on the action of synthetic drugs point to acute and long-term health risks, particularly where several psychoactive substances are used concurrently.

Apart from prevention-oriented approaches, assistance programs also must be further improved upon. The priority here must be to motivate the addict to undergo an abstinence therapy. Doing so requires a continuum of different, customized measures, from low-threshold assistance programs up to substitution programs.

In view of the need to make more efficient use of existing resources, assistance programs must be rendered more effective through cooperation projects designed to network and coordinate the services available in a region.

By contrast, experiments such as the supervised distribution of heroin to hard-core addicts provide no justifiable approach. The outcomes of this Swiss project are not nearly as positive as its advocates assert. Objectionable eligibility criteria, poor abstinence outcomes, heavy co-consumption of other drugs outside the program, and the resulting maintenance of contact with the destructive lifestyle are only some of the aspects that more than justify a critical assessment of the program.

The positive aspects of a physical and psychological stabilization and reintegration into everyday life and professional activity are in most cases essentially the result of an intensive medical and psychosocial care of the addicts, an insight that will ultimately prove to be the decisive, most promising avenue to take.

Eduard Lintner is drug commissioner of the federal government and parliamentary state secretary at the Federal Ministry of the Interior in Germany.

THE BUZZ ON DRUGS

The Miami bust and the rumblings on the campaign trail are only background noise. The real issue is whether the nation's whole war against drugs needs some serious rethinking.

BY JONATHAN ALTER

AN AMERICAN AIRLINES PILOT COMplained that his coffee "tasted weird." It turned out to be mixed with heroin that had been smuggled aboard along with cocaine and marijuana in coffee containers, suitcases and baggage holds as part of an astonishingly brazen criminal operation run out of Miami International Airport. A two-year sting operation last week yielded indictments of 58 American Airlines baggage handlers and food contract workers, as well as three law-enforcement officials.

Predictably enough, the drugs were from Colombia, a nation whose economy is now essentially run by narcotics traffickers. Interdiction is proving to be a Vietnam-style quagmire, sucking billions into an increasingly militarized fiasco. Meanwhile, heroin use in the United States has spiked so much that it recently passed cocaine as the second most common reason (behind alcohol) for users to check into treatment centers.

Grim news, yes, though the overall drug picture in the United States is not as dark as the legalizers would have it. In fact, there are nearly 10 million fewer drug users than in 1985, when the crack epidemic ripped through urban America. "We know what works in terms of prevention," says James Burke, who heads the Partnership for a Drug-Free America. "As perception of risk and social disapproval go up, usage goes down across every ethnic and age group." That decline in demand has in turn driven a decline in crime rates, which are closely related to drugs.

Even so, the collateral damage of the drug war has been immense, and it may yet reverberate through American politics. The reason Gov. George W. Bush isn't being held to account for refusing to answer questions about using cocaine in his 20s is that Ameri-

cans are basically fair-minded; it was a long time ago. But that same sense of fairness might now, ironically, put the whole subject of drugs back on the table for some serious rethinking—about the glaring injustices of the criminal justice system; the moral ambiguities of baby-boomer parenting; the twists of fate that can leave one man a prisoner, another a possible president.

The drug war can't be abandoned—too many lives are destroyed by drugs—but it can be fought without savage inequities and mindless human warehousing. The U.S. prison population—now at 1.8 million—has nearly quadrupled since the early 1980s. More than half of all American prisoners are nonviolent offenders—usually small-time drug dealers who need help with their own addictions. Many learn in prison how to be real criminals. Their children, in turn, are likely to continue the cycle. (Half the prisoners in Kansas, for instance, have parents who have been imprisoned, too.) U.S. leaders know this. Gen. Barry McCaffrey, the nation's drug czar and an advocate of increased treatment, says "we cannot arrest our way out of the problem."

Yet the United States is still doing just that. While many neighborhoods are deeply grateful to have been cleared of drug dealers, the enforcement of drug laws remains patently unjust. "When it's a low-income kid, it's a criminal-justice problem," says Marc Mauer of the Washington, D.C.-based Sentencing Project. "When it is a suburban kid, it's a health issue."

That inequity began in the 1980s. In the wake of the 1986 death of basketball star Len Bias from a cocaine overdose, Congress and the country panicked. Federal sentencing guidelines, in place for only two years, were tossed aside in favor of extraordinarily rigid "mandatory minimums" that tie the

hands of judges in federal drug cases. Bias died from powdered cocaine, but it was crack—used mostly by minorities—that was the target of the new laws. Possession of five grams of crack (about the size of a pack of sugar) brings a mandatory five-year sentence. The same sentence for powdered cocaine requires possession of 500 grams—a 100-fold differential. Crack and coke are pharmacologically identical; only the delivery system (smoking versus sniffing) varies.

Judges, including Supreme Court Justice Anthony Kennedy, a Reagan appointee, have complained about mandatory minimums for years, but politicians won't listen. So the unfairness continues. California U.S. District Court Judge Terry Hatter explains how the system now works in federal cases: "It's all decided behind closed doors by the [prosecutors] and never heard before the public. Judges now have less authority than young lawyers fresh out of law school who are working at the U.S. Attorney's office."

THE PUBLIC WRONGLY ASSUMES that if it's a federal case, it must involve drug kingpins. But Department of Justice figures show that 36 percent of federal drug-law offenders are "low level" violators—small-time, nonviolent dealers and their sometimes unwitting friends. Judge Hatter says that many of them land in the federal system arbitrarily: "Police officers get angry with a particular person they arrest and then send them to federal court instead of state court."

Then there's the informant game. Those who implicate others get their sentences reduced, which in practice means that bigger fish—who can finger more people—sometimes get shorter sentences than defendants who are less involved in the drug scene.

Mandatory minimums can create maximum strangeness in sentencing. According

From *Newsweek*, September 6, 1999, pp. 25-28. © 1999 by Newsweek, Inc. All rights reserved. Reprinted by permission.

A System Under Stress

Drug use may be down, but drug offenders are helping to fill up prisons.

Behind Bars

▓ PRISONERS JAILED FOR DRUG OFFENSES

STATE PRISONS

6%
1980

23%
1996

FEDERAL PRISONS

25%
1980

60%
1996

Cocaine Use

MILLIONS

6
4
2

1979   98

Crack Cases

A person selling 5 grams of crack cocaine is subject to the same mandatory prison sentence as one selling 500 grams of powder cocaine

Punishments

FEDERAL SENTENCES, SIMPLE DRUG POSSESSION

Probation	56.5%
Prison	34.4%
Probation and Confinement	8.4%
Prison/Community Confinement	0.7%

SOURCES: U.S. SENTENCING COMMISSION, NATIONAL HOUSEHOLD SURVEY ON DRUG ABUSE

to the book "Shattered Lives," more than 2,000 "Deadheads" have been sent to expensive federal prison after undercover agents infiltrated Grateful Dead concerts. Small-time pot growers are often sent away for years, not months. Same with small-fry couriers. Because mandatory minimums are based on weight, LSD-laced sugar cubes automatically bring longer sentences than lighter but equally potent blotter acid.

Some state courts are even harsher than the Feds. In Texas, Melinda George, with no prior drug arrests, angered a jury by missing a court appearance. Jurors saw to it that she was sentenced to 99 years for possession with intent to distribute of one tenth of a gram of cocaine—the equivalent of one "line" of the drug. Besides making it easier to sentence first-time offenders to jail, Governor Bush signed a bill requiring stiffer penalties for dealers whose drugs lead to overdoses. That sounds sensible enough, but opponents say that in practice it means over-

dosing drug users and their friends will wait longer before going to the hospital for fear of arrest.

Other states are moving away from inflexible sentencing. "States are ahead of Washington on this," says Monica Pratt of Families Against Mandatory Minimums. Michigan last year repealed its "650-lifer" law, which required life sentences for anyone caught with 650 or more grams of hard drugs. Arizona is the first state to offer treatment instead of jail to all of its nonviolent drug offenders. The early results are promising, with more than 70 percent of those on probation testing clean. (Treatment is also much less expensive for the state than incarceration.)

Even in New York, home of the draconian "Rockefeller laws" that cracked down on drugs, first-time offenders arrested for possession rarely end up in jail. Repeat offenders are also offered a drug-treatment alternative to prison. Surprisingly, most offenders don't enroll; they fear automatic incarceration for as much as nine years if they fail the program. But the stick of jail time can also be helpful. Those who complete the New York program have a high success rate in staying off drugs.

Drug treatment often fails, especially when it's short-term. "A lot of these programs don't work," says Rep. John Mica. But they almost always save the government money. A State of California study showed that every dollar spent on treatment saved seven dollars in reduced hospital admissions and law-enforcement costs. That's because each day an addict is on the wagon is a day he's not draining money from society. A 1997 Rand Corporation study found that "treatment reduces about ten times more serious crime than conventional enforcement and 15 times more than mandatory minimums." In some places, the message is getting through. Special "drug courts," begun in Florida in 1992, are now in 400 locations nationally, with specially trained judges mixing treatment and jail as appropriate in individual cases.

Unfortunately, drug courts handle fewer than 2 percent of drug cases. And even as drug-treatment spending is rising overall, in-

jail treatment is actually declining. In 1997, only 15 percent of state and federal inmates received substance-abuse treatment during their current terms, down from one third getting help in 1991. This is especially damaging because, as the Columbia University Center on Addiction and Substance Abuse keeps proving, treating all addicted prisoners before release is essential. According to a Bureau of Prisons study, inmates who have received treatment are 73 percent less likely to be re-arrested in the first six months after release than those who have not.

There are other intriguing ideas coming to the surface of the drug debate. Former New York mayor Ed Koch, along with his old enemy Al Sharpton and Harvard Law School professor Charles Ogletree, has been circulating a "second chance" plan for some nonviolent drug felons (not those who, say, smuggle drugs aboard an airliner). If they complete their sentences, receive a high-school equivalency diploma and are certified drug-free a year or two after release, these ex-cons would be eligible for pardons that would expunge their felonies. This would allow them to vote, find better jobs and be more suitable marriage prospects. In other words, move on—just as the 70 million other Americans who were not punished for their youthful mistakes were able to do.

Can any of this pierce the drug-war platitudes of a presidential campaign? Of the major candidates, only Bill Bradley has said he would take a fresh look at mandatory minimums. So far, Bush's "compassionate conservatism" has not included any talk of compassionate treatment options for drug abusers. It's unclear whether the questions about his past will make Bush more likely to show leadership here—or less. "The 'I didn't inhale' led to such ridicule that Clinton was traumatized, and so he hasn't done any reform," says Michael Massing, author of "The Fix," a pro-treatment book. Bush says he's a different kind of baby boomer. Now he and the rest of the pack will have to show that they mean it—by thinking anew about drugs.

With Gregory Beals *in New York*

Governments and Drugs

The Netherlands: Let's Be Realistic

Drug use is a fact of life and needs to be discouraged in as practical a manner as possible.

HERBERT P. BARNARD

The Dutch policy on drugs is a disastrous mistake. The Netherlands regrets its liberal policy and is about to turn back the clock." "Drug use has increased by 250 percent in two years, armed robberies by 70 percent, shoot-outs by 40 percent, and car thefts by 60 percent." "In the Netherlands, 1,600 addicts receive daily injections of heroin on government orders." "In Amsterdam recently, a father who was addicted to cannabis massacred his whole family." "There's plenty of heroin for sale in every Dutch coffee shop."

Do you believe all this? I am quoting just a few statements by foreign politicians and other "experts" who disagree with the Netherlands' drug policy. There is evidently an audience willing to believe all this, which gives such critics a reason to continue spreading these stories. Aside from questioning the honesty of this approach, one should ask what purpose is served by repeating such nonsense. It is certainly not in the interest of drug users, their immediate neighbors, the government, or health-care and social service institutions.

The drug problem is too serious an issue to be used as a political football by ambitious politicians. Nor should it be the subject of speculations about reality, making the facts of the matter irrelevant. As a representative of the Netherlands government, I take this opportunity to present the facts.

To understand the Dutch drug policy, you need to know a little about the Netherlands and the Dutch people. After all, a country's drug policy has to fit in with the nation's characteristics and culture.

The Netherlands is one of the most densely populated countries in the world, with around 15.5 million people in an area one-quarter the size of New York State. Commerce and transport have traditionally been important sectors of industry in our country. Rotterdam is the busiest port in the world, handling almost 5 million containers a year. In fact, the Netherlands is generally seen as the gateway to Europe.

The Dutch have a strong belief in individual freedom. Government is expected to avoid becoming involved in matters of morality and religion. At the same time, we feel a strong sense of responsibility for the well-being of the community.

The Netherlands has a very extensive system of social security, while health care and education are accessible to everyone. What is the Dutch drug policy? The main objective is to minimize the risks associated with drug use, both for users themselves and those around them. This objective was formulated in the mid-1970s and can be characterized as harm reduction *avant la lettre*.

Many elements of the harm-reduction approach are very similar to Dutch drug policy. Our policy does not moralize but is based on the idea that drug use is a fact of life and needs to be discouraged in as practical a manner as possible. This calls for a pragmatic and flexible approach that recognizes the risks for both drug users and those around them.

Our policy focuses on reducing demand as well as supply. A combination of these two instruments requires close cooperation with public health and law enforcement authorities on all policy levels, Furthermore, we invest a lot of money in cure and prevention. Since the 1970s and early '80s, respectively, low-threshold methadone provision and needle exchange programs have been important elements in our harm-reduction approach.

Our policy is based on two important principles. The first is the distinction between types of drugs, based on their harmfulness (hemp products on the one hand and drugs with unacceptable risks on the other). The second legal principle is a differentiation according to the nature of the punishable acts, such as the distinction between the possession of small quantities of drugs for one's own use and possession with intent to deal. This makes it possible to pursue a finely tuned policy based on the application of criminal law.

The possession of up to 30 grams of cannabis is a petty offense punishable with a fine. The sale of small amounts of cannabis, through what are known as "coffee shops," subject to strict conditions, is not prosecuted. The idea behind the policy on coffee shops is that of "separating the markets." The reasoning is that if retailers of cannabis are not prosecuted under certain conditions, the experimenting user will not be forced to move in criminal circles, where higher profits are made by urging users to take more dangerous drugs (such as heroin).

People often think that drugs are available legally in the Netherlands and that we do not focus on combating the supply side of the drug market. Nothing could be less true. Aside from the retail trade in cannabis, a high priority is given to tackling all other forms of drug dealing. The police and customs authorities seize large consignments of drugs almost every week, working closely with other countries in the fight against organized crime.

Some people think that harm reduction and legalization are synonymous. I disagree and would like to emphasize that harm reduction is not legalization in disguise. Harm reduction is first and foremost concerned with reducing the risks and hazards of drug taking. Harm reduc-

tion is meant to reduce the risks for not only the drug user but the immediate environment (i.e., the public) and society as well. This implies that intensive cooperation at all times between those providing care for addicts, the criminal justice authorities, and the government is an essential element in the harm reduction approach.

What are the results of our policy? The Dutch government recently issued a document discussing its drug policy, evaluating the policy of the last 20 years, and mapping out approaches for the future. This paper can be compared with the yearly *National Drug Control Strategies of the White House Office of National Drug Control Policy*. I will summarize the main outcomes.

Regarding the evaluation of Dutch policy on hard drugs, the document makes the following points:

Our policy of harm reduction has been quite successful. Thanks to a high standard of care and prevention, including extensive low-level and nonconditional methadone prescription, social and medical assistance for drug users, and a large-scale free needle-exchange program, we have reached a situation that is matched by few other countries.

The number of addicts in the Netherlands is relatively low compared with that in many countries. This implies that harm-reduction measures do not increase the use of drugs.

The population of addicts is rather stable and rapidly aging. This suggests that few new users are joining in. Heroin is not fashionable among youngsters. The average age of Amsterdam methadone-provision clients increases by almost one every year, and the *number* of young heroin users using services like methadone provision has shrunk over the years to a handful. The average age of Amsterdam methadone-provision clients was 36.2 years in 1995. The average age of newly registered drug clients in the Netherlands was 32 years in 1995.

The mortality rate among drug users is low, due to the low-threshold methadone programs that provide protection against overdose.

The damage to health caused by the use of hard drugs has been kept within limits. The number of addicts infected with HIV is exceptionally low. In the Netherlands, the percentage of intravenous drug users (IDUs) among the total cumulative number of AIDS cases is low. In addition, the incidence of HIV infections among IDUs has decreased since 1986. An evaluation study concluded that a combination of harm-reduction measures (i.e., methadone provision, needle exchange, training, and counseling) has resulted in safer sexual and drug-taking behaviors. Safe sex practices among addicted prostitutes have increased as well.

Another result of our policy is that a comparatively large proportion of drug users in our country has been integrated into society to a reasonable extent.

The number of regular hemp smokers has gradually increased in recent years. Lifetime prevalence and last-month prevalence have increased substantially since 1984. An annual survey among older pupils in Amsterdam showed, however, that the prevalence of cannabis use has stabilized since 1993–94. This might indicate that we have reached the peak of the upward trend of the past years.

Can the increase in cannabis use, especially among students, be attributed to the existence of coffee shops in the Netherlands? An analysis of surveys shows an upward trend in many other European countries. Since the late 1980s, cannabis use among youngsters (as well as the general population) has increased in France, the United Kingdom, Germany, and the United States. Compared with the U.S. prevalence, the figures for the Netherlands are considerably lower. According to the results of the 1995 *Monitoring the Future Surveys,* published by the University of Michigan, cannabis use has increased tremendously among American youngsters. To my knowledge, this increase cannot be attributed to any significant change of policy.

The fact that the rate of cannabis use in the Netherlands is comparable with that in other countries (and even lower than in the United States) shows that government policy probably has less influence on use than we think. Other factors, such as trends in youth culture, social differences, and other social influences, probably play a far more important role. In our view, this does not mean that it makes no difference whether one pursues a liberal or a restrictive drug policy. The difference is that a tolerant policy prevents the marginalization of the user. A situation often encountered in other nations, where the user—in most cases a minor—runs the risk of getting into trouble with the police, is seen as highly undesirable in my country.

Some conclusions

1. Comparisons with other countries show no indications that our policy has led to an increase in the number of cannabis users. Therefore, there is no reason to change our policy on cannabis.

2. Our policy on cannabis has not led to an increase in the number of hard-drug users. In the Netherlands, the steppingstone hypothesis cannot be confirmed.

3. The wide range of provisions for care and prevention has held down the number of hard-drug users, and has ensured that the health of these users can be described as reasonable. Harm reduction actually works, if you invest in it.

4. By definition, the Dutch drug policy requires an integral cooperation with public health, law enforcement, and public order officials. The Dutch drug policy, therefore, is not a disastrous experiment but a serious effort to tackle a serious issue. Our policy has produced results that are demonstrably better than those in many of the countries criticizing us. While we realize that an ongoing dialogue with all those involved with the drug problem is a precondition for any progress, we are not going to change our policy on the basis of unjustified criticism.

Herbert P. Barnard is counselor for health and welfare at the Royal Netherlands Embassy.

Q: Would legalizing drugs serve America's national interest?

Yes: Take huge profits away from criminals and invest the money in harm reduction.

BY DIRK CHASE ELDREDGE

Eldredge served as co-chairman of Ronald Reagan's first California gubernatorial campaign and is author of Ending the War on Drugs—A Solution for America.

America's war on drugs is reminiscent of the Russian princess who wept profusely at the death of the hero in the opera, while, at the curb, her waiting carriage driver froze to death in a cruel Moscow ice storm. Policy makers are deeply preoccupied with waging the war on drugs. While they do, the destructive, albeit unintended, consequences continue to pile up like the icy snows of Moscow.

The world would be a much better place if illicit drugs didn't exist, but they do, so we must deal with them. Our challenge is to do so in a way that will advance our national interest. Our failed war on drugs is doing just the opposite; America must respond to that reality with a basic change in approach.

Legalization is the only practical way to bring about positive results. The money legalization would generate to fight drug abuse would make harm reduction—rather than the twice-failed policy of prohibition—the fulcrum of our drug policy. The failure of prohibition as public policy stems from its transformation of some citizens' cocktail-hour-like drug use and others' medical and psychological problems into crimes. It is no less devastating than if we made both possession and consumption of alcoholic beverages illegal. Social drinkers and alcoholics alike would suddenly be criminalized.

As it always does, prohibition has spawned a robust black market that inevitably has spun off other social pathologies such as violence and corruption. Furthermore, it is a policy that can only fail because its objective—a drug-free America—is unrealistic and unattainable.

Supporters of the drug war allege that we are winning, citing as proof a decline in drug use from the peak years of the 1970s, but that drop came to an abrupt end in 1992. The number of regular users has increased each year since then among several age groups.

Many argue against the decriminalization of drugs on the grounds that more people would abuse drugs than under prohibition. This politically popular theory is unsubstantiated and misleading. Within any group there are a certain number prone to abuse of mind-altering substances. This propensity for abuse has everything to do with the individual's personal value system and psychological stability and absolutely nothing to do with the legal status of drugs. Legalizing currently illegal drugs will neither increase nor decrease the number of people inclined toward, or indulging in, addictive behavior.

Those inclined to addictive behavior have that inclination independent of the law of the land and have ample opportunity to obtain drugs under existing laws and customs. They have two major mind-altering alternatives available that are legal: prescription drugs and alcohol. A third alternative is illegal drugs.

What effect will legalization have on the abuse of drugs? To answer that question intelligently we must understand that drug use is not necessarily drug abuse. The try-and-die concept promoted by the drug warriors simply does not square with the facts. The vast majority of drug users fall into the recreational category. For instance, less than 1 percent of those who try cocaine become daily users, and 74 percent of regular cocaine users use it less than once a month. Looked at in the context of these facts instead of the hysteria promoted by the defenders of the status quo, it is not surprising that three different studies have shown only 2 to 4 percent of respondents would try now-illegal drugs if they were legalized. Given the small percentage of drug users who lapse into abuse, this hardly suggests that legalization will trigger a mass movement into drug abuse. Legalization re-asserts the truth that we are all responsible for our own behavior.

The drug war, while barren of results, is rich in ironies. For example, increased law-enforcement pressure on smuggling encourages more concentrated drugs, leading to less bulk and reduced chance of discovery. Some recent samples of heroin are 90 percent pure, compared with 7 to 15 percent purity a few years ago. This greater potency has added to heroin's popularity, exactly the opposite of what law enforcement intends, because heroin is by far the most dangerous street drug.

Our national amnesia over alcohol prohibition destines us to repeat an unintended consequence from that era. During Prohibition, the consumption of lower-potency alcoholic beverages, such as beer, plummeted while the market share of moonshine and other strong distilled spirits soared. Soon after repeal, the consumption patterns of both high- and low-potency beverages returned to pre-Prohibition levels. From this experience, we can extrapolate that today's shift to more-potent drugs is directly related to drug prohibition.

Prohibition dictates that illicit drugs only can be obtained via the black market. Prices are whatever the market will bear, resulting in high prices and obscene profits. Because drugs are so expensive, many users recruit friends to become users so they can sell drugs to them and help defray their own costs. In fact, 70 percent of those who deal drugs also are users. This results in the drug market's version of a Mary Kay network. Think for a moment about the size and motivation of the resulting drug-sales force which would immediately be immobilized by legalization.

One of the most damaging aspects of the drug black market is the allure of the easy money it makes available

to our inner-city youth. A 16-year-old from Washington, virtually unemployable after having been arrested 12 times, manages to clear the heady sum of $300 to $400 a day selling crack. "I don't want to make this a life thing," he alleges. "Ill quit when I get out of high school." He then makes a telling and contradictory admission: "But when you start you really can't stop. The money is too good."

With drugs, corruption is the cancer and money the carcinogen. The corruption of public officials—police, judges, border and prison guards, customs inspectors and others in positions of public trust—is a destructive consequence of our prohibitionist drug policies. Bribery corrupts far and wide. A law-enforcement officer can provide protection against arrest. A drug-cash-laden defendant can purchase perjured testimony or bribe a judge. The wide availability of drugs inside even our most secure prisons is powerful testimony to the corruption drug money can buy.

> ## Misdirected public policy, always clad in the armor of good intentions, carries with it the very real threat of repression.

And America is exporting this corruption. Ask the police officials of Mexico, Colombia and other source countries. American narco dollars pay for drug-related murders, kidnappings and bribery in those countries. Instead of owning up to the fact that our demand is the real cause of the problem, we try to export the blame as well. We indulge in the arrogant charade of certification, judging whether other nations are doing their part in fighting the drug problem, when we should be focusing on solving the problem, whose root cause lies directly at our feet. Without our demand there would be no supply.

Misdirected public policy, always clad in the armor of good intentions, carries with it the very real threat of repression wrought by the frustration-repression cycle of its own failure. As various drug-war tactics such as asset seizure and mandatory minimum sentences fail, policy makers can justify ever more desperate measures. The tight spiral of initiation, failure and more-desperate measures inevitably results in a creeping loss of civil liberties.

In response to the rising pitch of drug-war hysteria during the 1980s and 1990s, 28 states passed laws to tax the possession of illegal drugs, an idea that does violence both to the principle of fair taxation and respect for the rule of law. We have government declaring it illegal to possess marijuana and cocaine while simultaneously demanding payment of a tax for possession, a clear violation of the constitutional protection against self-incrimination. Despite court decisions overturning the laws, many states, most notably North Carolina, have tweaked their statutes to skirt the law and go right ahead collecting the tax. Not coincidentally, police and sheriff's departments get 75 percent of the take. This leads to the mixing of law enforcement with the profit motive, a recipe rife with opportunities for abuse. But never mind the danger to our civil liberties. This is war.

Because drug dealing and use are victimless crimes, the police must either personally observe the crime or participate in it in undercover mode to make a valid arrest. This makes drug-law enforcement doubly labor intensive. Those in law enforcement routinely estimate that more than half of today's crimes are drug-related, leading to the imprisonment of over 1 million citizens per year for drug-related crimes. This, in turn, has resulted in 40 states being placed under court order to end prison overcrowding.

A major cost of the drug war is the corrosive effect it is having on the confidence of black Americans in their government. A 1990 opinion poll of African-Americans in New York City showed 60 percent gave partial or full credence to the ludicrous charge that government deliberately makes sure drugs are easily available in poor, black neighborhoods in order to harm black people.

As demonstrated by the social pathologies enumerated above which derive directly from prohibition, like the Russian princess, America is so preoccupied with the show of prohibition it is oblivious to what is going on in the real world.

By legalizing drugs and selling them for about half the present prices through state-operated retail outlets similar to those in the 13 states that presently have state-controlled alcohol sales, we could produce profits of conservatively $21 billion per year to fund harm reduction. This money would be required, by law, to be used to buy the drugs for resale, run the outlets and fund treatment on demand ($12 billion), an anti-drug education program equal in cost to the combined advertising budgets of the big-three auto makers ($3.25 billion) and an AIDS-sized research budget ($1.3 billion) to find pharmacological solutions to drug addiction and dependence.

This would advance the national interest by making real progress against the drug problem, not through fear, coercion, and incarceration, but through education, treatment and research.

No: Don't wave the white flag yet, a true war on drugs has yet to be launched.

BY REP. BILL MCCOLLUM

McCollum, a Florida Republican, is chairman of the House Subcommittee on Crime and vice chairman of the Banking and Financial Services Committee.

No discussion on the merits of drug legalization is legitimate unless it is prefaced by these alarming, undisputed facts:

- Teen drug use has doubled since 1992;
- Nearly half of all 17-year-olds say they could buy marijuana within an hour;
- The number of heroin-related emergency-room admissions jumped 58 percent between 1992 and 1995;
- and, most shockingly, illegal drugs and drug-related crime and violence kill 20,000 Americans a year, at a cost of $67 billion.

If thousands of young Americans were killed in Bosnia or in any other place across the globe, there would be riots in the streets.

And yet, even with these troubling statistics as a backdrop, a small, vocal minority are advocating drug legalization as the cure for our nation's drug crisis. I can't think of a more grim proposal for our children and our nation.

Many legalization advocates argue that if drugs were legalized, crime and violence would decrease. The commonsense response to that argument is that the already unacceptably high level of teen drug use undoubtedly would soar even higher, dragging in its wake the societal problems that accompany drug use. The reality is that drug use is almost always a contributing factor to criminal behavior.

According to a survey of state prison inmates, 28 percent of prisoners convicted of murder, 20 percent of inmates convicted of sexual assault and 23 percent of inmates convicted of assault were under the influence of drugs when they committed their crimes. Another study indicated that drug users were 10 times more likely to commit a violent act than non-drug users. Drug use and crime go hand in hand—it is that simple. In fact, history has demonstrated the reverse effect drug legalization would have on crime rates. When California attempted to decriminalize marijuana in 1976, arrests for driving under the influence of drugs rose 46 percent among adults and 71.4 percent among juveniles within the first six months.

Another myth often associated with the legalization movement is that revenue and taxes from the sale of drugs would help boost the economy. This claim is flawed at best and unsubstantiated by facts. The economic benefit, if any, would be eclipsed by the billions spent treating the societal ills caused by drug abuse. The Drug Enforcement Administration, or DEA, estimates drug legalization would cost society between $140 billion and $210 billion a year in lost productivity and job-related accidents.

For instance, total tax revenue from the sale of alcohol is $13.1 billion a year, but alcohol extracts more than $100 billion a year in social costs such as health care and lost productivity. There is no evidence that taxing narcotics such as cocaine, heroin and marijuana would bolster revenues any more than alcohol does. And the expected revenue certainly would not offset the social and medical costs.

With 90 percent of the public against drug legalization, proponents have masked their tactics with phrases such as "drug reform," "medicalization" and "harm reduction." In an effort to chip away at our nation's drug laws, groups are promoting the adoption of loosely worded state ballot initiatives that would legalize marijuana for "medicinal use."

With clear evidence of marijuana's gateway effect—12 to 17-year-olds who use marijuana are 85 times more likely to use cocaine than those who abstain—these efforts are quite troubling. The cavalier labeling of a dangerous and highly addictive drug as "medicine" sends the wrong message to our youth.

An initiative that was proposed for this fall's ballot in Washington, D.C.—where 96 percent of all youth arrested for crime test positive for marijuana—would permit individuals to legally use marijuana for medical treatment when recommended by a licensed physician. No written prescription would be required. Like its highly publicized predecessors in California and Arizona, this initiative would have made growing, trafficking and possessing marijuana legal for almost any ailment. Unlike all other drugs used to treat illness or pain, no Food and Drug Administration, or FDA, approval would be necessary. When almost anyone could find a physician to recommend smoking marijuana for any ailment, policing illegal use and trafficking would become a practical impossibility.

While I do not possess the medical or scientific expertise to pass judgment on whether marijuana is a medicine, the FDA does. So do the National Institutes of Health, the American Medical Association, the American Cancer Society and the National Multiple Sclerosis Association. Yet, each and every one of these esteemed organizations has concluded marijuana has no medicinal value. The collective expert judgment of these organizations and the long-established FDA drug approval process cannot be ignored

simply because some people want to label marijuana "medicine." Science cannot be based on opinion polls.

For three decades, marijuana has been classified as a Schedule I drug, meaning it has a high potential for abuse, lacks any currently accepted medical use and is unsafe, even under medical supervision. According to the National Institute of Allergy and Infectious Diseases, HIV-positive smokers of marijuana progress to full-blown AIDS twice as fast as nonsmokers and have an increased incidence of bacterial pneumonia.

There is no doubt that these campaigns are more about drug legalization than about providing relief for the sick and dying. In 1993, Richard Cowen, director of the National Organization for the Reform of Marijuana Laws, declared " . . . medical marijuana is our strongest suit. It is our point of leverage which will move us toward the legalization of marijuana for personal use, and in that process we will begin to break down the power of the narcocracy to wage a war of terror over things."

I can think of no political strategy more unseemly than drug legalization masquerading as compassion. Voters and, more importantly, the seriously ill, deserve the facts, not emotional half-truths.

Legalization advocates point out that despite ongoing efforts, drug use is up. So why not wave the white flag in the drug war? While it's true that drugs are cheaper and more plentiful than ever before on the streets of America, now is not the time to abandon our efforts. The truth is, America has not been waging a true war on drugs. The lack of a balanced anti-narcotics strategy has played a key role in the rise in drug use. Not a single U.S. military airplane or warship is assigned to interdiction efforts in the Eastern Pacific between Colombia, Mexico and the United States. The number of flight and steaming hours spent patrolling the Caribbean Sea and Gulf of Mexico has been cut by two-thirds since 1992. With the exception of the U.S.-Mexico border effort, resources to intercept drugs entering the country from source countries and the transit zone have also been cut by two-thirds since 1992.

Despite clear evidence that a balanced approach to the drug war achieved real success (from 1988 to 1991, cocaine use dropped by 35 percent and marijuana use dropped by 16 percent), in mid-1993 the Clinton administration made a very public, "controlled shift" in its drug strategy. This shift resulted in increased funding for prevention and treatment efforts at the expense of interdiction efforts. Since 1993, funds dedicated to international interdiction efforts have continued to languish around 13 percent of total federal expenditures on the drug war, as opposed to the 33 percent allotted in 1987.

> **Prevent drugs from entering the country and you drive up the price of drugs. Drive up the price of drugs and you save lives.**

The result? Quantity is up, price is down and more kids are becoming users. Let's not kid ourselves. Drug trafficking is a business. The less it costs to grow and transport illegal drugs into this country, the lower the price of drugs on the street. Therefore, reducing the flow of drugs entering the United States must be a top priority. Until the availability of drugs is dramatically reduced and the price driven up, education and law-enforcement efforts cannot be expected to succeed in any meaningful way.

All the cocaine entering the United States originates in Colombia, Peru and Bolivia. Most of the heroin in the country is grown and produced in Colombia. When I visited these countries earlier this year, key U.S. antinarcotics personnel told me that the supply of drugs leaving those countries could be reduced by 80 percent in only a couple of years if our government would commit the necessary resources and adjust its policies in cooperation with the source-country governments.

Peru, which already has adopted more aggressive tactics, is producing results. In the two years since Peruvian President Alberto Fujimori implemented a get-tough, antitrafficking and crop-eradication program—including shooting down drug smugglers' aircraft—cocaine production in Peru has dropped 40 percent. With more U.S. support, victory over the narcotics trade in Peru is within reach. The same could be accomplished in Bolivia and Colombia with the cooperation of their governments and a continued U.S. effort to keep radar and tracking planes in the air 24 hours a day.

A continued investment in demand-reduction strategies is critical. I strongly support finding ways to persuade Americans that doing drugs is wrong—that it destroys lives, families, schools and communities. But we need a comprehensive counter-drug strategy that addresses all components of this problem. The lesson of the past decade is simple: Prevent drugs from entering the country and you drive up the price of drugs. Drive up the price of drugs and you save lives.

Unfortunately, a lot has changed in recent years. Instead of a comprehensive drug-education effort in our schools, homes and workplaces, we see attitudes of indifference and ambivalence. The legalization movement is but one reason why the message that drug use is both destructive and wrong has been lost. Sadly, today's youth increasingly see no harm in using drugs.

This dramatic reversal in trends spells grave harm for both the present and the future. We owe it to our kids to wage a true war on drugs.

Industry foes fume over the tobacco deal

They insist it won't slow teenage smoking

BY JOSEPH P. SHAPIRO

The massive $206 billion settlement between the states and cigarette makers may accomplish many things, but deterring people—especially teens—from smoking is not likely to be among them. The deal contains few fresh approaches to solving one of the nation's most intractable health care dilemmas. Just how stubborn the problem is became clear last week in a new study that surprised even the most experienced public health experts: It showed a sharp rise in smoking among college students, the one group of teens that in the past had resisted tobacco's temptations.

Despite that blunt reminder of tobacco's lure, few chapters in the history of America's smoking wars were more consequential than a four-day stretch last week. On Monday, a group of state attorneys general at a crowded Washington press conference released details of the deal they had negotiated with cigarette makers to settle state lawsuits to recover the health costs of treating smokers. The money on the table—to be paid out over 25 years—was a tempting jackpot for governors. But, like hungry salesmen of timeshare condos, the negotiators gave other states just four days to analyze 146 pages of legalese and decide whether to sign on or to gamble on grabbing more money by pursuing individual suits. Former Surgeon General C. Everett Koop and former Food and Drug Administration chief David Kessler were among public health officials urging rejection of the deal, accusing the states of selling their "virtue if the price is right" to give Big Tobacco protection against future lawsuits. Still, by week's end, no state took a pass on the largest civil settlement ever. (Four states settled

New study shows young people are lighting up more than ever these days.

earlier suits.) Tobacco firms will ink the deal this week.

State officials, President Clinton, and even tobacco industry representatives hailed the agreement as a milestone for fighting teen smoking. But the rhetoric that this was all for the kids was belied by what the deal left out. Unlike the $368.5 billion settlement between states and tobacco—which crumbled in June when Congress failed to approve it—the new pact is softer on tobacco. There's no federal regulation of nicotine, as the original bargain stipulated. (As a result, Congress won't have a say in this deal.) Also missing this time: penalties for tobacco companies if teen smoking rates do not drop, and an end to cigarette vending machines, the easiest place for kids to buy cigarettes. Public health groups vowed to ask Congress for such tools to fight tobacco. The American Heart Association's Cass Wheeler summed up the public health community's mixed reaction to the settlement: "Perfect? No. A beginning? Yes."

Nipped in the butt? Even the weapons provided may do little to discourage smokers. Tobacco companies will be banned from using cartoon characters—which attract young smokers—in ads.

But R. J. Reynolds, under public pressure, already killed its Joe Camel ads. And the Marlboro Man and other appealing tobacco symbols stay. Clothes and merchandise with tobacco logos will be barred, but stores can still post cigarette ads. About $2 billion will be set aside for antismoking research and ad campaigns. Nothing in the agreement requires states to spend any of the settlement to reduce tobacco use.

Perhaps the best way to deter smoking is simply to raise the price of cigarettes. Various studies show that a 10 percent increase could reduce overall smoking rates by about 4 percent—and smoking among teens even more. (But other studies show black-market sales burgeon as the nicotine-addicted seek cheaper alternatives.) Tobacco industry analysts expect the price of a pack of cigarettes to rise 35 cents over the next few years, as tobacco makers look to recoup the settlement costs. But even that is far less than the $1.10 federal excise tax that Congress sought last spring.

Yet it was the study of college-student smokers that mocked the celebration over the tobacco settlement. Harvard School of Public Health researchers, publishing in the *Journal of the American Medical Association*, reported smoking jumped 28 percent among college students between 1993 and 1997. The authors blamed cigarette marketing. But researchers know that even in California, a state considered a model for its aggressive antismoking advertising and school programs, teen smoking is peaking again. Peer pressure seems to trump even the best-thought-out antismoking strategies. And that's something that no tobacco deal can touch.

COLOMBIA

The Narco-Guerrilla War

A mysterious U.S. Army plane crash highlights the Pentagon's biggest covert operation in Latin America

By JOSHUA HAMMER AND
MICHAEL ISIKOFF

WHEN A U.S. ARMY PLANE went down in the jungles of southern Colombia, American officials sought to downplay it as a routine anti-narcotics patrol. But this was guerrilla country, a stronghold of the Marxist Revolutionary Armed Forces of Colombia (FARC). And the U.S. Army DeHavilland RC–7 was packed with sophisticated intelligence equipment for the interception of radio and mobile-phone communications—just the sort of equipment that would be useful in tracking guerrilla movements. "This had to do with surveillance," said one source familiar with the flight's mission. "We're not supposed to be monitoring guerrillas, but that's what they were doing." American officials in Colombia are only supposed to be fighting drugs. But as Colombia's guerrillas turn to drug trafficking to finance their 40-year-old struggle, the war against drugs becomes a war against them too.

The crash of the U.S. spy plane was only the most recent example of the Pentagon's rapidly expanding role in Colombia's civil war. NEWSWEEK has learned that more than 300 American personnel are in the country, 200 of them soldiers and more than 100 Drug Enforcement Administration and CIA operatives. Already the United States is pouring $250 million into Colombia, making it the third-biggest recipient of U.S. aid, after Egypt and Israel. The White House drug czar, Barry McCaffrey, visited the country last week and proposed doubling that amount. McCaffrey arrived just as Colombian and American search and rescue teams reached the wreckage of the RC–7 plane containing the bodies of five American soldiers—including a woman pilot—plus two Colombians. Nor were these the first Americans to die. Since 1997 three American pilots flying drug-interdiction missions for Dyn-

Corp, a private U.S. military contractor, have been killed. Some U.S. officials are wary. "What you have here is a 1964 model of Vietnam," said one congressional staffer.

So far the largely covert effort, easily the biggest U.S. military mission in Latin America, has had little effect. Buoyed by an estimated $600 million in annual profits from the drug trade, the FARC has built up its armory and extended its control. "There are armed organizations with more automatic weapons than the Colombian Army," McCaffrey told NEWSWEEK. In early July the FARC launched its biggest offensive in 40 years, seizing 15 villages, including one just 30 miles from Bogotá. The assault sent a terrifying message that the insurgents could assemble in large numbers and attack nearly anywhere in Colombia. Last Friday the Army accused FARC of setting off a car bomb in front of its offices in Medellín, killing 10 persons.

Until recently Colombia's drug war has been fought by its national police, not the Army. The police force sprays fields with chemical defoliants in conjunction with DynCorp, and conducts helicopter raids on drug laboratories—mostly carried out in aging Vietnam-era A1–H1 "Hueys." But the police lack the arms and the training to battle an increasingly aggressive guerrilla force. "The police are getting their a—s kicked," says a top-ranking U.S. military source in Colombia. "They go in with two helicopters, they run into a hundred FARC on the ground and they get chewed up."

That may soon change, thanks to prodding from the Pentagon and conservative congressmen. This September the national police will receive six Black Hawk attack helicopters, high-altitude fliers that can provide protection to planes defoliating mountainside poppy fields. By December the U.S. Special Forces will have finished training a

special anti-narcotics battalion of the Colombian Army, a 980-man, rapid-reaction force capable of taking on the FARC on its own turf. Some congressmen worry, though, about the deplorable human-rights record of the Colombian military, which often actively cooperates with right-wing paramilitaries. In the first four months of this year, the paramilitaries killed or "disappeared" 400 suspected guerrilla sympathizers. "Every soldier in that counterterrorism battalion has been cleared by the U.S. State Department," insists one high-ranking U.S. official. There are also doubts that targeting the coca fields makes sense. The areas of cultivation are vast, bigger than Switzerland. "There are not enough chemicals in the entire United States to kill the s— down there," says a U.S. military source in Bogotá. Areas of cocaine cultivation have actually increased by 50 percent in the past two years, according to a congressional report.

American officials say that taking no action against the FARC will invite a widening of the civil war, and a flood of cocaine and heroin onto America's streets. "There is no desire in the United States to send troops to Colombia to fight a guerrilla war that Colombians themselves have—until recently—not committed themselves to fighting," says one U.S. government source. He insisted, though, that only military hardware—not men—will be dispatched to Colombia's guerrilla-ruled jungles. That promise sounded somewhat hollow as Capt. Jennifer Odom, 29, the pilot, and the four other U.S. crew members were flown back in body bags to Dover Air Force Base in Delaware at 2 a.m. Saturday, for a ceremony closed to the public. At the rate things are going, they may not be the last ones to make that sad journey.

With MARK DUFFY *in Bogotá and*
JOHN BARRY *in Washington*

Unit 8

Key Points to Consider

❖ How effective are drug education and prevention programs? Are they too generic? How are they assessed and evaluated?

❖ Does the responsibility for drug education and prevention programs lie with the family, the schools, the police, or the federal government? Explain. Who is willing or unwilling to get involved?

❖ How effective is drug treatment? Do you agree or disagree that providing free, publicly sponsored drug programs would be one way to greatly reduce America's drug problem?

❖ What must treatment programs and treatment philosophy consider when providing services to a diverse population of clients? If an addicted friend or loved one asked your advice on finding treatment, how would you respond? What are your options?

❖ How does the prevailing American attitude toward drug addiction reflect an uncomfortable resistance toward becoming involved?

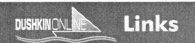 **Links**   **www.dushkin.com/online/**

These sites are annotated on pages 4 and 5.

There are no magic bullets for preventing drug abuse and treating drug-dependent persons. As one commentator stated, "Drug addicts can be cured, but we're not very good at it!" History is replete with accounts of the diverse attempts of frustrated societies to reclaim or reject their fallen members. Addicts have been executed, imprisoned, and treated with ambivalent indifference. In some circles, the debate still rages as to whether addicts suffer from a pernicious disease or simply a weak character. The evolution of processes used to rehabilitate addicted persons and prevent future abuse has been slow and filled with paradox. Yet the case is not lost. On the contrary, great new strides have been made in not only understanding the various genetic, physiological, psychological, and environmental frameworks that combine to serve as a basis for addiction but in using these frameworks successfully to treat and prevent dependency. Research continues to establish and strengthen the role of treatment as a critical component in the fight against drug abuse. Some drug treatment programs have been shown to reduce dramatically the costs associated with high-risk populations of users. For example, recidivism associated with drug abuse has been shown to decrease 50 percent after treatment. Treatment is a critical component in the fight against drug abuse but it is not a panacea. Society cannot "treat" drug abuse away just as it cannot "arrest" it away.

Drug prevention and treatment philosophies subscribe to a multitude of modalities. Everything seems to work a little and nothing seems to work completely. The following articles illustrate the diversity of methods utilized in prevention and treatment programs. Also illustrated is the struggle in which prevention and treatment programs compete for local, state, and federal resources.

Prevention

A primary strategy of drug prevention programs is to prevent and/or delay initial drug use. A secondary strategy is to discourage use by persons minimally involved with drugs. Both strategies include: (1) educating users and potential users, (2) teaching adolescents how to resist peer pressure, (3) addressing problems associated with drug abuse such as teen pregnancy, failure in school, and lawbreaking, and (4) creating community support and involvement for prevention activities.

Prevention programs are administered through a variety of mechanisms. Schools are an important delivery apparatus, as are local law enforcement agencies. Over 10 thousand police officers are involved in the Drug Abuse Resistance Education program (D.A.R.E.), provided to over 5 million students each year. Other prevention programs are community-based and sponsored by civic organizations, church groups, and private corporations. All programs pursue funding through public grants and private endowments. Federal grants to local, state, and private programs are critical components to program solvency.

The multifaceted nature of prevention programs makes them difficult to assess categorically. School programs that emphasize the development of skills to resist social and peer pressure produce generally varying degrees of positive results. Research continues to make more evident the need to focus prevention programs with specific populations in mind.

Treatment

Like prevention programs, drug treatment programs enlist a variety of methods to treat persons dependent upon legal and illegal drugs. There is no single-pronged approach to treatment for drug abuse. Treatment modality may differ radically from one user to the next. The user's background, physical and mental health, personal motivation, and support structure all have serious implications for treatment type. Lumping together the diverse needs of chemically dependent persons for purposes of applying a generic treatment process provides confounding results at best. In addition, most persons needing and seeking treatment have problems with more than one drug—polydrug use. Studies have shown that 54 percent of drug abusers and 37 percent of alcohol abusers have, in addition to their drug problem, at least one serious mental illness. Identifying a user's drug and associated mental health problem is referred to as dual diagnosis. The implications of such a diagnosis are serious, as it is estimated that there are 30 to 40 million chemically dependent persons in this country. The popularity of cocaine and methamphetamine use is felt to have increased the percentage of dually diagnosed persons because of the potential of these drugs to alter negatively neurochemical balance, pushing already troubled persons into the realm of mental illness. Providing treatment services to dually diagnosed persons is one of the most difficult and troubling aspects of the treatment equation. Historically, drug treatment programs have avoided or denied services to addicts suffering from psychological disorders such as schizophrenia. Mental health service providers have responded similarly due to their inability to treat drug addiction.

Although treatment programs differ in methods, most provide a combination of key services. These include drug counseling, drug education, pharmacological therapy, psychotherapy, relapse prevention, and assistance with support structures. Treatment programs may be outpatient-oriented or residential in nature. Residential programs require patients to live at the facility for a prescribed period of time. These residential programs, often described as therapeutic communities, emphasize the development of social, vocational, and educational skills.

The number of available treatment programs is a continual political controversy with respect to federal and state drug budget expenditures. The current trend is toward increasing the availability of treatment programs. The best evidence suggests that while providing drug treatment is costly, not providing it is more costly.

The Tenacity of Error in the Treatment of Addiction

by

Michael J. Lemanski

It was a hot, humid July evening and I knew that the room wouldn't be air conditioned. I also knew that the atmosphere would be stuffy and repressive. It had been more than a decade since I'd been to an Al-Anon meeting but, strangely drawn to return, I walked in and was handed an information packet for newcomers. Then, as the group members went through the ritual of their readings, I went through the printed materials. And there it was: the very same pamphlet I'd found so offensive my first visit. I'd come back for one last look to see if anything had changed, but it was just as I'd remembered. The message was clear and essentially as before. The same, it turns out, can be said of the larger twelve-step movement and the addictions field in general: the message has developed little in the last six decades.

William Griffith Wilson, the founder of Alcoholics Anonymous, was born November 26, 1895, in East Dorset, Vermont. When he was nine, his parents divorced, apparently because of his father's drinking, and he was left in the care of his grandparents. In 1918, Wilson married Lois Burnham and began a career as a stockbroker; he also continued his father's career of drinking.

Later, after years of alcohol abuse and its associated miseries, Wilson began admitting himself to the Charles B. Towns Hospital in Manhattan. On December 11, 1934, he admitted himself for the fourth time and was treated by a neurologist named William Duncan Silkworth. Dr. Silkworth sedated Wilson and began administering treatment with belladonna. What happened next can best be described in Wilson's own words from his book *Alcoholics Anonymous Comes of Age:*

> My depression deepened unbearably and finally it seemed to me as though I were at the very bottom of the pit. I still gagged badly on the notion of a Power greater than myself, but finally, just for the moment, the last vestige of my proud obstinacy was crushed. All at once I found myself crying out, "If there is a God, let Him show Himself! I am ready to do anything, anything."
>
> Suddenly the room lit up with a great white light. I was caught up into an ecstasy which there are no words to describe. It seemed to me, in a mind's eye, that I was on a mountain and that a wind not of air but of spirit was blowing. And then it burst upon me that I was a free man. Slowly the ecstasy subsided. I lay on the bed, but for a time I was in another world, a new world of consciousness. All about me and through me was a wonderful feel-

From *The Humanist*, May/June 1997, pp. 18-23. © 1997 by Michael J. Lemanski. Reprinted by permission.

ing of Presence, and I thought to myself, "So this is the God of the preachers!"

Wilson's psychic conversion was accomplished. On the surface, at least, he was a changed man.

This experience kept him sober for five months. Then, while on a business trip in Akron, Ohio, he was overcome by the fear of relapse and panicked. It was here that he came into contact with a doctor named Robert Smith, who was also a drinker, and the two men had what has been regarded as the first Alcoholics Anonymous meeting.

Nan Robertson, in her book *Getting Better Inside Alcoholics Anonymous,* suggests that Wilson's deep religious experience at Towns Hospital may have been the result of hallucinations during his withdrawal, induced or precipitated by his medication. Belladonna is an atropine powder derived from the leaves and roots of *Atropa belladonna,* a poisonous Eurasian plant popularly known as "deadly nightshade." In any event, Wilson was apparently never able to recapture his original high (which he in his later years would call his "hot flash") and continued to seek some form of spiritual transformation. His pursuit of spirituality through séances and experiments with LSD, as well as megavitamin therapy, ultimately scandalized AA.

3. Made a decision to turn our will and our lives over to the care of God as we understood Him.
4. Made a searching and fearless moral inventory of ourselves.
5. Admitted to God, to ourselves, and to another human being the exact nature of our wrongs.
6. Were entirely ready to have God remove all these defects of character.
7. Humbly asked Him to remove our shortcomings.
8. Made a list of all persons we had harmed and became ready to make amends to them all.
9. Made direct amends to such people wherever possible, except when to do so would injure them or others.
10. Continued to take personal inventory and when we were wrong promptly admitted it.
11. Sought through prayer and meditation to improve our conscious contact with God, as we understood Him, praying only for knowledge of His will for us and the power to carry that out.
12. Having had a spiritual awakening as the result of these steps, we tried to carry this message to alcoholics, and practice these principles in all our affairs.

> **Frank N. D. Buchman's religious ideas of human powerlessness, redemption from above, the value of taking a moral inventory of oneself, and the value of making amends to others inspired AA's "Twelve Steps of Recovery."**

But AA was the result of more than just a hot flash and a chance meeting. Its basic philosophy was derived from the Oxford Group Movement, founded in 1921 by Frank N. D. Buchman, a spirited evangelist and self-proclaimed "soul surgeon." Smith introduced Wilson to the Oxford Group Movement. Buchman's religious ideas of human powerlessness, redemption from above, the value of taking a moral inventory of oneself, and the value of making amends to others inspired Wilson to develop the "Twelve Steps of Recovery," which, referring to alcoholism only twice, reads:

We:

1. Admitted we were powerless over alcohol—that our lives had become unmanageable.

2. Came to believe that a power greater than ourselves could restore us to sanity.

Wilson started his recovery program in 1935 as part of the Oxford Group but broke from the movement to form Alcoholics Anonymous in 1936. Beyond his assimilation of many of Buchman's ideas, Wilson developed a formula that was remarkably egocentric. The basic concepts of AA embody the parochial singularities of his own recovery experience and are spelled out in his book *Alcoholics Anonymous*—nicknamed "The Big Book"—which is essentially the bible of AA.

The first such concept is that of "hitting bottom": reaching a state of total emotional collapse and depression. He viewed this as an essential component to the recovery process: emotionally, you have to feel as though you are "at the bottom of the pit."

The second concept is that of "deflation of ego in depth": essentially, the admission and acceptance of defeat. Desperation is viewed as an essential component with Wilson saying that "proud obstinacy" has to be "crushed." Desperation is necessary for a "conversion experience."

The third concept is that of a "higher power": the turning of one's life and will over to an external entity that is more powerful and capable of managing one's life. In essence, this entails psychic surrender—turning one's life and will over to "the God of the preachers" or at least to the group pressure and collective belief system of AA.

Because AA came into being at a time when modern methods of medical therapy, clinical psychology, clinical sociology, and professional counseling were all but nonexistent in the field of addictions treatment, AA filled a vacuum. The medical and psychological communities had failed to provide appropriate and adequate care for those addicted to alcohol, and so AA got the franchise. This meant that, for decades after AA's founding, expensive and lengthy addictions treatment programs adopted and offered essentially the same basic philosophy and methodologies as AA.

In 1951, the organization known as Al-Anon was founded. It follows the same basic philosophy of AA, utilizing the twelve-step approach, but provides a support network for the recovering alcoholic's family and friends. In 1953 came Narcotics Anonymous, a twelve-step program and support network of recovering drug addicts. Then, through the 1970s and into the 1980s, there was an explosion of twelve-step recovery programs. New organizations emerged until the self-help domain had expanded to include just about every compulsive or self-defeating behavior one could think of. It was like an evangelical movement: each program was a part of the larger AA religion, each one reframing reality to conform to the same monolithic culture and belief system. The growth was therefore lateral instead of vertical—a widening application of a single set of ideas rather than a progressive, research-oriented development of new ideas and improvements. With its one-size-fits-all approach, this larger AA movement was entirely formulaic; any self-defeating or compulsive behavior called for the same prescription, the formation of yet another twelve-step program.

A simple listing of existing groups is instructive: Adult Children of Alcoholics, Al-Anon, Alcoholics Anonymous, Alcoholics Victorious of the Institute for Christian Living, ARTS (Artists Recovering Through the Twelve Steps) Anonymous, Augustine Fellowship: Sex and Love Addicts Anonymous, Calix, Cocaine Anonymous, Codependents Anonymous, Codependents of Sex Addicts, Debtors Anonymous, Drug-Anon Focus, Dual Disorders Anonymous, Emotional Health Anonymous, Emotions Anonymous, Ethics Anonymous, Gamblers Anonymous, Incest Survivors Anonymous, Naranon, Narcotics Anonymous, Nicotine Anonymous, Obsessive-Compulsive Anonymous, Overcomers Outreach, Overeaters Anonymous, Pill Addicts Anonymous, Pills Anonymous, Prostitutes Anonymous, Sex Addicts Anonymous, Sexaholics Anonymous, Survivors of Incest Anonymous, and Workaholics Anonymous. Though some of these groups offer their own minor variations of the twelve steps, all have the same spiritual-religious orientation.

The general nature of all these groups is best seen in the pamphlet *Al-Anon Spoken Here,* which I found so objectionable at my first Al-Anon meeting. In it, guidelines

> **The twelve-step philosophy is essentially static and resistant to change. New ideas aren't readily embraced and new methodologies from outside are viewed as a threat.**

for the operation of the meetings are provided. The reader is told that, within meetings, only Al-Anon "conference approved" literature can be read and discussed; sources of information from outside the program are not to be used because they "dilute" the spiritual nature of the meetings. Therapy, therapists, and professional terminology are also taboo topics of discussion, as are other recovery or treatment programs.

Such limitations on freedom of inquiry and discussion are common throughout the wider movement. The twelve-step philosophy is essentially static and resistant to change. New ideas aren't readily embraced and new methodologies from outside any given program are viewed as a threat. The peculiar thing about this is an ironic relationship to the "denial" that is so often discussed within meetings. When AA-style programs discourage objective and critical thinking, as well as new information, they essentially embrace a blatant and collective denial system of their own.

Worse, if an individual in AA, for one reason or another, doesn't make adequate progress, the typical view is that he or she isn't adequately "working the program." The usual prescription, then, is to attend more meetings. This is another form of denial: the program can never be the problem.

In 1983, therapist Janet Geringer Woititz published a book entitled *Adult Children of Alcoholics,* which describes the syndrome associated with individuals raised in an alcoholic family. This book became a best seller. After its success, a number of other authors began publishing on adult children of alcoholics, as well as on codependence in general. Within the framework of the twelve steps, both the ACoA and codependence movements grew rapidly, gaining considerable media attention.

Of course, true to form for any AA movement, acceptance of these new ideas was not easy or immediate. Within Al-Anon, for example, a large proportion of the membership banded together to resist incorporating ACoA groups into their program. Though this incorporation eventually occurred, it was only after the twelve steps had been safely imposed upon the membership within the newly formed meetings.

The next development occurred in 1986 when therapist Anne Wilson Schaef, in her book *Codependence Mistreated-Misunderstood,* expanded the concept of codependence from its original clinical application—involving the spouse of an alcoholic—to declare "that it includes the majority of the population of the United States." Along the same line, Herbert Gravitz and Julie Bowden prefaced

> ## Donald Goodwin charges that "therapists 'invented' the concept that adult children of alcoholics have special problems that can be treated through therapy. It was a way for therapists to tap into a new market and make money."

their 1987 book *Recovery: A Guide for Adult Children of Alcoholics* with the statement, "Children of alcoholics are but a visible tip of a much larger social iceberg which casts an invisible shadow over as much as 96 percent of the population."

The next logical step was reported in an article entitled "Healing Ourselves and Our Planet" in the winter 1992 issue of *Contemporary Drug Problems,* in which Robin Room, vice-president for research and development at the Addiction Research Foundation in Toronto, described the way in which many individuals within the growing twelve-step movement—particularly in Northern California—moved between programs for a variety of life problems. He then warned of the potential emergence of "a generalized twelve-step consciousness" with a "sociopolitical agenda." The message was clear: if a majority of the world's population could be described as essentially codependent or dysfunctional, the global solution was simple and obvious: therapy for everyone in conjunction with the twelve steps.

The first important challenge to this growing absurdity came from psychologist Stanton Peele in 1989. His book *Diseasing of America* questioned the efficacy of the proliferating twelve-step programs and described the movement within the addictions field as "out of control." He included an important quote from Donald Goodwin, pioneering researcher in the inheritance of alcoholism, who charged:

> Therapists "invented" the concept that adult children of alcoholics have special problems that can be treated through therapy. They were able to sell this concept to the public and now they are eligible for reimbursement from insurance companies. In short, it was a way for therapists to tap into a new market and make money.

And so, in the fall of 1991, at the national conference of the American Association for Marriage and Family Therapy, psychiatrist Steven J. Wolin, a keynote speaker, publicly denounced the ACoA and codependence movements, declaring that "the recovery movement and its lopsided counsel of damage has become dangerous." After this

statement, he received a standing ovation from the five thousand members in attendance. When a ranking member of the ACoA movement was later asked by a reporter from *USA Today* to respond, he answered, "They're just jealous of all the money we're making."

In 1992, Terence Gorski, a prominent spokesperson within the field of addictions, addressing a conference of the National Association of Alcoholism and Drug Abuse Counselors, stated:

> If I were hired by the enemies of the chemical dependency field . . . I couldn't give them a better strategy [to destroy the field] than the adult children of alcoholics movement and the codependency movement. When we as a field expanded addictions to include all compulsive disorders we destroyed our constituency base . . . destroyed our funding base . . . destroyed our economic stability.

The paradox to all this is that one limited segment of the population to which these syndromes actually do apply has not been appropriately addressed or effectively handled. This population was identified by therapist Paul Curtin at both the 1986 and 1987 conferences of the National Association for Children of Alcoholics. Citing the work of Stephanie Brown—who had related the ACoA syndrome to the framework of eight stages of childhood development, as formulated by psychologist E. H. Erickson—Curtin applied the patterns of behavior encompassed within the syndromes to the actual professionals within the addictions field, saying:

> Right now when we talk about an impaired professional in the alcoholism field, we mean a counselor who is a recovering alcoholic and who has relapsed. If her work is true, would we not have to say that the impaired professionals in the alcoholism field are also untreated adult children of alcoholics and untreated codependents. The implications of this are enormous.

About that time, other researchers were coming to the same conclusion. Addictions professional Susan Nobleman, conducting a survey on how addictions counselors enter the field, learned that 71 percent of the professionals she surveyed had entered as a result of a personal need for addictions treatment. "The vast majority of the sample simply did not plan in the sense of any schooling or special training for this job," she reported. They had simply entered into a treatment program and were later recruited into the profession by other recovering professionals within the field.

Joseph C. Kern, director of Alcoholism Treatment Services in Nassau County, New York, surveyed his own staff and discovered that at least 80 to 85 percent were raised in alcoholic homes. Within the agency structure, most of his staff replicated in their behavior patterns the life-style of their dysfunctional families of origin. Kern also noticed that many of the professionals within the addictions field were as psychologically unhealthy as their clients.

In this context, it was no surprise that the response of most of Kern's staff to those staff members who didn't conform to the norms of the twelve-step belief system, or who attempted to expose and correct obvious flaws, was to engage in a variety of passive-aggressive behaviors, avoiding direct confrontation, until the nonconformers were "frozen out" and induced to resign. Criticism of the belief system wasn't tolerated; maintenance of the status quo was more important than efficacy.

Emil Chiauzzi and Steven Lilijegren, in a 1993 article appearing in the journal *Substance Abuse Treatment,* took note of this problem, calling the treatment of addictions within the health care field an "anomaly." They named several topics of inquiry considered taboo among health care providers, one of the most predominant being to question either the efficacy or necessity of AA and the twelve steps.

This is the nature of the "anomaly." The addictions field is one of the few areas of professional endeavor where the counselors and the patients are drawn from the same constituency, hence the twelve-step bias. It's not just what these individuals embrace in terms of a belief system that's important; it's *how* they believe it. Their faith in the twelve-step approach is quite literally as if their lives depended on it. True believers recruit other true believers, and the belief system perpetuates itself. This creates an obvious resistance to any other treatment possibilities that might be proposed.

Not surprisingly, because so many addictions professionals are as dependent upon the twelve steps as their clients, it is not at all uncommon at professional addictions conferences, workshops, and seminars for twelve-step support groups to be made available for the benefit of the professionals in attendance. This is almost always done to the exclusion of any other type of support group with a differing philosophy.

All this calls into question the health of the addictions field. With the majority of its professionals having had a personal and intimate relationship with addiction, either through their own or through parental addiction within their families of origin, they often lack the emotional and psychological detachment necessary to maintain objectivity when providing treatment and open-mindedness when assessing new scientific data.

Is such therapeutic distance and new scientific data actually needed? After all, one could argue that just because the AA movement has a religious origin and nature, the features of which are significantly tied to the singularities of the founder's recovery experience;

> **Comparative analysis of treatment outcomes places Alcoholics Anonymous, lectures and films, counseling, and psychotherapy at the very bottom of the list in terms of effectiveness.**

just because it is a one-size-fits-all dogma that is offered as a panacea for so broad a range of problems that nearly everyone in the world is thought to need it; and just because most of the people who administer its treatments are also among the treated, that doesn't logically prove that there's anything wrong with it. The AA method could be wonderfully effective nonetheless.

But it is not. It suffers from two central problems: it scarcely works, and its cure is almost as bad as the malady.

George E. Vaillant, in his 1983 landmark book *The Natural History of Alcoholism,* describes the natural healing process associated with individuals addicted to alcohol. Without AA, therapy, or any other outside intervention, a certain percentage of the population addicted to alcohol will reach a point when they will, of their own volition, choose to abstain from the drug. Vaillant's question was: does the AA modality improve on this percentage? Compiling forty years of clinical studies, including an eight-year longitudinal study of his own, he was able to determine that this treatment approach produces results no better than the natural history of the malady.

Initially such programs do produce dramatic results, as the testimonials attest. However, over the long run, the "cured" population, through relapse, like water seeking its own level, asymptotically approaches the low water mark. With or without the AA approach, approximately 5 percent of the alcoholic population Vaillant surveyed managed to achieve *sustained* abstinence. Subsequent studies have produced similar results. Therefore, to the extent that AA and other twelve-step programs work, they do so for only a tiny percentage of the addicted population.

Overall, the best hard research evidence available indicates that the most commonly employed addiction treatment modalities in the United States and Canada have questionable efficacy and consistently produce negative treatment outcomes. Extensive research in a comparative analysis of treatment outcomes, conducted and compiled by Reid K. Hester and William R. Miller at the Center on Alcoholism, Substance Abuse, and Addictions—places Alcoholics Anonymous, educational lectures and films, general alcoholism counseling, and psychotherapy at the very bottom of the list in terms of effectiveness. On the other hand, modalities which include brief intervention, coping and social skills training, motivational enhancement, community reinforcement, relapse prevention, and cognitive therapy—when employed within the context of a client-to-program matching system typically found in Europe—consistently produce positive treatment outcomes. A statement by Miller in the September/October 1994 issue of *Psychology Today* puts it best: "The drug treatment community has been curiously resistant to using what works."

In fact, it has been curiously attached to that which is harmful. Twelve-step groups offer what is, in reality, the antithesis of therapy. There is no cure; the solution provided by such programs entails an endless attendance at meetings. An old slogan says it best: "You never graduate from Al-Anon." And you don't; you become addicted to it, desperately hanging on to the program like a spiritual lifeline in a sea of sin and death.

Somewhere within the quagmire of the AA movement and all of the twelve-step programs associated within it, the meaning of *recovery* was lost. By definition, recovery is a retrieval and reclamation process, not a surrender and abdication. The process of recovery or emotional balance and psychological well-being entails independence from addictive chemicals, compulsive behaviors, therapists, and recovery groups. To transfer dependence on chemically addictive substances to emotional or psychological dependence on a group or recovery program is not recovery in the true sense of the word.

Looking back to William Wilson, we might do well to describe him as an untreated adult child of an alcoholic and an untreated codependent. Given the patterns of his behavior and life-long spiritual quest for an external solution to an internal problem, he effectively institutionalized both syndromes into his twelve-step program.

This can be readily seen by returning to the original definition of the term *codependence*. Prior to having been expanded, convoluted, and rendered empty, the term had meaning in a limited clinical setting for a specific population. In her book *Choice-making*, Sharon Wegscheider-Cruse quotes Robert Subby, director of Family Systems, Inc., of Minneapolis, who defined *codependency* as "an emotional, psychological, and behavior condition that develops as a result of an individual's prolonged exposure to, and practice of, a set of oppressive rules—rules which prevent the open expression of feelings, as well as the direct discussion of personal and interpersonal problems." Using this as a base, Wegscheider-Cruse expands her own definition: "Codependency is a specific condition that is characterized by preoccupation and extreme dependence (emotionally, socially and sometimes physically) on a person or object. Eventually, this dependence on another person becomes a pathological condition that affects the codependent in all other relationships." These definitions are significant in that they describe so well both the nature of twelve-step programs and the relationship of the participants in these programs to their groups.

Alternative Recovery Programs

- **Drinkwise**
  University of Michigan Medical Center
  527 East Liberty, Suite 209, Ann Arbor, MI 48104–2242
  1–313–747–9473; 1–800–222–5145

- **Moderation Management**
  P.O. Box 6005, Ann Arbor, MI 48106–6005
  1–810–788–8040; kishline@ic.net
  http://comnet.org/mm/

- **Rational Recovery Systems, Inc.**
  P.O. Box 800, Lotus, CA 95651
  1–916–621–2667; rr@rational.org
  http://www.rational.org/recovery

- **Secular Organizations for Sobriety**
  5521 Grosvenor Boulevard, Los Angeles, CA 90066
  1–310–821–8430; sosla@loop.com
  http://www.codesh.org/sos

- **Self-Management and Recovery Training [SMART]**
  24000 Merchantile Road, Suite 11, Beachwood, OH 44122
  1–216–292–0220; srmaill@aol.com
  http://home.sprynet.com/sprynet/mike888/

- **Women for Sobriety/Men for Sobriety**
  P.O. Box 618, Quakertown, PA 18951–0618
  1–215–536–8026; wfsobriety@aol.com
  http://www.mediapulse.com/wfs/

And if the problem of AA addiction isn't bad enough on its own, there's an economic incentive to keep it going. Since twelve-step recovery programs admittedly offer no cure—only a lifetime of participation in a recovery group—the advantage to the professionals is obvious. Each new client can be viewed as offering the potential financial equivalent of an annuity. People looking to break a dependency on alcohol may find greater success as a participant in one of the many nonspirituality-based treatment programs which, although not as widely publicized, are available as alternatives to AA-style programs.

Michael J. Lemanski is a member of the National Association for Children of Alcoholics and has been active in the ACoA movement since its inception in the early 1980s. He currently serves as coordinator for Self-Management and Recovery Training (SMART) in Massachusetts.

OUTPATIENT DETOXIFICATION FROM ALCOHOL, OPIATES, AND STIMULANTS

Marc A. Schuckit, M.D.

ABSTRACT

There are three classes of drugs that can cause clinically relevant withdrawal syndromes after repeated heavy use. They are the depressants (including alcohol, the benzodiazepines, and the barbiturates), the opiates (heroin, methadone, codeine, and so on), and the stimulants (including all forms of amphetamines and cocaine). This issue of the newsletter reviews the withdrawal syndromes associated with each of these three classes of drugs, describes the treatment (called detoxification or detox) appropriate for each syndrome, and evaluates whether the treatment can be safely and effectively carried out in an outpatient (as opposed to an inpatient) setting. The major conclusion of this review is that outpatient detox is a safe and effective option for some, but not all, patients.

I. INTRODUCTION

A withdrawal (or abstinence) syndrome can develop when a person takes increasing doses of a drug over an extended period of time and then cuts back (or abstains) from use. For drugs that stay in the body for short periods of time (like alcohol or heroin) the symptoms usually begin within two to eight hours after stopping the substance, with a longer delay for drugs like Valium (diazepam) or methadone with very long periods of action. The symptoms observed are like a rebound because they are often the opposite of those that develop during intoxication. What appears to be occurring during withdrawal is that the body has changed in an effort to resist the effects of the drug during intoxication, so that when the person stops or cuts back on the drug, the body is no longer normal and can take days to weeks or more to return to a state of comfort.

Mild rebound symptoms can be seen after long-term exposure to almost any substance, even aspirin. However, for three classes of drugs, clinically important symptoms can occur during withdrawal, problems that both cause discomfort and increase the chances of relapse as the person recognizes that one way to get rid of the symptoms is to take more of the drug again. The classes are the depressants, the opiates, and the stimulants. This issue of the newsletter briefly reviews these withdrawal syndromes and asks if they can be safely treated in an outpatient setting.

II. THE WITHDRAWAL SYNDROMES

The most potentially dangerous of the withdrawal pictures can occur after repeated intake of brain depressants such as alcohol, the Valium-type drugs (the benzodiazepines), or the barbiturates (such as Seconal or secobarbital). The intoxication experienced with all depressants is similar, and is likely to include a feeling of relaxation, sleepiness, and some changes in physical functioning (e.g., decreases in heart rate, blood pressure, and any symptoms of hand tremor). Therefore, the withdrawal from depressants involves high levels of anxiety, insomnia, and increases in those same areas of physical functioning. For shorter-acting drugs, such as alcohol, Serax (oxazepam) or Ativan (lorazepam) the symptoms begin within six hours or so, peak in intensity on Day 2, and are likely to markedly improve by Day 5. For longer-acting drugs such as Valium or Librium (chlordiazepoxide) symptoms might not begin for several days to a week, and might linger for two to three weeks. Unlike other drug withdrawal states, abstinence syndromes associated with depressants such as alcohol can include physical symptoms of convulsions and severe confusion in perhaps 3% or so of patients (a larger proportion for those withdrawing from benzodiazepines or barbiturates).

The next most physically taxing withdrawal is associated with opiates such as heroin, methadone, codeine, and almost all prescription pain pills. Being the opposite of the symptoms seen during intoxication, these abstinence symptoms are likely to include a general feeling of discomfort, pain almost everywhere, along with sweating, a runny nose, and a cough. Opiate withdrawal is not associated with any severe symptoms such as convulsions. For most

From *Drug Abuse and Alcoholism Newsletter*, August 1997, pp. 1-4. Reprinted with the permission of Vista Hill Foundation, San Diego, California.

people, the symptoms are most intense on Day 1 or 2, and are markedly improved by Day 5. However, if someone was physically addicted to a long-acting opiate such as methadone, the time course can last several weeks.

Finally, withdrawal from stimulants (such as all forms of amphetamines, cocaine, and most weight reducing pills) is associated with two to five days or so of eating too much, sleeping too much, and feeling depressed, with few physical signs and symptoms. Other drugs of abuse such as nicotine, caffeine, and marijuana have withdrawal symptoms that can be psychologically disturbing but are usually relatively mild, and for some of these drugs (such as marijuana), even these are relatively rare. Other types of drugs (such as inhalants, hallucinogens, PCP, and so on) have not been shown to be associated with clinically relevant withdrawal pictures.

The treatments of the withdrawal syndromes for depressants, opiates, and stimulants is called detoxification or detox. The therapies are based on the specific symptom pattern and the time course over which the problems occur. The next section briefly reviews the treatment approaches from the perspective of the potential appropriateness of carrying out these procedures in an outpatient environment.

III. CAN DETOX BE EFFECTIVELY AND SAFELY CARRIED OUT WITH OUTPATIENTS?

A. A general description of detox

The goals of detoxification are fairly straightforward. They include the need to optimize the level of physical functioning, to minimize the psychological and physical symptoms of withdrawal, and to begin to prepare patients for the level of work required in the rehabilitation phase of care. The safest, most intensive, and perhaps most effective way to carry out detoxification is in an inpatient setting. Here, physiological symptoms can be monitored, medications (if needed) can be adjusted within a short time of any change in symptoms, and patients can be regularly reassured that they are going to be fine.

For all types of withdrawal, treatment involves a careful physical examination to identify physiological problems that need correction, offering good nutrition including supplemental vitamins, and giving individuals an opportunity to rest and recuperate. For withdrawal from depressant drugs such as alcohol, optimal care involves readministering a depressant on Day 1, using doses that markedly decrease symptoms, and then diminishing the level

of medication to zero over the subsequent four or five days (using a longer time if patients are withdrawing from a long-acting drug such as Valium). For opiate withdrawal, the optimum medication regimen would involve administering an opiate such as methadone, using doses that markedly diminish symptoms on Day 1, and then gradually reducing the dose over the next five days or so. However, because of legal restrictions on the use of these opiate drugs, most programs invoke a mixture of nonaddicting medications that help with the symptoms of pain, diarrhea, a runny nose and cough, and so on, often including the drug Catapres (clonidine) to help settle down the nervous system. There are no data that the stimulant withdrawal syndrome is significantly aided by any specific medication.

B. Application of this approach to outpatients

Financial resources don't always allow detoxification to be carried out in an inpatient setting. However, most authors agree that outpatient detox is not appropriate for individuals who are pregnant, those with specific medical conditions (such as asthma or high blood pressure), or people with severe psychological problems such as high levels of depression or confusion. For withdrawal from depressants, it is generally felt unwise to use an outpatient setting if the individual has a history of epileptic seizures, or has had convulsions in prior withdrawal states. Of course, to participate in an outpatient detox program, the individual must have some level of life stability, and be able to travel to the clinic almost daily.

Similar to inpatient detox, the core of outpatient programs involves efforts to educate individuals about the problems that they are facing, reassure them regarding the help to be offered, and the implementation of behavioral and cognitive approaches to help them to relax and begin their recovery. In an outpatient arena individuals must also be warned about the potential dangers of mixing street drugs with any medications they might receive, and should be offered the opportunity of calling the clinic and/or visiting the emergency room if withdrawal symptoms markedly increase.

A cornerstone of outpatient detox is regular, often daily, clinic visits. Thus, a patient is only given one day's supply of medications (slightly longer if over a weekend), and a quick physical evaluation is made daily before the next day's dose of medication is prescribed. While attending the clinic, patients can be encouraged to listen to educational lectures, view videotapes, read educational materials, and to participate in some brief counseling sessions aimed at trying to increase motivation for continued abstinence and for entering

a longer-term phase of care. Similar to inpatient procedures, any medications that are used are usually decreased to zero over the three to five days of detox, or the first several weeks of treatment if longer-acting drugs such as Valium or methadone were involved in the addiction.

C. Outpatient detoxification for alcohol

Studies indicate that between 70% and 90% of alcohol dependent individuals might be appropriate for outpatient detox, as they have no history of recent seizures or a seizure disorder, and can travel to the clinic daily. Similar to inpatient settings, in our own program we usually use medications for alcohol detox, beginning, for example, with 25 mg of Librium by mouth three to four times a day. We ask patients to skip a dose if they feel very sleepy, and give them the opportunity of taking up to two extra doses on that first day if they feel very shaky. Individuals are given only a one day supply, and return to the clinic the next day for evaluation, with the goal of decreasing the doses to zero by Day 5. Other clinicians report using 30 mg of Serax every six hours and at bedtime on Day 1 (for a total of approximately 120 mg the first day), with subsequent decreases, or have prescribed a total of 30 to 40 mg of Valium on Day 1 with a five-day taper. Less data are available regarding the use of other brain depressant drugs such as Tegretol (carbamazepine) or the drug Catapres, and it is likely that these medications offer no advantages over the usual benzodiazepines.

Outpatient alcohol detox does seem to work. One author estimated that patients kept about 90% of their clinic visits, and others have reported that about 70% complete the five plus days of more intensive care. Other indicators of the potential usefulness of outpatient alcohol detox include a shorter length of treatment (an average of 6.5 days vs. 9.2 days for inpatient detox in one study), and reports that between 50% and 90% of those who undergo outpatient detox follow through with at least one clinic visit for rehabilitation. However, a direct comparison of outpatient and inpatient detox revealed that even better figures were likely to be seen for inpatient procedures.

D. Outpatient detox for other drugs

Less data are available regarding outpatient opiate detoxification. Theoretically, this procedure has both good news and bad as compared to alcohol. On the positive side is the almost complete absence of severe physical consequences such as convulsions for opiate withdrawal. On the negative side, however, is the inability of a clinician to use opiates to ease patients through this difficult period of time. Thus, most outpatient detox protocols use a combination of medications aimed at controlling symptoms over those first five days or so. They often depend upon Catapres (up to 1 mg or so on the first day in divided doses), along with decongestants, nonopiate pain pills, antidiarrheal medication, and sometimes the short-term use of benzodiazepines (e.g., Serax 15 mg every six hours on Day 1 as needed). In a variation of this approach, some research programs also incorporate an opiate antagonist such as Trexan (naltrexone) to speed the recovery process along. In one trial between 50% and 90% of opiate dependent outpatients completed the detox procedure, and of these approximately 75% entered a rehabilitation phase of outpatient care.

While outpatient detox from depressants such as benzodiazepines and barbiturates or from stimulants would be feasible, there are few systemic studies. Anecdotally, however, many clinicians report using education, reassurance, frequent clinic visits, and appropriate behavioral or cognitive approaches for the outpatient treatment of the withdrawal phase associated with amphetamines or cocaine.

IV. CONCLUSIONS

As is true of most things in life, outpatient detoxification has both assets and liabilities. From my reading of the literature, I am impressed by the study of Hayashida and colleagues (1989) showing that a higher proportion of individuals with inpatient alcohol detoxification complete the procedure and enter rehabilitation. That same study, however, also demonstrated the substantially lower cost of outpatient treatment when compared to inpatient care (an average of about $400 per patient for outpatient alcohol detox versus over $3,000 for inpatient care). While not as dramatic, the potential financial benefits of outpatient detox have also been documented in Australia and in the United Kingdom. Outpatient detox has the additional advantage of not separating a patient from his or her family or other sources of social support. However, it is apparent that the price one pays with outpatient treatment is a lower completion rate, a greater probability of the concomitant use of alcohol or street drugs during detox, less rigorous clinical supervision, and less complete compliance with treatment procedures, including medications.

It seems to me that this review of the literature has indicated a "general truth" that applies to the alcohol and drug fields overall. Not everyone requires inpatient care, but there are individuals for whom psychological and/or medical impairments make the inpatient environment optimal. However, even for those individuals in the middle ground, there is a significantly higher level of attrition from treatment when the less intensive outpatient approach is used. Thus, I believe that these data strongly support the need for a continuum of care from inpatient to outpatient in order for us to best serve our clients and patients.

This review is based on a large number of studies. Those of you who wish additional readings might consider beginning with: Abbott, P. J., et al. Ambulatory medical detoxification for alcohol. *American Journal of Drug and Alcohol Abuse* 21:549–563, 1995; Alterman, A., et al. Treatment response and safety of ambulatory medical detoxification. *Journal of Studies on Alcohol* 49:160–166, 1988; Fishbain, D. A., et al. Opiate detoxification protocols: A clinical manual. *Annals of Clinical Psychiatry* 5:53–65, 1993; Hayashida, M., et al. Comparative effectiveness and costs of inpatient and outpatient detoxification of patients with mild-to-moderate alcohol withdrawal syndrome. *New England Journal of Medicine* 320:358–365, 1989; Kleber, H. D., et al. Clonidine in outpatient detoxification from methadone maintenance. *Archives of General Psychiatry* 42:391–394, 1985; Klijnsma, M. P., et al. Outpatient alcohol detoxification—outcome after two months. *Alcohol and Alcoholism* 30:669–673, 1995; O'Connor, P. G., et al. Ambulatory opiate detoxification and primary care: A role for the primary care physician. *Journal of General Internal Medicine* 7:532–534, 1992; and Schuckit, M. A. Drug and Alcohol Abuse. Fourth Edition. New York: Plenum, 1995.

The Peer Principle: The Key to Addiction Treatment

Frank Riessman

On the surface, there seem to be competing orthodoxies in the field of addiction treatment:

- You are an alcoholic so you must be abstinent. Alcoholics can drink socially.
- You must turn your problem over to a higher power. You can quit on your own.
- You need to get into residential treatment. You can overcome your addiction while maintaining your work and personal life.
- Young people must just say no. Youth need lots of social support to avoid early addiction.

So, it was surprising to read an article in the *New York Times,* by Denise Grady ("Hardest Habit to Break," 10/27/98), that proclaimed, "Compared with people who have other mental or physical disorders, addicts have few treatments to choose from."

Actually, there is an array of treatment modalities to suit the temperament of the addict and the type of addiction (simple or complex). But the key element in all of them, whether it is emphasized or not, is the power of the peer principle.

Frank Riessman is a founder of *Social Policy* and executive director of the National Self-Help Clearinghouse.

From *Social Policy,* Winter 1998, pp. 10-12. © 1998 by Social Policy Corporation. Reprinted by permission.

The best statement of the peer principle came from Bill Wilson, the legendary Bill W., co-founder of Alcoholics Anonymous: "Drunks don't need a drink," he said, "they need a drunk." This mutual aid concept became the basis of a worldwide movement that has spread to many groups beyond AA. In essence, people are influenced and can best be helped by others who share their condition or problem.

Peer drug education programs for youth are far more effective than bringing adult role models (such as athletes who have quit drugs) or law enforcement officers into classrooms to prevent drug use. Young people are more likely to listen to their peers on the subject of drugs—for good or for ill. And the young people who volunteer to educate their peers gain a special benefit. Their advocacy for not using drugs has a profound impact on their own ability to stay away from illicit and damaging substances. In applying the helper-therapy principle, the helper (in this case, the peer educator) gains more from involvement in the program than the people being helped (other students).

The Partnership for a Drug Free America and other campaigns directed primarily at parents will fail because they violate the peer principle.

The Therapeutic Community (TC) approach to treating addiction has had notable successes, but often at such great cost that there is a severe shortage of treatment slots. TCs make tremendous use of recovering drug addicts to help users seeking recovery, another excellent application of the peer principle.

Alternative medical approaches to end addiction are also gaining ground, notably acupuncture programs such as Michael Smith's at the Lincoln Hospital Center in the Bronx, New York. Rather than relying on ear acupuncture alone, Smith combines a Narcotics Anonymous chapter in his program along with professional counseling. This triple treatment approach has been replicated in over 30 US cities.

Most addicts who seek to deal with their problem through professional treatment are referred to self-help groups for supplemental and ongoing support. It is hard to get away from the power of the peer principle.

A New Intensive Self-Help Approach

At the National Self-Help Clearinghouse, we are seeking to develop self-help groups for addicts that go beyond the traditional approach of Narcotics Anonymous where the stress is on social support and the 12-Steps. We propose to add the self-help ethos and the helper-therapy principle, that is, more emphasis on a person's strengths and more stress on the healing power of helping. And we would also remove the religious overtones found in 12-Step programs.

To test the effectiveness of what we propose, longitudinal and retrospective research would be a part of the program. We would treat simple and complex addicts differently. Our entire approach, in contrast to the biodetermined model promoted by Denise Grady and Bill Moyers, stresses what can be learned in treating addiction to one substance from the practice of treating another—a cross-addiction analysis.

We are interested in answers to questions such as the following:

1. Why were addicts—such as many soldiers involved in the Vietnam War—able to break their heroin addictions relatively easily on their return to the US?
2. What is the difference between the 56 million people who have quit smoking on their own and those who have not despite repeated efforts?
3. Why are some diabetics able to control their sugar intake relatively easily while others violate their diets with life-threatening indulgence?
4. Why is addiction a major mode of disturbance in our society?
5. Is alcohol addiction unique?
6. When does simple addiction (relatively easy to give up) cross over into complex addiction (bound up with emotions and psychology)?
7. How are process addictions such as gambling, sex, compulsive eating, work, and spending different from substance addictions like sugar, alcohol, and hard drugs?
8. How does changing the condition in which the addict lives help control his or her addiction?
9. What are the cost benefits of diagnosing addicts as simple or complex?
10. What is the relationship of the new genetic theory of addiction and traditional approaches?

We have more questions than answers when it comes to addiction. But we have learned that the peer principle plays a powerful role in making and healing addicts.

Needle exchanges: Prevention or problem?

Are needle exchanges a successful HIV prevention tactic or do they only exacerbate existing illegal drug problems?

BY MATTHEW A. BOWDY

Matthew A. Bowdy is a health policy analyst for The Council of State Governments.

Despite increasing support, needle exchange programs are not yet being touted as a panacea for HIV prevention among intravenous drug users.

In the quest to stop the spread of HIV, the virus that causes AIDS, state and local officials face a decision that may make the difference between life and death for some of their constituents. One way people spread HIV infection is through sharing tainted needles during drug use. This has created a demand for programs to supply clean needles to intravenous drug users. In response, there are at least 113 needle exchange programs operating within 80 cities in 30 states.

Until now, the Clinton administration and Congress have agreed that state and local officials should decide which HIV prevention strategies to implement. Some, however, see needle exchange programs as the wrong solution.

For example, the federal budget signed into effect last October includes a ban on federal and District of Columbia funding for needle exchange programs within the district. The budget provision also calls for revoking all federal funding to any agency in the district that trades needles, even if the agency does so with private funds. The provision of the budget only applies to the district and not to programs operating in some 30 states. States, however, are experiencing problems of their own.

African-Americans in New Jersey are not seeing the same rapid decline in HIV infection rates as other groups in the United States are. In an effort to curb rates of infection, New Jersey's Senate Health Committee in September approved two bills to establish a needle-exchange program and authorize pharmacies to sell hypodermic needles without a prescription. Gov. Christine Todd Whitman promised to veto any bill the Legislature passes that promotes needle exchange.

States such as New Jersey are under immense pressure to decide on HIV prevention strategies. The decision is not easy when it comes to making a choice on needle exchange programs. Proponents and opponents each hold valuable resources and information in their corners.

No easy answer

States are left with the daunting prospect of finding, analyzing and evaluating numerous studies and viewpoints that both support and refute the success of needle exchanges.

The needle exchange debate raises two primary issues. First, some fear that needle exchanges will perpetuate the nation's drug problem. Second, HIV is spreading more rapidly than ever before among intravenous drug users. These two issues merge where the use of intravenous drugs not only creates HIV risk from injection with tainted needles, but also increases risk of contracting HIV and other sexually transmitted diseases through promiscuous sex, possibly related to drug use.

A plethora of research data, oftentimes conflicting, and opinion muddy the waters of definitive judgment on the issue. Experts disagree on the effectiveness of needle exchanges. Some maintain the programs might encourage drug use and sexual behavior that spreads HIV infection. Dr. Janet Lapey, former president of Drug Watch International, a volunteer nonprofit information network and advocacy organization, wrote in a 1998 report, "Any societal intervention which encourages drug use will also result in increased AIDS rates. It is important to note that needle sharing is not the only way drug users are infected with AIDS since they are at high risk for acquiring AIDS sexually through promiscuity or prostitution."

A 1998 article in *The American Journal of Public Health* discussed the relationship between drug use and HIV. One of its findings noted that stimulants such as cocaine are reported to increase sexual drive and may delay satisfaction. Thus, illicit drug use may prolong and increase frequency of sexual episodes, which increases exposure to sexually transmitted diseases such as HIV.

Other study results, conducted in 1997 and published in the British medical journal *The Lancet*, found that worldwide in 29 cities with needle exchanges, HIV infection dropped by an average of 5.8 percent a year among drug users. In 51 cities without needle exchanges, drug-related HIV rates rose by 5.9 percent a year.

> "A comprehensive approach that includes needle exchange, health care, treatment, social support and counseling is also needed."

Middle ground may exist. Julie Bruneau, assistant professor of psychiatry at the University of Montreal, and Martin Schechter, professor of epidemiology at the University of British Columbia, suggest a balanced approach. *The New York Times* quoted them as saying, "A comprehensive approach that includes needle exchange, health care, treatment, social support and counseling is also needed." Perhaps this is a merger of strategies, from both opponents and proponents of needle exchanges, to contain drug-related HIV infection.

Accessing all research studies and their data is a huge undertaking and deciphering often confounding results is an arduous process. A study

of intravenous drug users in Montreal found that drug addicts participating in needle exchanges are 2.2 times more likely to contract HIV than addicts not participating in such programs.

The authors of the Montreal study, Julie Bruneau and her colleagues, hypothesize that needle exchanges might have attracted existing groups of marginalized individuals who were engaging in more high-risk activities. Bruneau said, "We caution against trying to prove directly the causal relation between [needle exchange program] use and reduction in HIV incidence. Evaluating the effect of [needle exchange programs] per se without accounting for other interventions and changes over time in the dynamics of the epidemic may prove to be a perilous exercise."

Leaving it to the states

Early last year, President Bill Clinton opposed a congressional proposal, H.R. 3717, to ban use of federal funds for the distribution of needles or syringes for the hypodermic injection of illegal drugs. He called the ban "unnecessary and unwarranted."

The White House said the secretary of Health and Human Services should have the authority to determine the scientific and public health merit of needle exchange programs as they affect rates of HIV transmission and injection drug use. Additionally, the administration said the decision on which HIV prevention strategies to use should rest with state and local officials.

Other organizations also opposed H.R. 3717. Chris Lanier, of the National Coalition to Save Lives Now, an advocacy group for access to clean needles for IV drug users, called the legislation damaging. "First, it takes the authority for decision-making on needle exchange out of the hands of the administration and the Department of Health and Human Services. Second, it makes the ban we already have a permanent

one, which would require more action by Congress to reverse."

Another important issue to consider is public opinion of needle exchange programs. Some popular media outlets condone these programs, but the public is less supportive. In 1997, The Family Research Council, a nonprofit organization that strives to reaffirm and promote the traditional family unit, polled 1,000 registered voters to examine their views on needle exchanges. Most (62 percent) opposed exchanges, thinking that federal funding of these programs condones illegal drug use. Additionally, most voters (64 percent) believed government-funded needle exchanges encourage illegal drug use among teen-agers.

The 1997 Family Research Council poll results also document that nearly nine of 10 Americans are concerned that needle exchanges will result in increased crime and create public health hazards due to tainted and discarded needles. Six in 10 want their members of Congress to terminate needle exchanges and focus on abstinence and drug rehabilitation.

States are searching for definitive answers. U.S. Reps. Maxine Waters, D-Calif., and Xavier Becerra, D-Calif., called upon Donna E. Shalala, secretary of the Department of Health and Human Services, "to make an immediate determination that [needle exchange programs] reduce the risk of HIV transmission and do not promote the use of illegal drugs."

Shalala on April 20, 1998, answered the call, stating that "needle exchange programs can be an effective part of a comprehensive strategy to reduce the incidence of HIV transmission and do not encourage the use of illegal drugs."

Shalala and the Department of Health and Human Services strengthen support for the idea that needle exchanges can be effective in prevention of HIV. The question now is what the states will do with the information that is sitting before them.

Can Addiction-Related Self-Help/Mutual Aid Groups Lower Demand For Professional Substance Abuse Treatment?

Keith Humphreys

Keith Humphreys is a research psychologist and consulting assistant professor of psychiatry at the Veterans Affairs Health Care System and Stanford University School of Medicine in Palo Alto, California. Preparation of this article was supported by the VA Health Services Research and Development Service. Opinions expressed here do not necessarily reflect policy positions of the VA or Stanford University School of Medicine.

Professional substance abuse treatment in the United States grew extensively through the 1970s and 1980s, becoming literally a billion dollar annual enterprise. In recent years, however, the professional treatment network has contracted due to the arrival of managed health care and to recent public sector disinvestment. Clinicians and health policy planners now face the difficult challenge of attempting to care for addicted individuals within increasingly tight fiscal constraints. But there is a potential bright spot in the current gloomy addiction care picture—the possibility that self-help/mutual aid organizations can help substance abusers recover, while at the same time lowering demand for scarce formal health care resources.

The self-help/mutual aid group movement covers a vast range of health, social, and political concerns, but the largest and probably best-established component of the movement focuses on addiction. Alcoholics Anonymous (AA), Moderation Management, Narcotics Anonymous (NA), and Women for Sobriety (WFS) are among the many self-help organizations that help addicted individuals live productive, substance-free lives. These organizations differ from professional services in many ways—peer control, an emphasis on personal experience rather than credentials and training, informality, mutual rather than one-way helping—but in this context their most important defining quality is that they are essentially free of charge. Many of them "pass the hat" for small, voluntary contributions, but this is a trivial cost compared with those of professional addiction services.

The Impact of Self-Help Groups on the Demand for Treatment

In a national, representative survey of US adults, Kessler and colleagues (*Social Policy*, Spring 1997) found that individuals who attend self-help groups were more likely than non-attenders to have been treated by a professional for substance abuse problems. Perhaps surprisingly, this positive correlation neither detracts from nor supports the hypothesis that self-help groups lower demand for professional addiction treatment. As this reasoning might not be intuitively clear, consider an example that is a bit more down-to-earth.

If we surveyed all Americans about the restaurants they had patronized in the past year, we would find that the frequency of eating at Wendy's, Burger King, and McDonald's were all positively correlated (i.e., people who ate at one of the chains some of the time were more likely to also eat at the other two chains). Yet we know for a fact that these chains are in competition with each other, and when one of them opens new stores the others lose business. This apparent contradiction between our cross-sectional correlation and what we know to be true comes about because underlying common factors influence eating at all three chains: a tendency to eat out rather than cook and a preference (by taste or economic necessity) for fast-food restaurants over other types of restaurants. Hence, the three restaurant chains can share customers yet be in competition at the same time.

Similarly, the positive cross-sectional correlation between self-help group involvement and utilization of professional addiction treatment services is likely attributable to common factors, namely having a substance abuse problem and being comfortable seeking help from others outside of one's immediate family and social circle. These common factors produce the positive correlation noted in Kessler's survey but, as with the example of the fast-food chains, they cannot tell us one way or the other whether self-help group participation lowers demand for addiction-related health care. The only way to answer that question is to conduct studies that examine patterns of health care utilization and self-help groups over time.

For example, a study of 227 alcohol-abusing workers randomly assigned participants either to an inpatient treatment program followed by AA meetings or to community-based AA meetings only. The research team monitored substance abuse and job-related outcomes (e.g., absenteeism), as well as alcohol-related health care costs over the two-year period. At the conclusion of the study, the average participant assigned to AA only had consumed $8,840 in alcohol-related health care resources versus $10,040 for the inpatient treatment participants. This amounts to a savings of $1,200/person or 10 percent. However, although the two groups fared equally well on job-related outcomes, the AA group had more relapses over the course of the study. Hence, potential health care cost savings from self-help have to be considered in light of whether outcomes will be compromised, producing additional suffering and health harms.

Although the reconceptualization of the role of addiction professionals that I have outlined would serve the public interest, it might put professionals in a difficult position.

Following up on this research, a colleague and I studied 201 alcohol-abusing individuals who sought help either from AA or a professional outpatient treatment service provider. Over the ensuing three years, both groups of individuals improved substantially, reducing, for example, their daily alcohol consumption by 70 percent on average. Unlike in the study of inpatient treatment, AA attendees' outcomes were just as positive as those of individuals who had received professional services. Importantly, those in AA consumed 45 percent less alcohol-related health care resources over the three years of the study (about $1,800 less/person). This study indicates that self-help group involvement can lower demand for professional treatment without compromising health outcomes. My colleagues and I are now at-tempting to replicate this finding in a different sample of patients, and initial results confirm the findings of the first study.

These studies, considered together with the research literature showing that self-help groups for psychiatric problems seem to lower demand for professional mental health services, coalesce in support of the proposition that self-help groups can lower the demand for addiction-related professional services. This finding becomes more believable and more understandable when we recognize that both self-help organizations and professional treatment services are networks. Most helpers are more comfortable referring an addicted individual to someone in their own network than to an outside network. For example, when people go to their first AA meeting, they are likely to hear about other AA meetings and potential AA sponsors, whereas when they go to a professional, they are likely to hear about other professionals and the services that they can provide.

Other research projects currently underway will provide more definitive evidence on whether and to what extent addiction-related self-help groups can lower demand for formal health care while promoting positive outcomes. In the meantime, it is worth speculating on what it would mean for substance abuse treatment policy if future studies replicate the findings reviewed above.

Rethinking the Relation between Professional Services and Self-Help Groups

Addiction treatment professionals and self-help groups currently collaborate and intersect in many ways. Many "recovering" individuals, for example, work as counselors in treatment programs and many professionals refer their patients to self-help groups. At the same time, many if not most professionals think of this relationship in professionally-centered terms. Professionals often conceptualize self-help groups as an "adjunct" or "aftercare" intervention that can play a supportive role to the "real" intervention provided by professionals.

This perspective is partially attributable to professional socialization and training that, across fields, inculcate a bias that professionals are better at a wide range of tasks than are nonprofessionals. The now collapsing system of fee-for-service health care, however, also played a role by giving professionals a financial disincentive to "lose" patients to self-help groups. Under the fee-for-service system, a patient who elected to attend Women for Sobriety instead of a four-week inpatient treatment program represented a loss of several thousand dollars to the professional program. Hence, even if such an intensive intervention were unnecessary, the incentives were clearly to discourage self-help group involvement except as an adjunct or aftercare component to the costly professional program.

In contrast, under most managed care arrangements, a professional or health care plan is financially better off when an addicted individual who does not really need hospitalization or another professional treatment seeks out a free self-help group instead. From a cost-conscious point of view, self-help groups should be the first option evaluated when an addicted individual makes initial contact with professional services (e.g., in a primary care appointment or a clinical assessment at a substance abuse agency or employee assistance program).

No one should be forced to attend a self-help group, but the risk to an addicted person of trying out a few meetings is sufficiently slight (and the payoffs in terms of outcome and health care cost savings sufficiently large) that a recommendation to visit a few groups should be standard practice among health care professionals. In this framework, self-help groups would move from being the "junior partner" of professionals to being "the first line of defense." In contrast, the role of addiction treatment professionals would be redefined from treating as many individuals as possible (including individuals who could recover without treatment) to treating that subset of individuals who do not benefit from self-help groups. Such patients

might include addicted individuals who also have severe comorbid psychiatric and medical problems that require close monitoring, as well as patients who have tried self-help groups and found them unhelpful.

Were this arrangement consistently adopted, scarce professional services would be better targeted to individuals with more severe problems. Further, health care costs would likely drop because many individuals who initially sought professional treatment would ultimately rely more on self-help groups than on professional services. From the point of view of wise and socially just resource allocation, this seems an ideal arrangement. Nevertheless, some professional organizations may resist such a change.

Without besmirching any particular helping professional (I am one, after all), it is safe to say that professions pursue their own guild interests, even when they are not in line with the public interest. Although the re-conceptualization of the role of addiction professionals that I have outlined would serve the public interest, it might put professionals in a difficult position. For example, the more avaricious managed care companies may overreach from the evidence and refer all addicted patients to self-help groups, regardless of need or preference, and then stop reimbursing professional treatment services. Faced with this legitimate fear,

professionals may resist becoming secondary to self-help groups because they understandably do not want to be put out of business.

Bringing professionals on board will require both education and advocacy. The education component is necessary for those professionals who still conceptualize their work in terms appropriate for the old fee-for-service model (i.e., that they are competing to provide more services to more patients). These professionals would benefit from learning the workings and underlying logic of newer capitated managed care models, in which everyone "wins" when an addicted patient who recovers with the aid of a self-help group relies less on professional services. In terms of advocacy, either through the pending federal HMO legislative process or as part of individual contracts negotiated through employers, addiction professionals and payers will need to work together to ensure that the benefits and cost savings of self-help groups are not used as a rationale to eliminate professional services. If addiction professionals have assurance that a greater emphasis on self-help groups in the US system of formal and informal care for addiction will not result in the elimination of professionals, they will be more likely to implement the model proposed here, and that should result in better allocation of our addiction-related health care resources.

The Glass Half Empty

It's easy to scoff at the notion that
alcoholics can be cured with a pill.
Maybe because we don't think
they deserve to be.

By Caroline Knapp

ALCOHOL IN AMERICA: DATA

Since 1977, per capita consumption of alcohol in the U.S. has dropped 17 percent. Beer consumption is down a few percentage points, wine has stayed about the same and hard-alcohol is off by 39.6 percent.

Beer is the most popular alcoholic beverage. The typical American drinks 32 gallons of it a year (nearly one 12-ounce can a day), which makes it the nation's fourth most popular beverage (trailing soft drinks, coffee and milk).

According to The Journal of Substance Abuse, 44 percent of American adults are drinkers, 22 percent are former drinkers and 34 percent are lifetime teetotalers.

Nearly 14 million adult Americans have alcohol-abuse problems. Alcohol abuse figures in half of American homicides and about a third of suicides.

My approach to well-being, circa 1990: Scotch, chardonnay. Very direct, very effective.

My approach today: A.A., Zoloft, therapy, exercise, relationships. Very elusive, hard to maintain, but ultimately more rewarding.

A new approach, coming soon to a pharmacy near you: antiaddiction drugs, designed to tamper with the circuitry of dependence. Efficacy as yet unknown.

The neuroscientists are at it again. Having already amassed a sizable arsenal of drugs against miseries like depression and obsessionality, researchers have turned to the battlefront of chemical dependence. Drugs with names like Naltrexone and Campral, which diminish the highs of substance abuse and dampen the cravings of withdrawal, are on the market or are soon to be. Before long, we may well have pharmaceuticals that mop up cocaine before it hits the brain, even drugs that trigger the body's immune system to produce antibodies against addictive substances.

Drugs to get us off drugs? Just imagine—a generation of Americans trading in martinis for meds, swapping dependencies like baseball cards, bantering at cocktail parties in the new millennium: "Alcohol? How 20th century! Forget the Campari—bring me a Campral!"

Such scenarios are fun and easy to indulge in, in part because it's so tempting to overstate the promise of drugs, to see them as neurological super-heroes, poised like Prozac to swoop down and rescue us from the jaws of addiction. The idea, of course, is as illusory as it is seductive. Having been desperate enough to quit drinking five years ago—and scared, willing and lucky enough to stay that way—I don't put much stock in magic bullets. I tend to believe that recovery is, as the expression goes, an "inside job," a matter not just of switching off the urge to drink or take drugs but also of understanding and addressing the feelings behind that urge. This is one reason recidivism rates among addicts are so high: getting sober is hard, life-altering work, and the payoffs come at a glacial pace. All that in pill form? Forget it.

And yet my own knee-jerk skepticism feels a bit dangerous, a product, perhaps, of the stigma that still surrounds addiction. Despite our growing acceptance of the idea that alcoholism is a disease, drunks and addicts still make us very uncomfortable. We judge them harshly; we find it far harder to address the murky and multiple roots of addic-

---

Caroline Knapp is the author of "Drinking: A Love Story" and "Pack of Two."

tion (social, psychological and physical) than its tangible results. And so we read news reports about Darryl Strawberry, nabbed in Tampa with cocaine in his wallet, and we think, How stupid, how pathetic, what a complete failure of will. There may be elements of truth to that, but such swift judgment also betrays the limits of our compassion. People who overcome their problems once and for all are redeemed; those who relapse are reviled. Missing from view is the vast middle ground of addicts, of people who live out complicated, shame-ridden cycles of sobriety and relapse that can go on for years.

The bias isn't limited to addicts. We harbor similar suspicions about the mentally ill, secretly (and sometimes not so secretly) linking Prozac use with weakness, superficiality, lack of moral fiber. We have next to no sympathy for the obese; greater understanding of the genetics of obesity—and a newly approved pill to combat extreme cases—will probably do little to dampen the deeper sentiment that corpulence is really a prod-

uct of gluttony and laziness. When it comes right down to it, biology be damned; whether it's food, drink or despair, solving these problems ought to be a test of our values and determination. It ought to be hard.

Indeed, the automatic criticism of meds—that they're a quick fix, avoidant and simplistic—reflects a general suspicion not only that problems like addiction can't be fixed with drugs but also that they shouldn't be. It indicates that for all our nods to the disease model of alcoholism, we continue to believe that it's actually a moral problem, the result of deep and frightening character flaws. Treat addiction medically? Like a "real" disease? Better to keep drunks hidden in church basements, where they belong.

Church basements, of course, may be precisely the place to find enlightenment, for both individuals and the larger culture. At an A.A. meeting not long ago, I heard a young woman, just out of rehab, talk about how it felt to be home alone, dying for a drink. She described quite eloquently the tapes-

try of feeling behind that craving— threads of loneliness and boredom, of sorrow and inexplicable need, the whole range of sensation that addiction so effectively, if temporarily, keeps at bay.

As I listened, I thought about this body of drug research, about how science might serve her. It's doubtful that meds alone could ease the tangle of longing that led her, like so many, to self-medicate in the first place. Not even neuroscience can come up with a shortcut across the minefield of sober human emotion. But it's possible that medication could ease the specific craving, mitigate the discomfort long enough to get her to the next meeting, and then the next. That's promising: if a drug can give you an edge, provide enough relief and agency to help you start fighting back, there's no reason to be against it. Very gradually, neurology has helped coax depression out of the closet, destigmatizing it enough to help countless Americans seek help. Perhaps antiaddiction pills will have a similar effect, easing not just cravings but shame.

DARE (Drug Abuse Resistance Education)

Very Popular but Not Very Effective

Richard R. Clayton

Carl G. Leukefeld

Nancy Grant Harrington

Anne Cattarello

The purpose of this chapter is to review and examine what is known about the most widely distributed school-based drug abuse prevention program in the world, DARE (Drug Abuse Resistance Education). It is likely that you know about DARE; you have seen the T-shirts, the bumper stickers, floats in Independence Day parades, DARE cars, and the hundreds of other ways that this program has been marketed. Perhaps you yourself were in a class or school that received the DARE curriculum in the fifth or sixth grade.

DARE is a social phenomenon (Wysong, 1993). In the 1983–84 school year, it was delivered to about 8,000 elementary school students in Los Angeles. Today, DARE is found in more than one half of all school districts in the United States and reaches at least 25 million students each year (Ennett, Tobler, Ringwalt, & Flewelling, 1994). Although the numbers are difficult to confirm, it is estimated that $750 million is spent on DARE each year in the United States. DARE can also be found in Australia, Canada, Mexico, New Zealand, Norway, and Sweden.

AUTHORS' NOTE: This study was funded by Grant No. DA–05312 from the National Institute on Drug Abuse to the Center for

The DARE Program

DARE began in Los Angeles in 1983–84 as a school-based drug prevention program. The curriculum is a result of the joint efforts of the Los Angeles Police Department and the Los Angeles Unified School District, one of the country's largest.

Unlike most other school-based prevention programs, which are taught by teachers, DARE is taught by uniformed police officers who must undergo 80 hours of rigorous training before they can teach the program (Falco, 1989).

The stated purpose of DARE is to "prevent substance abuse among school children." The principal way it seeks to achieve this goal is to teach students the skills for recognizing and resisting social pressures to experiment with tobacco, alcohol, and other drugs. The 17 DARE lessons also focus on enhancing students' self-esteem, decision making, coping, assertiveness, and communication skills and on teaching positive alternatives to substance use. The curriculum and basic goals and structure of the DARE program have remained essentially the same since its beginnings. However, in 1992–94, additional lessons were added to place greater emphasis on the prevention of tobacco use and a new and enhanced focus was placed on violence prevention and conflict resolution. In addition, the actual classroom style became more "interactive" rather than one-directional from officer to student. The revisions were phased in during 1993–94, and beginning January 1, 1995, all DARE officers were required to use the "new" program.

The original DARE program was targeted at students in the fifth or sixth grade, preferably the grade immediately prior to entering junior high or middle school. Now there are DARE programs for kindergarten through third-grade students, middle-school students, and high school students (Kochis, 1995).

Being at the Right Place at the Right Time

National political interest in the drug problem was focused in 1986 with President Reagan's "War on Drugs" address to the nation. This led to broad support from both the Democratic and Republican parties and the passage of the Anti-Drug Abuse Act of 1986 (Falco, 1989). In both the Bush and the Clinton administrations, there was increasing recognition of the complexity of the problem and the requirements that law enforcement/supply reduction and prevention-treatment/demand reduction efforts be coordinated. The Office of National Drug Control Policy (ONDCP) is responsible for this coordination and has placed increasingly strong emphasis on prevention and drug education programs. In fact, federal spending for all "educational" prevention activities rose from $230 million in 1988 to $660 million in 1995.

DARE was at the right place at the right time, with just the right types of political support to become what the Justice Department called the "long term solution to the drug problem." In fact, the congressional testimony of Los Angeles Police Chief Daryl Gates and support from powerful members of Congress and President Bush led in 1990 to an amendment to the 1986 Drug Free Schools and Communities Act. This amendment mandated federal funding for DARE. The Drug Free Schools Act divided money given to the states into two parts: 70% of the money went to the departments of education in the states, and 30% went to the governor. The amendment required that 10% of the governor's portion be used to fund programs such as Project Drug Abuse Resistance Education (DARE). In fact, DARE was the only school-based prevention program singled out for mandated funding.

Congressional and other support for DARE continued into the mid-1990s, when it was again singled out for federal funding through a renewed commitment in Congress to what was now called the "Safe and Drug Free Schools and Communities Act."

DARE: More Than Just a Drug Prevention Program

One of the reasons DARE has been so successful in spreading across the country is organizational. DARE America is a private, nonprofit corporation organized in 1987 with a goal of getting the program into all states and communities, developing and supporting a national DARE instructor training program, and getting funding nationally.

Training

The Bureau of Justice Assistance (BJA) within the Department of Justice started funding DARE in 1986 with a BJA grant of $140,000. In the late 1980s, BJA funded five regional DARE training centers. As part of the funding agreement, BJA appoints 5 of the 15 members of the DARE training center policy advisory board.

Additional Funding and Support

DARE America has been successful in attracting major corporate sponsors such as Bayliner, Herbalife, Kentucky Fried Chicken, Kimberly-Clark, McDonalds, Packard Bell, Security Pacific National Bank, and Warner Brothers. At the local and state level, there are thousands of large and small firms contributing to the program.

Inconsistency: DARE's Popularity and its Effectiveness

The principal purpose of DARE is to reduce substance abuse among school children. About the only way to determine if DARE has achieved success (i.e., "works") is to conduct research on students who receive DARE and those who do not receive DARE. Both the experimental group (received DARE) and the control group should be examined prior to the start of the prevention effort and followed for 1 to 5 years to see if differences persist. DARE is the most widely research-evaluated school-based prevention program in the United States. There have been at least 15 evaluation studies conducted (Ennett et al., 1994), several of which followed DARE and non-DARE students for up to 4 or 5 years (Clayton, Cattarello, & Johnstone, 1996). Although the results from various studies differ somewhat, all studies are consistent in finding that DARE does not have long-term effects on drug use (Kochis, 1995). It does seem to have some effects on knowledge and attitudes toward drugs, but even these effects diminish over time. In fact, two long-term follow-up studies show that after 3 or more years, students who received DARE do not even have more positive attitudes toward the police than students who did not receive DARE (Clayton et al., 1996; Wysong, Aniskiewicz, & Wright, 1994).

Why Is DARE So Popular If It Is Not Effective?

This is an important question because it reveals so much about the United States and its approach to social problems (Aniskiewicz & Wysong, 1990).

Police

DARE is popular among police for two reasons. First, it puts police officers into community institutions previously "off limits" to them. Before the advent of DARE, there was a widespread and deep-seated mistrust of police officers by school officials. In fact, police were seen by many community members and organizations as generally less educated and brutish. By entering school systems to teach DARE, police can change these stereotypes. Second, it allows police officers to do things that are seen as "positive." In most police departments prior to the mid-1980s, absolutely the worst assignment was what was then called "community relations." No police officer wanted that assignment. Now police officers are standing in line for an opportunity to be a DARE officer. Police officers perceive a different response to them from the public if they are involved with DARE. In fact, it could be said that DARE has had a major effect on the relationship between police departments and other community-based organizations. Police are now active players in a wide variety of positive community projects and initiatives.

Parents

DARE is popular among parents for at least two reasons. First, they are extremely concerned about drug abuse and violence, and most feel helpless in dealing with either. Therefore, if there is a police officer in the school teaching the DARE program, it might protect their child from being victimized by violent predators or by drug dealers. Second, most Americans have a naive and false sense of confidence in the power of "education." It is the panacea brought out to "solve" all our problems: If people just know the "facts," they will make rational choices. The DARE officer represents authority, and parents have faith that children will listen to and heed the advice of an authority. Besides, the prevailing orientation to drugs in this society is primarily concerned with legality/illegality—a law enforcement perspective. The DARE officer represents the prevailing perspective held by parents.

Teachers

DARE is also quite popular among teachers, and for two very good reasons. First, teachers, just like the parents, perceive the school to be a safer place when DARE officers are in the school. Second, the DARE officer teaches the drug prevention curriculum, which means that the teachers do not have to teach the lessons. In fact, although the teachers are required to be "in the classroom" during the drug prevention lessons, they get a respite from their work, a break of sorts. This second reason is very important as an unintended consequence of how far and how quickly DARE has diffused across the country. At present, no colleges of education require preparation of teachers to deliver substance abuse prevention curricula. Even so, a significant proportion of fifth- and sixth-grade teachers in the United States could probably teach the DARE curriculum because they have seen and heard it taught one or more times. If the education establishment had been called on to provide 80 hours of training to teach a drug prevention curriculum such as DARE, it would have cost billions of dollars. Instead, such a curriculum has been provided at no cost to the education establishment in the course of the spread of DARE across America.

Administrators

School administrators, the principals and superintendents, seem to like DARE because it provides a sense of extra security at the school, it provides a respite for the teachers which makes them happy, it is generally very popular among parents and gets them more involved with the school than would otherwise be likely, and it links the school with another important institution of the community, the police department. A number of principals regularly request that the DARE officer be in the school on Mondays because attendance is noticeably higher when the DARE officer is in the school (Clayton, Cattarello, Day, & Walden, 1991).

The "Feel-Good" Approach to Drug Prevention

Someone might wonder: If everybody likes DARE and it makes students, teachers, administrators, parents, police, and politicians "feel good" because something is being done about drug abuse, why should we be worried by lack of evidence that it delays the onset or inhibits the continuance of drug use by adolescents? The answer to this question is quite simple and has three parts. First, publicly funded programs should be accountable for what they achieve. If they do not achieve their stated goal (in this instance, a reduction in drug use), how can further expenditure of public funds be justified? Second, other similar programs consistently show some effects in the desired direction, although the effects are not huge (Botvin, Dusenbury, Botvin, & Diaz, 1995). Why should the American public pay for a program that has proven to be ineffective when programs that have proven to be successful exist? Third, a principal reason for evaluation research is to examine the effectiveness of public programming that may seem sound on the surface but is unsound in practice. The evidence for the lack of sustained effectiveness of DARE is strong, consistent, and impressive.

Why, then, the continued strong support of DARE? The answer to this question must be: Because it makes all the important groups (parents, teachers, administrators, police, politicians) "feel good." It is sad to say, but an overwhelming majority of people in the United States have a rather naive view of the world and how to solve social problems such as drug use and abuse by adolescents. DARE seems to reflect most of these naive notions and in some ways to exploit them.

Drug use is *not* a simple phenomenon. It will not be solved by simple slogans and bumper stickers and T-shirts and a bunch of people believing that DARE is "the" answer to drug abuse in America. If anyone really and truly believes this is true, we have some swamp land in Florida we would like for them to buy.

The "scientific" research on the effectiveness of DARE is clear. DARE does not produce sustained effects on drug use or on even attitudes toward police (Clayton et al., 1996). Furthermore, the most recent data suggest that drug use (marijuana, inhalants, LSD, stimulants, cigarettes) began to rise significantly among 8th, 10th, and 12th graders beginning in 1992 and continuing through 1994. The cohorts in which drug use began to rise for the first time since 1979 would have been 6th graders in 1990, 8th graders in 1992, and 10th graders in 1994. If we assumed that DARE had spread all across America by 1990, these would be the students who would have been most affected by the diffusion of DARE.

To be fair, DARE could not be expected to produce miracles and wipe out drug use among adolescents entirely. Many forces in society promote drug use or dilute efforts to fight drug use among adolescents. However, DARE could be expected to produce some reduction in drug use, or at the very least positive and sustained effects on attitudes toward drug use by adolescents. Instead, as has been shown, there are *no* sustained effects from the DARE program on attitudes or behavior. In fact, it is probably naive to think that any *universal* (one size fitting all students) type of school-based, curriculum-driven drug prevention program could exert enough influence to counter the forces driving youth toward experimentation with various drugs. These types of programs are simply not powerful enough, do not provide enough exposures to the intervention, and may not even directly address the primary causes of drug use by youth. For example, one entire lesson in the DARE curriculum is designed to heighten self-esteem. However, the extensive research literature on the relationship between self-esteem and drug use among adolescents indicates very little correlation between drug use and self-esteem. Therefore, even if the lesson helped to improve self-esteem for some of the students, that improvement would probably not be translated into a lower probability of drug use. So although DARE is very popular, it is not very effective. Therefore we as a nation should be ready to accept that fact and deal with its implications if we *really* want to have an effect on drug use among youth.

References

Aniskiewicz, R., & Wysong, E. (1990). Evaluating DARE: Drug education and the multiple meanings of success. *Policy Studies Review, 9,* 727–747.

Botvin, G. J., Dusenbury, L., Botvin, E. M., & Diaz, T. (1995). Long term follow-up results of a randomized drug abuse trial in a white middle class population. *Journal of the American Medical Association, 273,* 1106–1112.

Clayton, R. R., Cattarello, L., Day, E., & Walden, K. P. (1991). Persuasive communication and drug prevention: An evaluation of the DARE program. In H. Sypher, L. Donohew, & W. Bukoski (Eds.), *Persuasive communication and drug abuse prevention.* Hillsdale, NJ: Lawrence Erlbaum.

Clayton, R. R. Cattarello, A. M., & Johnstone, B. M. (in press). The effectiveness of Drug Abuse Resistance Education (Project DARE): Five year follow-up results. *Preventive Medicine.*

Ennett, S., Tobler, N., Ringwalt, C., & Flewelling, R. (1994). How effective is Drug Abuse Resistance Education? A meta-analysis of Project DARE outcome evaluations. *American Journal of Public Health, 84,* 1394–1401.

Falco, M. (1989). *Winning the drug war: A national strategy.* New York: Priority.

Kochis, D. S. (1995). The effectiveness of Project DARE: Does it work? *Journal of Alcohol and Drug Education, 40,* 40–47.

Wysong, E. (1993, October). *The frontier of drug education: D.A.R.E. as a social movement.* Paper presented at the annual meeting of the Indiana Academy of Social Sciences, Hanover College, Hanover, IN.

Wysong, B., Aniskiewicz, R., & Wright, D. (1994). Truth and DARE: Tracking drug education to graduation and as symbolic politics. *Social Problems, 41,* 448–473.

Absorption: The passage of chemical compounds, such as drugs or nutrients, into the bloodstream through the skin, intestinal lining, or other bodily membranes.

Abstinence: The total avoidance of a specific substance, such as alcohol, tobacco, and/or drugs.

Acetylcholine: A cholinergic transmitter thought to be involved in the inhibition of behavior.

Acetylsalicylic acid (aspirin): A generic over-the-counter analgesic drug (painkiller).

Acupuncture: A traditional Chinese health care technique for treating illness or administering anesthesia by inserting needles into specific points of the body in order to stimulate the production of natural endorphins.

Addiction: Use of a substance in a chronic, compulsive, or uncontrollable way.

Adrenergic system: The group of transmitters, including epinephrine, norepinephrine, and dopamine, that activates the sympathetic nervous system.

Alcohol abuse: See Alcoholism

Alcoholics Anonymous (AA): A voluntary organization founded in 1935, consisting of individuals seeking help for a drinking problem. The AA program is based on total abstinence, achieved by following a 12-step process.

Alcoholism: Any use of alcoholic beverages that causes damage to the individual or to society. See also Disease Model.

Amotivational syndrome: Apathy and loss of motivation that is believed to occur in long-term marijuana users.

Amphetamine psychosis: A psychotic disorder characterized by loss of contact with reality and hallucinations brought on by the stopping or cutting back of doses of amphetamines by an amphetamine-dependent person.

Amphetamines: A class of drugs, similar in some ways to the body's own adrenaline (epinephrine), that act as stimulants to the central nervous system.

Anabolic steroids: Synthetic derivatives of the male hormone testosterone.

Analgesics: Drugs that relieve pain.

Anesthetic: A medication that produces an artificial loss of sensation in order to relieve pain.

Angel dust: Slang term for phencyclidine (PCP), a synthetic depressant drug.

Anorectic: A drug that decreases appetite.

Antianxiety tranquilizers: Tranquilizers, like Valium and Librium, used to relieve anxiety and tension, sometimes called minor tranquilizers.

Anticholinergics: Drugs that block the transmission of impulses in the parasympathetic nerves.

Antidepressants: Synthetic drugs used to relieve or prevent psychological depression by increasing the activity of the neurotransmitter norepinephrine in the brain. See also Depression.

Antihistamines: Drugs that relieve allergy or cold symptoms by blocking the effects of histamine production.

Atropine: An alkaloid derivative of belladonna and related plants that blocks responses to parasympathetic stimulation.

Axon: The core of the nerve fiber that conducts impulses away from the nerve cell to the neurons and other tissue.

Barbiturates: Drugs used for sedation and to relieve tension and anxiety.

Benzodiazepine: A minor tranquilizer; the best-known brand name for benzodiazepine is Valium.

Bipolar disorder: A mental illness characterized by intense mood swings of extreme elation and severe depression. Also known as manic depression.

Blood level: The concentration of alcohol in the blood, usually expressed in percent by weight.

Brain stem: The region of the brain that links the cerebrum to the spinal cord.

Caffeine: An alkaloid found in coffee, tea, and kola nuts that acts as a stimulant.

Cannabis: See Marijuana.

Central nervous system (CNS): The brain and spinal cord.

China White: A synthetic reproduction of fentanyl, a widely used anesthetic and depressant. China White is very similar to heroin in its duration, blockage of pain, and euphoric effect.

Chipping: Using narcotics occasionally without developing an addiction.

Chlorpromazine: An antianxiety tranquilizer, manufactured under the name of Thorazine, used for treating severe psychoses. Also used as an antagonist to LSD panic reactions.

Choline: A transmitter, part of the cholinergic system.

Cocaine: A white, crystalline narcotic alkaloid derived from the coca plant and used as a surface anesthetic and a stimulant.

Codeine: A narcotic alkaloid found in opium, most often used as an analgesic or cough suppressant.

Coke: Slang term for cocaine.

Cold turkey: Slang expression for abrupt and complete withdrawal from drugs or alcohol without medication.

Contraindications: A condition that makes it inadvisable or hazardous to use a particular drug or medicine.

Controlled substances: All psychoactive substances covered by laws regulating their sale and possession.

Controlled Substances Act of 1970: Federal act that classifies controlled substances into five categories and regulates their use. Schedule I drugs are those most strictly controlled; they include heroin, marijuana, LSD, and other drugs believed to have high abuse potential. Schedule II drugs are also strictly controlled but have some medicinal uses; these drugs include morphine, methadone, and amphetamines. Schedule III, IV, and V substances include drugs that have increasingly less abuse potential; over-the-counter medicines not subject to any refill regulations fall into Schedule V.

Crack: A drug made by mixing cocaine, baking soda, other chemicals, and water, heating the mixture, and letting it solidify into "rocks" that are smoked.

Crisis intervention: The process of diagnosing a drug crisis situation and acting immediately to arrest the condition.

Decriminalization: The legal process by which the possession of a certain drug would become a civil penalty instead of a criminal penalty. See also Legalization.

Deliriants: Substances, like some inhalants, that produce delirium.

Delirium: State of temporary mental confusion and diminished consciousness, characterized by anxiety, hallucinations, and delusions.

Delta-9 tetrahydrocannabinol (THC): A psychoactive derivative of the cannabis plant.

Dependence: A state in which one cannot readily give up or stop the use of a drug; there are two types of dependence—physical and psychological.

Dependence, physical: The physical need of the body for a particular substance such that abstinence from the substance leads to physical withdrawal symptoms. See also Addiction; Withdrawal symptoms.

Dependence, psychological: A psychological or emotional reliance on a particular substance; a strong and continued craving.

Depressants: Also known as sedative-hypnotics, depressants produce a state of behavioral depression while also depressing chemical transmission between nerve cells in the brain. Effects of depressants include drowsiness, some behavioral excitation, and loss of inhibition. Alcohol, barbiturates, and antianxiety drugs are depressants.

Depression: A mental state characterized by extreme sadness or dejection far out of proportion to the reality of the situation over which the sufferer is depressed. Depression can be a neurosis or psychosis, depending on its severity or duration.

Designer drug: Any drug that is designed to match a client's desired effect and manufactured by chemists in illicit laboratories. Ecstasy and China White are examples of designer drugs.

Detoxification: Removal of a poisonous substance, such as a drug or alcohol, from the body.

Disease model: A theory of alcoholism, endorsed by AA, in which the alcoholism is seen as a disease rather than a psychological or social problem.

DMT: Dimethyltryptamine, a psychedelic drug.

DNA: Deoxyribonucleic acid, the carrier of chromosomes in the cell.

Dopamine: A neurotransmitter that helps control and coordinate movement.

Downers: A slang term for drugs that act to depress the central nervous system.

Drug: Any substance that alters the structure or function of a living organism.

Drug abuse: The taking of a drug in a manner that causes bodily or mental harm.

Drug paraphernalia: Materials, like hypodermic syringes, that are used for the preparation or administration of illicit drugs.

Duster: A PCP-laced joint.

DWI: Driving while intoxicated.

Dysphoria: Emotional state characterized by anxiety, depression, and restlessness, as opposed to euphoria.

Ecstasy: A derivative of nutmeg or sassafras, causing euphoria and sometimes hallucinations; also known as XTC, Adam, or MDMA.

Employee assistance program (EAP): A program offered as a workplace benefit by an employer, providing counselling and referral services to employees with personal problems, including substance abuse.

Endogenous drugs: Drugs that are produced inside the body.

Endorphins: Any group of hormones released by the brain that have painkilling and tranquilizing abilities.

Epinephrine: An adrenal hormone that acts as a transmitter and stimulates autonomic nerve action.

Ethical drugs: Drugs dispensed by prescription only.

Euphoria: Exaggerated sense of happiness or well-being.

Experimental drug use: According to the U.S. National Commission on Marijuana and Drug Abuse, the short-term non-patterned trial of one or more drugs, either concurrently or consecutively, with variable intensity but maximum frequency of ten times per drug.

Fetal alcohol syndrome (FAS): A pattern of birth defects, cardiac abnormalities, and developmental retardation seen in babies of alcoholic mothers.

Fix: Slang for a mood-altering drug dosage; an intravenous dose of an opiate.

Flashbacks: Spontaneous and involuntary recurrences of psychedelic drug effects after the initial drug experience.

Food and Drug Administration (FDA): Agency of the U.S. Department of Health and Human Services that administers federal laws regarding the purity of food, the safety and effectiveness of drugs, and the safety of cosmetics.

Freebase: A prepared form of cocaine that can be smoked.

Gas: Slang term for nitrate oxide.

Generic drugs: Prescription drugs manufactured to match the chemical composition of brand name drugs after their copyrights have expired.

Glass: See Ice.

Habituation: Chronic or continuous use of a drug, with an attachment less severe than addiction.

Hallucination: A sensory perception without external stimuli.

Hallucinogenic drugs: Drugs that cause hallucinations. Also known as psychedelic drugs.

Harrison Narcotics Act: Federal act passed in 1914 that controlled the sale and possession of prescription drugs, heroin, opium, and cocaine.

Hashish: The dried resin of the marijuana plant; often smoked in water pipes.

Head shops: Stores that sell drug-related products.

Herb: Commonly, any one of various aromatic plants used for medical or other purposes.

Heroin: An opiate derivative of morphine.

High: Intoxicated by a drug or alcohol; the state of being high.

Hog: Slang for PCP (pencyclidine).

Ibuprofen: An over-the-counter pain reliever that is an alternative to aspirin and acetaminophen; the active ingredient in Motrin, Advil, and Nuprin.

Ice: A smokable form of methamphetamine.

Illicit drug: An illegal drug; any drug or substance whose distribution to the general public is prohibited by the federal Controlled Substances Act of 1970.

Illy: Marijuana and mint leaves soaked in a deadly combination of embalming fluid and PCP.

Inhalants: Substances that emit fumes or gases that are inhaled and have the effect of psychoactive drugs. Also known as deliriants.

Interferon: A group of protein factors produced by certain cells in response to the presence of viruses.

Interleukin 2: A group of protein factors that acts as a messenger between white blood cells (leukocytes) involved in immune responses.

Intoxication: Medically, the state of being poisoned. Usually refers to the state of being drunk, falling between drunkenness and a mild high.

Intravenous (IV) drug users: Drug users who use hypodermic needles as a means of administering drugs; among the drugs normally administered in this manner is heroin, which may be injected either directly into a vein ("mainlining") or just under the surface of the skin ("skin popping").

Joint: A marijuana cigarette.

Junkie: A heroin addict.

Ketamine: A close relative of PCP, it is a legally prescribed drug for use as an anesthetic.

Legalization: The movement to have the sale or possession of certain illicit drugs made legal.

Limbic system: A set of structures in the brain that influences motivation and emotional behavior.

LSD: Lysergic acid diethlamide-25, a hallucinogen.

Ludes: Tablets of methaqualone (Quaalude).

Mainline: To inject a drug intravaneously.

Marijuana: A preparation of the leaves and flowering tops of the cannabis plant, the smoke of which is inhaled for its euphoric effects. Also spelled: marihuana.

MDMA: See Ecstasy.

Medical model: A theory of drug abuse or addiction in which the addiction is seen as a medical, rather than a social, problem.

Mescaline: A hallucinogenic alkaloid drug, either derived from the peyote plant or made synthetically.

Methadone: A synthetic opiate sometimes used to treat heroin or morphine addiction.

Methamphetamines: Stimulant drugs derived from and more potent than amphetamines. Also known as speed.

Methaqualone: A nonbarbiturate sedative/hypnotic drug, used to bring on feelings of muscular relaxation, contentment, and passivity. Also known as quaaludes.

Methylphenidate: Also known as Ritalin, its most popular brand name, methylphenidate is a stimulant used in treating hyperkinetic children (children who are hyperactive but have no academic difficulties).

Morphine: An organic compound extracted from opium; a light anesthetic or sedative.

Multimodality programs: Programs for the treatment of drug abuse or alcoholism involving several simultaneous treatment methods.

Narcotic: A drug that has both a sedative and a pain-relieving effect. Opiate drugs are narcotics.

Narcotics Anonymous (NA): An organization modeled after Alcoholics Anonymous to assist recovering drug dependents.

Neuroleptic: Any major, or antipsychotic, tranquilizer.

Neuron: The basic element responsible for the reception, transmission, and processing of sensory, motor, and other information of physiological or psychological importance to the individual.

Neurotransmitters: The chemicals that transmit messages from one neuron to another.

Nicotine: The main active ingredient of tobacco, extremely toxic and causing irritation of lung tissue, constriction of blood vessels, increased blood pressure and heart rate, and, in general, central nervous system stimulation.

Norepinephrine: Hormone found in the sympathetic nerve endings that acts as an adrenergic transmitter and is a vasoconstrictor.

Opiate narcotics: A major subclass of drugs that act as pain relievers as well as central nervous system depressants; includes opium, morphine, codeine, and methadone.

Opiates: The class of drugs that include opium, codeine, morphine, heroin, methadone, and other drugs derived from or chemically similar to opium; opiates are primarily used for pain relief.

Opium: A bitter brown narcotic drug that comes from the dried juice of the opium poppy, and from which such narcotics as heroin and morphine are derived.

Opoids: The group of synthetic drugs, including Demerol and Darvon, that resemble the opiates in action and effect.

Overmedication: The prescription and use of more medication than necessary to treat a specific illness or condition.

Over-the-counter drugs: Drugs legally sold without a prescription.

Parasympathetic nervous system: The part of the autonomic nervous system that inhibits or opposes the actions of the sympathetic nerves.

Parasympathomimetics: Drugs that produce effects similar to those of the parasympathetic nervous system.

Parkinson's disease: A progressive disease of the nervous system characterized by muscular tremor, slowing of movement, partial facial paralysis, and general weakness.

Peyote: A drug derived from either the peyote or the mescal cactus, possessing hallucinogenic properties.

Phencyclidine (PCP): A synthetic depressant drug used as a veterinary anesthetic and illegally as a hallucinogen.

Phenylpropanolamine (PPA): A medication used to prevent or relieve nasal and upper respiratory congestion. PPA is also used as an appetite suppressant.

Phobias: Persistent, intense fears of specific persons, objects, or situations, accompanied by a wish to flee or avoid the fear-provoking stimulus.

Physical dependence: A form of dependence in which the body's physical need for a particular substance is such that stopping use leads to physical withdrawal symptoms.

Placebo: An inactive substance used as a control in an experiment.

Polyabuse: Abuse of various drugs simultaneously.

Pop: To swallow a drug in pill form.

Poppers: Slang for amyl nitrate.

Pot: Slang term for marijuana.

Potency: Term used to compare the relative strength of two or more drugs used to produce a given effect.

Potentiate: To augment a depressant's effect by taking a combination of two or more depressants.

Prescription drugs: Drugs dispensed only by a physician's prescription.

Primary prevention: Efforts designed to prevent a person from starting to use drugs.

Proprietary drugs: Patent medicines.

Psilocybin: A naturally occurring psychedelic agent derived from the *Psilocybe Mexicana* mushroom.

Psychedelic drug: A drug that causes hallucinations; a hallucinogen.

Psychoactive: Affecting the mind or behavior.

Psychological dependence: A form of dependence in which the user's attachment to the emotional or psychological effects of a drug is such that he or she finds it difficult or impossible to stop use voluntarily; may or may not be accompanied by physical dependence.

Psychopharmacology: The study of the effects of drugs on mood, sensation, or consciousness, or other psychological or behavioral functions.

Psychosis: Severe mental disorder, characterized by withdrawal from reality and deterioration of normal intellectual and social functioning.

Psychosomatic: Describing a variety of physical reactions that are assumed to be closely related to psychological phenomena.

Psychotherapeutic drugs: Drugs that are used as medicines to alleviate psychological disorders.

Psychotomimetics: Drugs that produce psychosis-like effects.

Recidivism: Return to former behavior.

Recombinant DNA: DNA prepared in the laboratory by the transfer or exchange of individual genes from one organism to another.

Recreational drug use: Drug use that takes place in social settings among friends who want to share a pleasant experience; characterized by less frequency and intensity than addictive drug use. Also called social-recreational drug use.

Rehabilitation: Restoration of a person's ability to function normally.

Reinforcement: A stimulus that increases the probability that a desired response will occur.

Reticular activating system: A cluster of cell groups located in the upper part of the brain stem that controls the flow of information from the sensory organs to the cerebral cortex.

Reyes syndrome: An often fatal childhood disorder whose cause is unknown, but has been associated with the use of aspirin as a treatment for chicken pox.

Rush: Slang term for an immediate feeling of physical well-being and euphoria after the administration of a drug.

Schedules: Categories of drugs as defined in the Controlled Substance Act of 1970.

Scopolamine: Poisonous alkaloid found in the roots of various plants, used as a truth serum or with morphine as a sedative.

Score: To obtain a supply of drugs.

Secondary prevention: Early treatment of drug abuse to prevent it from becoming more severe.

Sedative: A drug that depresses the central nervous system. Also known as sedative-hypnotics, sedatives include barbiturates, antianxiety drugs, and alcohol.

Sedative/hypnotics: A more technical term for depressants, drugs that are used for general anesthesia, induction of sleep, relief from anxiety, and recreational disinhibition (alcohol).

Serotonin: A neurotransmitter that is produced in the brain stem and is involved in sleep and sensory experiences.

Set: The combination of physical, mental, and emotional characteristics of an individual at the time a drug is administered.

Setting: The external environment of an individual at the time a drug is administered.

Side effects: Secondary effects, usually undesirable, of a drug or therapy.

Sinsemilla: High-grade, flowering, seedless tops of marijuana.

Snort: To inhale a powdered drug.

Snuff: A preparation of pulverized tobacco that is inhaled into the nostrils.

Sobriety: The quality of being free from alcohol intoxication.

Social-recreational drug use: *See* Recreational drug use.

Socioeconomic: Both social and economic.

Somatic nervous system: That part of the nervous system that deals with the senses and voluntary muscles.

Speed: Slang term for methamphetamine, a central nervous system stimulant.

Stereospecificity: The matching of both electrical and chemical characteristics of the transmitter and receptor site so that binding can take place.

Stimulants: Chemical compounds that elevate mood, induce euphoria, increase alertness, reduce fatigue, and, in high doses, produce irritability, anxiety, and a pattern of psychotic behavior. Stimulants include amphetamines, nicotine, caffeine, and cocaine.

STP: Early slang term for phencyclidine.

Subcutaneous: Beneath the skin.

Substance abuse: Refers to cigarette smoking, alcohol abuse, or drug abuse.

Super K: Slang term for ketamine.

Sympathetic nervous system: The part of the nervous system that carries neural signals that stimulate the body and prepare it for action.

Sympathomimetic: Any drug that produces effects like those resulting from stimulation of the sympathetic nervous system.

Synapse: The space, or gap, between two neurons.

Synesthesia: The blending of the senses so that two or more are perceived in combination in reaction to one stimulus.

Tars: The dark, oily, viscid substances created by burning tobacco, known to contain carcinogenic agents.

Temperance: The practice of moderation, especially with regard to alcohol consumption. The Temperance Movement was a popular movement in the nineteenth and twentieth centuries to restrict or prohibit the use of alcoholic beverages.

Tertiary prevention: Treatment to prevent the permanent disability or death of a drug abuser.

THC: Tetrahydrocannabinol, a psychoactive derivative of the cannabis plant.

Therapeutic community: Setting in which persons with similar problems meet and provide mutual support to help overcome those problems.

Titration: The ability to determine desired drug dosage.

Toke: An inhalation from a pipe or cigarette.

Tolerance: The capacity to absorb a drug continuously or in large doses with no adverse effect.

Trance: Dazed or hypnotic state.

Tranquilizers: Drugs that depress the central nervous system, thus relieving anxiety and tension and sometimes relaxing the muscles, divided into the major tranquilizers, or anti-psychotics, and minor tranquilizers, or antianxiety tranquilizers.

Treatment: Drug treatment programs can be drug-free or maintenance, residential or ambulatory, medical or non-medical, voluntary or involuntary, or some combination of these.

Uncontrolled substance: Any chemical or drug whose distribution to the general public is unrestricted by governmental regulations (controls) other than those rules that apply to any similar consumer item.

Uppers: Slang term for amphetamines, and, sometimes, cocaine.

Valium: A brand name for benzodiazepine, a minor tranquilizer.

Withdrawal symptoms: The (usually unpleasant) set of physical symptoms experienced by the user as a result of stopping use of a drug upon which he or she has become dependent; these may include anxiety, insomnia, perspiration, hot flashes, nausea, dehydration, tremors, weakness, dizziness, convulsions, or psychotic behavior.

SOURCE
Drugs, Society, and Behavior (Wellness), 1992. Dushkin/McGraw-Hill, Guilford, CT 06437.

AE Article Review Form

We encourage you to photocopy and use this page as a tool to assess how the articles in **Annual Editions** expand on the information in your textbook. By reflecting on the articles you will gain enhanced text information. You can also access this useful form on a product's book support Web site at **http://www.dushkin.com/online/.**

NAME: _____ DATE: _____

TITLE AND NUMBER OF ARTICLE:
_____

BRIEFLY STATE THE MAIN IDEA OF THIS ARTICLE:
_____

LIST THREE IMPORTANT FACTS THAT THE AUTHOR USES TO SUPPORT THE MAIN IDEA:

_____

WHAT INFORMATION OR IDEAS DISCUSSED IN THIS ARTICLE ARE ALSO DISCUSSED IN YOUR TEXTBOOK OR OTHER READINGS THAT YOU HAVE DONE? LIST THE TEXTBOOK CHAPTERS AND PAGE NUMBERS:

_____

LIST ANY EXAMPLES OF BIAS OR FAULTY REASONING THAT YOU FOUND IN THE ARTICLE:

_____

LIST ANY NEW TERMS/CONCEPTS THAT WERE DISCUSSED IN THE ARTICLE, AND WRITE A SHORT DEFINITION:

_____

ANNUAL EDITIONS revisions depend on two major opinion sources: one is our Advisory Board, listed in the front of this volume, which works with us in scanning the thousands of articles published in the public press each year; the other is you—the person actually using the book. Please help us and the users of the next edition by completing the prepaid article rating form on this page and returning it to us. Thank you for your help!

ANNUAL EDITIONS: Drugs, Society and Behavior

ARTICLE RATING FORM

Here is an opportunity for you to have direct input into the next revision of this volume. We would like you to rate each of the 57 articles listed below, using the following scale:

1. Excellent: should definitely be retained
2. Above average: should probably be retained
3. Below average: should probably be deleted
4. Poor: should definitely be deleted

Your ratings will play a vital part in the next revision. So please mail this prepaid form to us just as soon as you complete it. Thanks for your help!

RATING	ARTICLE	RATING	ARTICLE
	1. Opium, Cocaine, and Marijuana in American History		31. Border Trafficking: Where the U.S. and Mexico Meet, the Drug Smugglers Are Riding High
	2. A Drug Trade Primer for the Late 1990s		32. Raising the Stakes in U.S.–Mexico Drug Wars
	3. A Hundred-Year Habit		33. The Charm City Blues
	4. One Nation under the Table		34. Drugs, Crime, Prison and Treatment
	5. New Museum Traces History of Drugs in the U.S.		35. Doping Kids
	6. Just Don't Say No, Not Us		36. Editorial: Substance Abuse and Addiction—the Need to Know
	7. America's Altered States		37. Visualizing America's Drug Problems: An Ethnographic Content Analysis of Illegal Drug Stories on the Nightly News
	8. Addiction and the Brain—Part I		
	9. A Little Help from Serotonin		38. The Casualties of War
	10. Cocaine Wreaks Subtle Damage on Developing Brains		39. Pregnant, Hooked & Booked
	11. What Type of Addict Are You?		40. Alcoholism in Women
	12. Alcoholism: Character or Genetics?		41. The Facts about Women, Alcohol
	13. New Pieces Filling in Addiction Puzzle		42. Medical Care of Heroin Users
	14. Taping the Horror		43. America's Drug Problem and Its Policy of Denial
	15. Resisting Cocaine's Tragic Lure		44. Strange Bedfellows: Ideology, Politics, and Drug Legalization
	16. Heroin High		
	17. Heroin and Cocaine—A Global Threat		45. Germany: A Strict Approach
	18. The Drinking Dilemma		46. The Buzz on Drugs
	19. Generation Wired: Caffeine Is the New Drug of Choice for Kids		47. The Netherlands: Let's Be Realistic
	20. Opium as Cash Crop Is Still Difficult to Beat		48. Q: Would Legalizing Drugs Serve America's National Interest?
	21. Hidden Dangers of Over the Counter Drugs		49. Industry Foes Fume over the Tobacco Deal
	22. Big Tobacco Rides East		50. The Narco-Guerrilla War
	23. High in the Heartland		51. The Tenacity of Error in the Treatment of Addiction
	24. Dying for a Drink		52. Outpatient Detoxification from Alcohol, Opiates, and Stimulants
	25. College Students Drunk on Campus Drinking Lore, Tradition		
	26. Party Politics		53. The Peer Principle: The Key to Addiction Treatment
	27. The Real Scandal		54. Needle Exchanges: Prevention or Problem?
	28. Sex Sells: Viagra Heats Up Market for Sexual Supplements		55. Can Addiction-Related Self-Help/Mutual Aid Groups Lower Demand for Professional Substance Abuse Treatment?
	29. Pain Breakers		
	30. New Date-Rape Drug Emerges: Metro Parents Worry Legal Product Touted by Health Stores, Internet Threatens Teens		56. The Glass Half Empty
			57. DARE (Drug Abuse Resistance Education): Very Popular but Not Very Effective

(Continued on next page)

We Want Your Advice

ANNUAL EDITIONS: DRUGS, SOCIETY AND BEHAVIOR 00/01

NO POSTAGE
NECESSARY
IF MAILED
IN THE
UNITED STATES

BUSINESS REPLY MAIL
FIRST-CLASS MAIL   PERMIT NO. 84   GUILFORD CT

POSTAGE WILL BE PAID BY ADDRESSEE

Dushkin/McGraw-Hill
Sluice Dock
Guilford, CT 06437-9989

Illrrrllrrrlrrlrrlllrrrlllrlrlrlrlrlrlrlrrrlrlrl

ABOUT YOU

Name _____   Date _____

Are you a teacher? ☐   A student? ☐
Your school's name
_____

Department
_____

Address _____   City _____   State ___   Zip ___

School telephone #
_____

YOUR COMMENTS ARE IMPORTANT TO US !

Please fill in the following information:
For which course did you use this book?
_____

Did you use a text with this *ANNUAL EDITION*? ☐ yes ☐ no
What was the title of the text?
_____

What are your general reactions to the *Annual Editions* concept?
_____

Have you read any particular articles recently that you think should be included in the next edition?
_____

Are there any articles you feel should be replaced in the next edition? Why?
_____

Are there any World Wide Web sites you feel should be included in the next edition? Please annotate.
_____

May we contact you for editorial input? ☐ yes ☐ no
May we quote your comments? ☐ yes ☐ no